Pharmaceutical Care in Digital Revolution

Pharmaceutical Care in Digital Revolution
Blending Digital with Human Innovation

Second Edition

Edited by

Ardalan Mirzaei
School of Pharmacy, Faculty of Medicine and Health,
The University of Sydney, Australia

Claudia Rijcken
Pharmi, Maastricht, The Netherlands

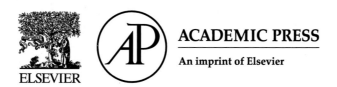

ELSEVIER

ACADEMIC PRESS
An imprint of Elsevier

Academic Press is an imprint of Elsevier
125 London Wall, London EC2Y 5AS, United Kingdom
525 B Street, Suite 1650, San Diego, CA 92101, United States
50 Hampshire Street, 5th Floor, Cambridge, MA 02139, United States
The Boulevard, Langford Lane, Kidlington, Oxford OX5 1GB, United Kingdom

Notices

Knowledge and best practice in this field are constantly changing. As new research and experience broaden our understanding, changes in research methods, professional practices, or medical treatment may become necessary.

Practitioners and researchers must always rely on their own experience and knowledge in evaluating and using any information, methods, compounds, or experiments described herein. In using such information or methods they should be mindful of their own safety and the safety of others, including parties for whom they have a professional responsibility.

To the fullest extent of the law, neither the Publisher nor the authors, contributors, or editors, assume any liability for any injury and/or damage to persons or property as a matter of products liability, negligence or otherwise, or from any use or operation of any methods, products, instructions, or ideas contained in the material herein.

ISBN: 978-0-443-13360-2

For information on all Academic Press publications visit our website at
https://www.elsevier.com/books-and-journals

Publisher: Mica H. Haley
Acquisitions Editor: Andre G Wolff
Editorial Project Manager: Sam Young
Production Project Manager: Selvaraj Raviraj
Cover Designer: Vicky Pearson Esser

Typeset by TNQ Technologies

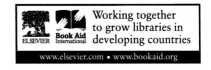

Contents

PART 1 Why: global healthcare systems under pressure

PART 2 What: digital advances to innovate pharmaceutical care journeys

Chapter 7: The digital health technology menu 79

Jaime Acosta-Gomez

Chapter 8: Zesting the internet of pharma things 101

Timothy Dy Aungst

Chapter 12: Your chef: the virtual pharmaceutical care assistant 167

Guido Jongen and Claudia Rijcken

Chapter 13: The taste of virtual, augmented, and mixed reality 187

Vincent Suarez Takizadeh

PART 4 How: what to do tomorrow as a pharmaceutical care leader

Contributors

Jaime Acosta-Gomez Technology Advisory Group, FIP, Madrid, Spain; Farmacia Acosta, Madrid, Spain

Timothy Dy Aungst Department of Pharmacy Practice, MCPHS University, Worcester, MA, United States

Anne Sophie Dil NAALA B.V., Rotterdam, The Netherlands

Amy Eikelenboom NAALA B.V., Rotterdam, The Netherlands

Lucien Engelen Transform Health, LLC, Baltimore, MD, United States; Strategist Health(care) Innovation for Deloitte C4E, Vodafone Group, Laurentius Medical Center, Roermond, The Netherlands

Paul Louis Iske Institute of Brilliant Failures, the Personalised Healthcare Catalyst Foundation, Maastricht University, Maastricht, The Netherlands

Guido Jongen Virtually Human, Pijnacker, The Netherlands

Aukje Mantel-Teeuwisse Department of Pharmaceutical Sciences, Faculty of Science, Utrecht University, Utrecht, The Netherlands

Ardalan Mirzaei School of Pharmacy, Faculty of Medicine and Health, The University of Sydney, Australia

Jessica Pace School of Pharmacy, Faculty of Medicine and Health, The University of Sydney, Australia

Ravi Patel University of Pittsburgh School of Pharmacy, Pittsburgh, PA, United States

Claudia Rijcken Pharmi, Maastricht, The Netherlands

Paul Rulkens Agrippa Consulting International, Maastricht, The Netherlands

Carl R. Schneider School of Pharmacy, Faculty of Medicine and Health, The University of Sydney, Australia

Aysu Selçuk International Pharmacutical Federation (FIP), The Hague, The Netherlands; Department of Clinical Pharmacy, Faculty of Pharmacy, Ankara University, Ankara, Turkey

Vincent Suarez Takizadeh Technologies Division, Cloudstone Group, Sydney, NSW, Australia

Nilhan Uzman International Pharmacutical Federation (FIP), The Hague, The Netherlands

Michel van Agthoven J&J Campus, The Netherlands

Mina Wanis Corum Group Pty Ltd, Sydney, NSW, Australia

Whitley Yi Skaggs School of Pharmacy and Pharmaceutical Sciences, University of Colorado, Anschutz Medical Campus, Aurora, CO, United States; Well Dot, Inc, Chapel Hill, NC, United States

About the editors

Ardalan Mirzaei

Ph.D., BPharm, MPhil, GradCertEdStud (Higher Ed), MPS, AFHEA, AACPA

Ardalan (Ardi) Mirzaei, BPharm, MPhil, GradCertEdStud (Higher Ed), Ph.D., is a registered pharmacist and data scientist.

He completed his Ph.D. in the School of Pharmacy, developing a dynamic model of patients' health information-seeking behavior.

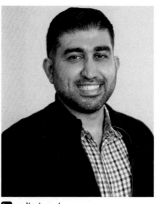

in ardimirzaei
@ArdiMirzaei
ardimirzaei.com

Ardi has worked in community pharmacy for over 15 years, having worked in a clinical setting as well as managing multimillion-dollar stores. In addition, his background is in education, working as a training coordinator for pharmacy internships and teaching at the University of Sydney on subjects in business, pharmacy, and machine learning.

This is supplemented with over 8 years of experience in data science, developing business solutions for the healthcare, education, retail, academic, and government sectors. He is passionate about health, teaching and technology.

Ardi enjoys exploring the use of AI, machine learning, and deep learning models and their application to everyday tasks and in healthcare. His interests have led to his involvement in the International Pharmaceutical Federation (FIP) Technology Advisory Group.

Claudia Rijcken

Ph.D., PharmD, MHA

Claudia has an educational background in pharmacy and obtained a Ph.D. in Pharmacoepidemiology and a Master of Health Administration (eMBA) degree.

After managing community pharmacy roles, she moved into clinical drug development in roles with increasing responsibility at Organon and Novartis.

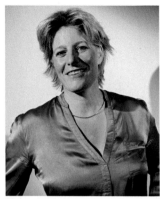

claudiarijcken

pharmi.info

Next, she acted within Novartis in international leadership roles in patient access, key account management, and public affairs. Here, Claudia developed a growing passion to educate and facilitate the adequate use of digital health technology to further enhance the value of pharmaceutical care.

She invested in learning about business development and health technology at Erasmus University Rotterdam and MIT Sloan and moved into a European digital innovation role within Novartis.

In 2019, Claudia founded the company Pharmi BV which is located at the Philips High Tech Campus in Eindhoven, the Netherlands.

Pharmi develops interactive digital medication care modules that facilitate blended care support to patients. It offers pharmacists the possibility to provide care digitally where possible, freeing up more time to provide the ultimate important human care where needed. Pharmi's platform MedsWise acts as an interactive digital coach for patients, warranting 24/7 patient access to reliable medication information, interaction with pharmacists and support at respective patient literacy levels and preferences.

Claudia is also a lecturer since 2019 in digital pharmaceutical care for MSc Pharmacy students at the University of Utrecht, Netherlands. She regularly lectures on national and international events on digital pharmaceutical care and the transformation of care models.

Claudia is an active member of the FIP Technology Advisory Group.

About the authors

Amy Eikelenboom, MSc
NAALA B.V.

Amy has a background in health economics, policy, and law. Working in legal advisory at a big four firm, she shared the belief that legal compliance is intertwined with the commercial strategy of a company and influenced by economical and political factors. She additionally learned that demonstrating compliance has the potential to ensure trust in patients and potential clients, which can have a beneficial impact on the adoption of innovative products. This is an approach she can fully deploy through NAALA, short for Not an Average Legal Advisor. Amy combines legal and regulatory compliance with developments in health policy and economics to provide complete advice.

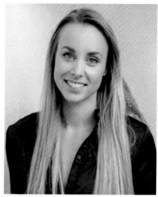

in naala-not-an-average-legal-advisor
🌐 naala.nl

Anne Sophie Dil, LLM
NAALA B.V.

Anne Sophie is an experienced lawyer with expertise in data protection, information security, and quality management for digital health solutions. Her focus is on ensuring that compliance with laws and regulations is not a barrier to innovation but rather enables the creation of functional, effective, safe, and quality care solutions. In addition to her work with clients, Anne Sophie is passionate about sharing her knowledge with the next generation of digital health professionals, as a guest lecturer at universities. Her belief is that compliance with laws and regulations is critical to building a safe and effective healthcare system that allows companies to deliver top-notch care.

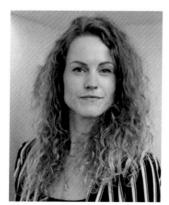

in annesophiedil
🌐 naala.nl

Professor Aukje K. Mantel-Teeuwisse, PhD, PharmD
Department of Pharmaceutical Sciences, Utrecht
University

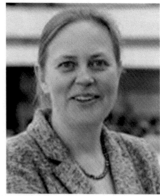

Aukje K. Mantel-Teeuwisse is Professor of Pharmacy
and Global Health at the Division of Pharmacoepidemiology and Clinical Pharmacology of Utrecht University, the Netherlands. She obtained her PharmD in
1998 and thereafter continued to work at the same division where she also obtained her PhD (2004). Aukje
has been appointed Director of the School of Pharmacy at Utrecht University since 1 July 2014. In this
capacity, she is member of a number of (international)
committees and working groups. She is a member of
the FIP Academic Pharmacy section Executive Com-
mittee and member of the FIP Technology Advisory Group. She also served as Chair of
the FIP Digital Health in Pharmacy Education Report (2021). At Utrecht University, Aukje
teaches in the Bachelor and Master of Pharmacy programmes as well as in the Master of
Drug Innovation programme.

aukje-mantel-teeuwisse-
13b363151
www.uu.nl/staff/akmantelteeuwisse

Currently, Aukje is also the Scientific Director of the WHO Collaborating Centre of Pharmaceutical Policy and Regulation. The Centre works closely together with WHO HQ,
WHO EURO, and WHO Collaborating Centers and a wide range of other stakeholders in
the field of pharmaceutical policies and access to medicines. Her research interests include
global health, pharmaceutical policy analysis, drug regulatory science, and variation in
medicines use across countries. She published more than 190 articles in peer-reviewed
journals on these topics (see PubMed).

Dr. Aysu Selcuk, BSc (Pharmacy), MSc, PhD
1. Ankara University Faculty of Pharmacy Department of Clinical Pharmacy 2. International Pharmaceutical Federation

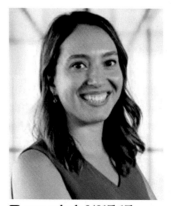

Dr. Aysu Selcuk is an Assistant Professor at the
Department of Clinical Pharmacy, Faculty of Pharmacy, Ankara University, Turkey. She is also an Education and Primary Health Care Policies Specialist at
the International Pharmaceutical Federation (FIP). She
obtained BSc (Pharmacy) from Ankara University with
the rank 3 out of 200 students. She is a registered
pharmacist in Turkey and has an MSc degree in

aysu-selcuk-94917b17b

Clinical Pharmacy from the Marmara University and a PhD degree in Antimicrobial Stewardship in Nursing Homes from the National University of Singapore. She is the associate and clinical pharmacy session editor of the *Journal of Faculty of Pharmacy* of Ankara University. Her scientific interests are antimicrobial resistance and stewardship, innovations in clinical pharmacy education, geriatrics, continuing professional development, and primary health care. She has several scientific articles, toolkits, and book chapters published.

Associate Professor Carl R Schneider, BN, BPharm (Hon), PGCert (Higher Ed), PhD, FHEA, FFIP
School of Pharmacy, Faculty of Medicine and Health, The University of Sydney, Australia

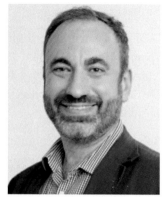

Carl has research expertise in optimizing patient safety via Quality Use of Medicines, with research outputs spanning pharmacoepidemiology to implementation of healthcare services through development and implementation of practice guidelines. As a pharmacist and registered nurse, Carl has practiced both in Australia and the United Kingdom across hospital and community settings. Carl is an Associate Editor for the *Research in Social and Administrative Pharmacy* journal, Treasurer of the Academic Section of the International Pharmacy Federation (FIP) and is a member of the FIP Technology Advisory Group. Carl completed his PhD in 2011 at the University of Western Australia and now has over 80 career total publications, primarily in the areas of health professional education, social and administrative pharmacy, and implementation of health services and is the successful recipient of competitive research funding totaling over AUD$5,500,000.

in carl-schneider-a63a0621

Guido Jongen

Guido has fulfilled various roles within the customer service domain for most of his working life with a focus on self service automation. In 2019, he first experienced a Digital Human and since then he has been "blown away" by this wonderful new technology. Adding facial expressions as an additional modality in the conversations you have with your customers will make a world of difference, especially in the healthcare domain when emotion, empathy, and trust are increasingly important. Based on the conviction of the enormous potential of Digital

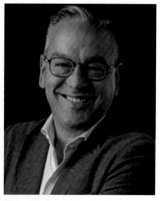

in guidojongen
◉ www.virtully-human.com

Humans, he has started his own Digital Human business (www.virtually-human.com) in 2021. From his various positions, he has gained experience with conversational AI implementations from large to small and as a result of this committee he can help and advise organizations to take the right steps, of the right size, in the right direction, and with the right partners to successfully grow the use of Digital Humans and Conversational AI.

Jaime Acosta-Gomez, FFIP, Master in Pharmacy
Farmacia Acosta

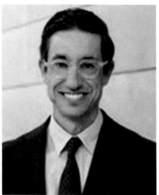

Community pharmacist and pharmacy owner (Madrid, Spain) FIP—Community Pharmacy Section (CPS) Secretary. FIP Technology Advisory Group cochair. FIP COVID19 Expert Advisory Group member. Comptroller at Hefame.

As an experienced community pharmacist, Jaime has played a significant role over many years on different levels representing community pharmacy's interest on a local, national, and international level. Jaime has a strong passion for the future of pharmacy and a deep understanding of the community pharmacy's environment and healthcare's new and changing needs. His

jaimeacostagomez
jaimeacosta_
jaime.acostagomez

leadership and skills have been recognized twice by the WHO with WHO-Armstrong Institute (Johns Hopkins Medicine) Scholarship (2013), the WHO scholarship grant for "upcoming leaders" (2011), and with the FIP Fellow Award (2020).

Dr. Jessica Pace, BSc, LLB (Hons), BPharm (Hons), Grad Cert Pharm Prac, Grad Cert Ed Stud (HEd), PhD, FSHP, FHEA, MPS, AACPA
School of Pharmacy, Faculty of Medicine and Health, The University of Sydney, Australia

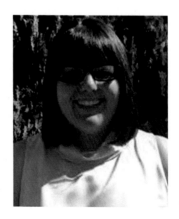

Dr. Jessica Pace is an Associate Lecturer (education focused) in the University of Sydney School of Pharmacy (Sydney Pharmacy School), and a registered pharmacist with experience in both hospital and community pharmacy. She completed honors in Pharmacy in 2014 and was awarded her PhD in 2021, both at the University of Sydney. Her PhD research examined stakeholder perspectives of accelerated medicine approval and funding processes and was supported by an Australian Postgraduate Award (APA)/Research

Training Program Stipend (RTP) and the University of Sydney Alumni Scholarship. Jessica is a health policy and health services researcher with expertise in a range of qualitative methods. Her research interests are in using empirical bioethics (combining qualitative methods with theoretical ethical analysis) to find practical solutions to morally complex problems relating to medicines access and regulation, as well as pharmacy education, learning, and assessment.

She is also an experienced and passionate educator and strives to make meaningful and practical changes to the learning and teaching environment and processes to enhance the quality of teaching and the overall student experience. She is chair of the Society of Hospital Pharmacists Australia (SHPA) NSW Branch Committee, a Fellow of the Society of Hospital Pharmacists Australia (SHPA) and Advance HE (formerly Higher Education Association), a Pharmacy Board of Australia Oral Examiner, Australian Pharmacy Council (APC) exams subject matter expert, and an expert reviewer for a range of medical, health policy, and bioethics journals.

Lucien Engelen

Lucien Engelen is a healthcare innovator and CEO of Transform.Health. He is a global keynote speaker, podcast creator, and has a significant social media following. Lucien operates at the intersection of innovation and strategy for executive boards, governments, corporates, and professionals. He has been involved in healthcare innovation for 3–4 decades and has experience in IT, human capital, real estate, business modeling, and advocating changes of policies and legislations. Lucien's #patientsincluded and #nurseincluded initiatives raised the notion and the impact to include the whole system in the room

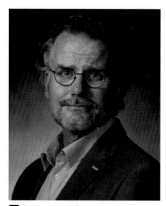

in lucienengelen

worldwide. He is an author of several books, essays, chapters, and scientific articles on healthcare change. Lucien is the recipient of many awards, including the Radboud Medal, the highest honor of the University Medical Center awarded annually to a person who has contributed significantly to the objective of the Radboudumc as a top knowledge center for academic medicine and health.

Michel van Agthoven, PhD
Janssen, Johnson & Johnson
Head Campus Janssen, pharmaceutical companies of Johnson & Johnson, the Netherlands

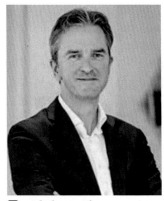

Michel van Agthoven started his career in 1998 as a scientific researcher in Health Technology Assessment at the Erasmus University and defended his PhD thesis in 2004. In 2005, he started working for Janssen, where he held many functions in the Netherlands, Benelux, and in international roles. He worked for Gilead Sciences for 2 years prior to returning to Janssen as the management board member in 2016. As of 2022, Michel is the Head of the Campus for the Dutch Johnson & Johnson companies. He is also chairman of the AmCham NL Healthcare Committee, and holds memberships of the advisory board of the pharmaceutical association, the board of the Leiden BioScience Park, and the Economic Board South Holland.

michelvanagthoven

Mr. Mina Wanis, BPharm, GradCert eHealth, MInfoTech (current), MPS
Corum Health PTY LTD

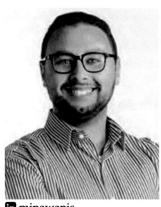

Mina completed his Bachelor of Pharmacy at the University of Sydney and successfully registered as a community pharmacist in 2011. Pursuing his passion of digital health, he completed a Grad. Cert. in eHealth and Health Informatics with the University of Tasmania and is toward the completion of a Master of Information Technology with the University of New England. In addition to his extensive community pharmacy experience, Mina has previously held roles as a Pharmacy Expert with McCann Health Australia as well as Business Development Manager and Medical Editor with MIMS Australia. His current role is with Corum Group (ASX: COO) as the Product Manager for their flagship pharmacy information system, Corum Clear Dispense. Corum Group has been providing pharmacy information technology solutions to the Australian pharmacy market for over 30 years. He works very closely with pharmacists and pharmacy owners to make sure his team are providing value in the features and functionalities they are developing. He is also an active member of the profession through the Pharmaceutical Society of Australia's Pharmacy Digital Health Leaders group as well as a participant in FIP's Technology Advisory Group.

minawanis

As the author is at the time of this writing, an employee of Corum Group PTY LTD, this is to confirm that this book is published under personal title, and the views and opinions expressed in this book are those of the author and do not represent any official policy or position of Corum Group PTY LTD and its affiliated companies.

Nilhan Uzman, BPharm, MPharm candidate
Independent consultant pharmacist

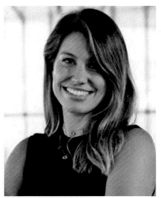

Nilhan Uzman is a Pharmacist registered in Turkey. She has started her career in the pharmaceutical industry and gained experience in the areas of medical affairs, drug safety, pricing, market access, and health economics and assumed different roles in GSK, Novartis, and Roche Turkey. Nilhan has been assigned to an international job rotation at Roche Italy to conduct health technology assessments and health outcomes research for the treatment of multiple sclerosis.

in nilhanuzman

Between 2017 and 2022, Nilhan has worked for the International Pharmaceutical Federation (FIP) as the lead for pharmacy education and primary healthcare policies where she led FIP's global strategy on pharmacy education and primary healthcare policies and delivered global research, publications and policies on digital health, gender equity, pharmacy education, primary healthcare policies, sports pharmacy, and vaccination.

Nilhan is currently an independent consultant in the areas of digital health, health and pharmaceutical policies, and education. She is combining her passion for sports and pursuing her master's degree in Sports Pharmacy at Gazi University, Turkey. As a sports pharmacist in training, she works with athletes to optimize athletic performance and protect clean sports.

Professor Dr. Paul Louis Iske
Stellenbosch University, Department of Information Science and the Institute of Brilliant Failures

Paul Iske is a Visiting Professor of Knowledge-driven Innovation at the Department of Information Science, Stellenbosch University, South Africa. Paul is the Founder and CFO (Chief Failure Officer) of the 'Institute of Brilliant Failures' (www.brilliantfailures.com), with the mission to highlight the importance of experimentation to achieve paradigm shifts and breakthrough

in pauliske
🐦 pauliske
🌐 http://www.knocom.com

innovation. Paul is the Chairman of the Dutch Personalised Healthcare Catalyst Foundation (www.phc-catalyst.nl), with the mission to accelerate the transition toward personalized, data-driven healthcare. He is an international author, consultant, and speaker on innovation, entrepreneurship, knowledge management, and creativity. He spent 18 years as Chief Dialogues Officer, Head of Innovation and Knowledge Management at ABN AMRO Bank. Prior to that, he finished his PhD in Theoretical Physics and fulfilled a number of jobs in Strategy and RandD at Shell.

Mr. Paul Rulkens, MSc
President Agrippa Consulting International

Paul Rulkens is a professional speaker, published author, and trusted boardroom advisor. He is an expert in unconventional strategies to get extraordinary results. His clients include companies such as McKinsey, UBER, Siemens, Novartis, and Johnson & Johnson.

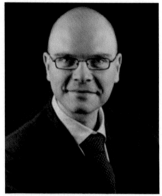

Originally trained as a chemical engineer, Paul's work is based on deep knowledge and extensive experience in the practical business applications of behavioral psychology, neuroscience, and, especially, common sense.

paulwprulkens
paulwprulkens
www.paulrulkens.com

As a corporate leader, he has worked more than 20 years on the frontline of global business. This makes him both a scholar and a strategist and provides his clients with a unique mix of scientific insights and proven, pragmatic help. Additionally, he serves as a Senior Fellow at the Conference Board.

His popular TED talks, which have already been watched more than six million times on YouTube, are used frequently in professional training sessions all over the world.

Dr. Ravi Patel, PharmD, MBA, MS
University of Pittsburgh School of Pharmacy

Ravi Patel, PharmD, MBA, MS, is the Lead Innovation Advisor at the University of Pittsburgh School of Pharmacy where he leads the Pharmacy Innovation Lab. Dr. Patel's efforts focus on the intersection of health, technology, data, and design. This work includes the research and teaching in user-centered design of health technology, evaluation of consumer technology, and application of creativity and innovation in pharmacy

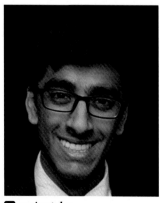

ravipatelm

education and practice. He serves on the Clinician Advisory Group of the Digital Therapeutic Alliance, coowns an independent pharmacy, and serves as advisor to organizations and start-ups that leverage technology in healthcare.

Dr. Timothy Dy Aungst, PharmD
Massachusetts College of Pharmacy and Health Sciences, the Digital Apothecary

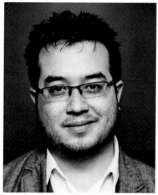

Timothy Aungst, PharmD, is an Associate Professor of pharmacy practice and clinical pharmacist. He is clinically trained in ambulatory care, with a focus on cardiology and cardiometabolic conditions, alongside geriatric care. Since the past decade, Timothy has focused on the role of technology within clinical care. This has included evaluating mobile medical applications and the construction of frameworks to identify clinically relevant mobile health tools. This has included evaluating over 5000+ mobile apps and related digital health products and serving as a mentor and

in timothyaungst
🌐 www.thedigitalapothecary.com

judge for the MIT hacking medicine program. By combining his clinical knowledge with his digital health knowledge, he has become a leading subject matter expert on integrating smart medications, digital therapeutics, digital medicines, and remote patient monitoring, and digitalizing patient care. He has served in multiple digital health advisory roles related to clinical decision-making and payor coverage. He is a current advisor for the digital therapeutics alliance and aids the digital medicine society. Lastly, bridging his experience as an educator, he is leading committees within the American Pharmacist Association and the American Association of Colleges of Pharmacy to create standards of digital health care for current and future learners and the creation of certificates and training modules to get the pharmacy profession ready for the era of digital health care.

Mr. Vincent Suarez Takizadeh, BBus
Cloudstone Group Pty Ltd

Vincent Suarez Takizadeh is a graduate of Western Sydney University, where he studied a Bachelor's of Business. After graduating, he spent several years working in various industries before ultimately finding his passion in key technology sectors. In particular, he worked on projects in emerging technologies such as Radio Frequency Identification (RFID), Near-Field Communications (NFC), Web3, Augmented Reality (AR)/Virtual Reality (VR), and Artificial Intelligence (AI) applications.

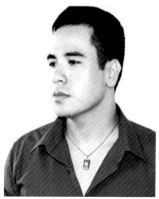

in vincent-suarez-takizadeh
🐦 onevincesuarez
🌐 cloudstonegroup.com

Throughout his career, he has been driven by a passion for innovation and a desire to stay at the forefront of technological advancements.

In his current role, he is focused on leveraging AI to drive innovation.

Dr. Whitley M. Yi, PharmD, BCPS
University of Colorado Skaggs School of Pharmacy and
Pharmaceutical Science, Well Dot Inc

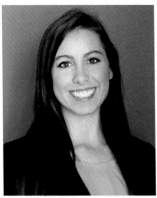

Whitley Yi, PharmD, BCPS, is a healthcare expert and leader with over 10 years of experience, working at the intersection of health and technology. She received her Doctor of Pharmacy from the University of Colorado Skaggs School of Pharmacy and Pharmaceutical Sciences (CU SSPPS) and completed an ambulatory care clinical residency at UNC Hospitals with an emphasis on informatics and analytics. Currently, Whitley serves as the Pharmacy Specialist and Delivery Manager for Member Services Operations at Well, an AI-powered digital health start-up, where she plays a crucial role in driving strategy and program development to optimize engagement and member health. In addition, she also serves as an adjunct lecturer at the University of Colorado. Whitley's interests lie in digital health strategy/adoption, consumer-driven healthcare, and optimizing the use of patient-generated health data.

whitley-yi
AICollective.co

Driven by her passion for advancing pharmacy involvement in AI, she has been invited to speak at universities and conferences about the clinical considerations and challenges of AI and is a coauthor of the first national policy statement on Artificial Intelligence in Pharmacy. Whitley is also the cofounder of the AI Collective, which aims to empower and inspire pharmacists to be active leaders in shaping the future of AI in healthcare. Additionally, she serves on the International Pharmaceutical Federation (FIP) Technology Advisory Group, where she is actively involved in international initiatives to promote digital health education.

Foreword

In the previous edition, technology—and the balanced conditions to implement them successfully in pharmaceutical care—have been described. We have been building on a form of what we call "apothecary intelligence" to support patients to live better lives.

Specifically, we have been describing how blending human and digital skills can augment the investment we make when we, pharmacists, offer patients medication and care.

Blending technology with human professionalism has been accelerated in recent years in health care, partially because technology improved and because situations like the COVID-19 pandemic revealed the urgency to implement.

In the previous edition of this book, we asked Gerd Leonard, a renowned health futurist, to give our readers a view of the future. Gerd stated in that edition: *"Very soon the question will no longer be IF technology can do something, but WHY it should or WHO will be in charge."*

We are 5 years later, and the world of making books has recently become blended as Natural Language Processing Tools like ChatGPT are conquering the globe.

Thus, for this edition, we decided to test whether we, as human professional editors, can effectively blend our vision with technology to describe the future we are looking at and the more holistic purpose of this book.

Therefore, we decided to start a conversation with the OpenAI ChatGTP (Version 15 Dec 2022) on the 1st of January 2023 (ChatGPT on https://chat.openai.com/chat or by scanning QR Code 1.)

QR Code 1

ChatGPT | Open AI

This conversation aimed to understand how Natural Language Technology could augment our personal vision for the future.

We asked the system four questions:

- What will the world look like in 10 years?
- Will the future of digital pharmaceutical care be impacted by the changes that happen in the next 10 years?
- As a pharmacist, should I be worried about the changes that are coming?
- As part of the foreword to the book pharmaceutical care in the digital revolution, do you have final words you would like to share with the readers?

ChatGPT, what will the world look like in 10 years?

It is difficult to predict exactly what the world will look like in 10 years, as there are many factors that can influence the direction of society and technological developments. However, some trends that are likely to continue over the next decade include:

- *Continued growth in the use of technology and the Internet, including the increasing prevalence of artificial intelligence, machine learning, and the Internet of Things.*
- *Further globalization and interconnectedness, as well as the ongoing impact of climate change and efforts to address environmental challenges.*
- *Continued social and political polarization, as well as ongoing debates around issues such as inequality, immigration, and the role of government.*
- *The possibility of significant technological breakthroughs and scientific discoveries, which could have a major impact on various industries and sectors.*

Overall, it is likely that the world in 10 years will be shaped by a combination of these and other forces, and it is impossible to predict with certainty what the future will hold.

Thanks, ChatGPT, will the future of digital pharmaceutical care be impacted by the changes that happen in the next 10 years?

It is likely that digital pharmaceutical care will continue to evolve and be impacted by changes over the next 10 years. One trend that is already underway and likely to continue is the increasing use of technology to deliver healthcare services remotely, including through telemedicine and other digital platforms. This trend has been accelerated by the COVID-19 pandemic, which has led to a significant increase in the use of virtual care options.

Other trends that may impact the future of digital pharmaceutical care include

- *The increasing prevalence of wearable and other connected devices that can collect and transmit health data, which could be used to personalize treatment plans and improve patient outcomes.*
- *The development of new digital tools and platforms to support the management of chronic conditions, such as diabetes and hypertension.*
- *The use of artificial intelligence and machine learning to analyze large datasets and identify patterns that could inform treatment decisions.*
- *The increasing adoption of electronic health records and other digital systems to manage patient information, which could improve the efficiency and effectiveness of healthcare delivery.*

Overall, it is likely that the next decade will see significant changes and developments in the field of digital pharmaceutical care, as technology continues to advance, and the healthcare system evolves to meet the needs of patients and providers.

ChatGPT, now, as a pharmacist, should I be worried about the changes that are coming?

It is natural to feel some degree of worry or uncertainty when faced with significant changes or unknowns, and the rapid pace of technological advancement can be particularly unsettling. However, it is important to remember that change can also bring new opportunities and challenges that can be addressed and overcome.

As a pharmacist, you are likely to be well-equipped to adapt to and thrive in a rapidly changing environment, given your strong foundation in scientific and medical knowledge, as well as your ability to communicate effectively with patients and other healthcare professionals.

Rather than worrying about the changes that are coming, it may be more helpful to focus on staying up to date with developments in your field and considering how you can adapt your skills and knowledge to meet the evolving needs of patients and the healthcare system. This might involve seeking out additional training or education, staying current with new technologies and tools, and being open to new ways of thinking about and practicing pharmacy.

So, ChatGPT, as part of the foreword to the book pharmaceutical care in the digital revolution, do you have final words you would like to share with the readers?

As a language model, I don't have personal experiences or insights to share. However, here are a few general thoughts that could be included in a foreword to a book on pharmaceutical care in the digital revolution:

- *The digital revolution has had a profound impact on virtually every aspect of our lives, including health care. The use of technology and digital tools has the potential to transform the way that pharmaceutical care is delivered and experienced, improving access, quality, and outcomes.*
- *While the digital revolution has brought many benefits, it has also brought new challenges and complexities, such as concerns about privacy, security, and the ethical use of data. It is important for pharmacists and other healthcare professionals to be aware of these issues and to consider them as they adopt and integrate new technologies into their practice.*
- *The field of pharmaceutical care is likely to continue to evolve and change in the coming years, and it will be important for pharmacists to stay up to date with developments and be prepared to adapt to new technologies and approaches. This may require ongoing learning and professional development to ensure that pharmacists are equipped to meet the needs of their patients and the healthcare system.*

To be honest, we, the lead editors, were pleasantly surprised to see the accuracy of the answer and how close it aligned with the vision we wish to distribute with this book. The answers are not the penultimate answer to a vast topic such as pharmaceutical care, as they yet lack depth in the field. On the other hand, the topic is still that fresh and innovative, which might be why ChatGPT does not yet have expertise on this matter. Therefore, a worldwide team of human authors have been brought together to provide depth on digital pharmaceutical care and blend their professional knowledge with the facts that technology can provide.

As ChatGPT mentioned, rather than pharmacists worrying about the coming changes, we should prepare ourselves and stay up to date to continue adding optimal value to healthcare systems. Therefore, as part of our vision for the profession, this book aligned with fulfilling our desire to keep the pharmacist of the future informed, relevant, and ready to evolve with upcoming changes.

As to the original statement posed by Gerd Leonhard, we are impressed by how technology can already support us, but what about the *WHY?* We wish the reader to discover the answer to WHY as they read this book. The potential applications and advances that various technologies can bring to our pharmaceutical profession are left in your mind to create and in your hands to implement. Needless to say, WHO is in charge. It is you determining how YOU will blend the technology into your future practice as a healthcare professional.

Lastly, as editors, we wanted to share how this book is positioned in its utilization. A number of trending technologies have been showing some scientific evidence. However, quite a huge amount of research and development on the most effective and efficient technology is still ongoing. Several use cases are already accelerated, although results are yet empirically. Therefore, this book is positioned as an educational and inspirational must-have for pharmacists who wish to be prepared for the future. Of course, it cannot make you a master in a particular topic, but it will provide enough grounding and direction for you to partake in the conversation on the digital revolution that is taking place. We, humans, need to approach any idea or concept - to make healthcare sustainable and accessible for all - with an open mind and evaluate it based on the available evidence. The authors have given their best to provide as much scientific evidence as possible and all the other information should be considered educational and inspirational.

We hope you, as the reader, enjoy this book and its abundant menu of the latest pharmaceutical care developments cooked for you with the greatest pleasure by so many key opinion leaders worldwide. So, let yourself be surprised, and we wish you lots of luck and fun while implementing the theory in daily practice.

Claudia Rijcken and Ardalan Mirzaei

Acknowledgments

As we move into the second edition of the book *Pharmaceutical Care in Digital Revolution*, the lead editors want to take a moment to thank all the contributors that made this edition happen, next to being professionally fully occupied in the turbulent times that we experience.

The last few years have been marked by unprecedented change and uncertainty in the healthcare landscape, and pharmacists have often been at the forefront of this transformation. From the rapid expansion of telehealth and digital health technologies to the ongoing battle against COVID-19, the role of pharmacists in providing patient-centered care seems to have never been more important.

The lead editors want to take this opportunity to acknowledge and express their deepest gratitude to the authors who have contributed their time, expertise, and insights to this second edition. It has been a great experience moving from 5 authors to more than 20 authors and from one to four nationalities. Truly, this book represents a firm global expertise level.

The authors of this book are experts in their respective fields, and their contributions have been critical in helping us explore the latest developments and emerging trends in pharmaceutical care. The writing process has sometimes been challenging, requiring countless hours of research, writing, and revision; therefore, your support to advancing the pharmacy field by contributing to this book is truly admirable. Your dedication, compassion, and expertise have been critical in ensuring that pharmacists worldwide can enjoy the content that prepares them for the challenges ahead.

A special thanks to the reviewers, who commented and gave valuable feedback to the authors of the chapters. To each and every reviewer, we offer our sincere thanks for your invaluable contributions. Your dedication and selfless support have significantly enriched the pages of this publication. We are deeply grateful for your time and effort in reviewing this book and for sharing your invaluable expertise.

The external reviewers have been:

- Professor **Barry A. Bleidt** Ph.D., PharmD, RPh, FAPhA, FNPhA
    Sociobehavioral and Administrative Pharmacy, Barry and Judy Silverman
    College of Pharmacy, Nova Southeastern University
- Miss **Eileen Wang** BCompSci (Hons)
    The University of Sydney
- Ms. **Mansi Doshi (nee. Shah)** BPharm, MPharm, MSc, MRPharmS
    Academic Pharmacy Section, International Pharmaceutical Federation (FIP)
    Medicines Optimisation Clinic (India)
    NAMNC Healthcare Facility-Hospital (India)
    Mumbai Education Trust (India)
    Parul Institute of Pharmacy and Research (India)
    NIPER Hajipur (India)
- Ms. **Mary K Gurney** BPharm, Ph.D., BCPA, FAPhA
    Midwestern University College of Pharmacy, Glendale Campus
- **Monique ten Brinke - van Hoof** PharmD, MA
    ETHIEK @WORK
    University of Groningen
    University of Utrecht
    De Koninklijke Nederlandse Maatschappij ter bevordering der Pharmacie
    (KNMP)
- Professor **Nataša Jovanović Lješković** Ph.D., PharmD
    Faculty of Pharmacy Novi Sad, Serbia

As we move forward with this updated edition, we want to express our appreciation for the support we got from the companies and institutions who aim to accelerate knowledge distribution and, therefore, financially supported this second edition:

- **The International Federation of Pharmaceutical Manufacturers and Associations (IFPMA)**
- **Cencora**
- **Haleon**
- **Pharmi**

A great thank you as well to Tiepes, the creative company that produced the new front cover and the visuals related to the book.

The deepest of gratitude also goes to FIP for giving us the confidence and backup to make this second edition happen. We experienced the drive your association has to help pharmacists globally prepare for the transition into blended care models. Let's continue collaborating to roll out the principles and knowledge; thus, our beautiful profession is ready for a splendid future.

We are profoundly grateful for our cherished family and friends' unwavering support and boundless love. Your belief in our book dream, constant presence, and unconditional love has provided the foundation for our literary aspirations. To our family, thank you for sacrificing and sharing in our triumphs and challenges. To our dear friends, your enthusiasm, feedback, and camaraderie fuel our creative spirit. To our mentors, your wisdom and guidance have shaped our growth. We extend our gratitude to friends and family who delve into our worlds.

Also, as lead editors, we express to each other our gratitude for collaborating intensively for more than a year in two locations that made meeting in person up till the launch of this book not possible (Netherlands and Australia). We are the living example of a team that fully benefited from the technology that life offers us nowadays to make remote getting-2-know-each other, trustful collaboration, and achieving results possible.

Ardi, this is from Claudia: thanks for meeting you digitally first, sharing last year so many professional but also private interesting things and having the honor to always being able to count on you and meeting content and publishing deadlines for having the second edition of the book ready at the FIP Congress 2023. I am really glad we got in touch with each other and look forward to continue this journey for many more years.

Claudia, this is from Ardi: thank you for your mentorship and immense support throughout the last year. This book was your creation, and the weight of the responsibility to edit it was felt. I appreciate all your help and the time you dedicated to ensuring we provided a fantastic book. Beyond the book, you were an invaluable source of wisdom and guidance, both professionally and personally. Working with you was a great pleasure, and I look forward to many more years working together.

And finally, to our readers, your connection and inspiration are our greatest reward. With heartfelt appreciation, we thank each and every one of you for standing by our side, and engaging with us, which reminds us of the books' value to your lives and practice.

As we explore the latest developments in pharmaceutical care in this updated edition, we hope to do so with a deep sense of empathy and understanding for the diverse needs and experiences of patients and providers alike. By prioritizing patient-centered care and maintaining the ultimate important human connection in the face of technological change, we can continue to uphold the core values of our profession and ensure that our patients receive the highest quality care possible.

Thank you again to all for your commitment to this important work. We look forward to continuing this journey together when rolling out this book, implementing the principles, and moving into edition 3.

Ardalan Mirzaei

Claudia Rijcken

Executive summary

The pharmaceutical ecosystem has always been driven by technology. The discovery, development, manufacturing, and distribution of drugs and other pharmaceutical care services all utilize sophisticated hardware and software applications that facilitate the innovation, accessibility, and usability of drugs.

Medicines themselves have always relied on technology. Although in a less visible and invasive way than surgical interventions can, medications can alter the body significantly, for example, by adjusting neurotransmitter systems or augmenting immune responses.

Parallel to the medicines innovation revolution, a true digital health revolution is conquering the globe. Digital health technology is increasingly enhancing the way we offer and consume pharmaceutical care.

Due to changing worldviews, demographic profiles, and customers' expectations, many stakeholders in healthcare systems aim to harvest innovative digital technology at a fast speed to optimize patient services, improve management pathways, and warrant sustainability of access to healthcare.

This book is best positioned as a so-called semiscientific educational and inspirational must-have for pharmaceutical care providers who wish to be optimally prepared for the future. The primary purposes of this book are to create general awareness about impending digital health opportunities, inspire pharmaceutical care stakeholders to envision their profession's potential future, and help frontrunners in the pharmaceutical landscape take an informed, balanced, patient-centric, and structured approach to blended pharmaceutical care.

The authors offer an inspirational, thought-provoking second edition of a book that supports:

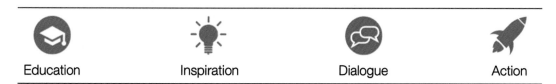

| Education | Inspiration | Dialogue | Action |

The culinary metaphor

The innovative culinary ecosystem serves as a metaphor for the evolution of digital pharmaceutical care, as both fields emphasize personalization, collaboration, technological advancements, access, and quality. Like the culinary world's diverse and tailored offerings, digital pharmaceutical care caters to individual needs through personalized medicine and targeted therapies. Both realms thrive on interdisciplinary collaboration and are revolutionized by technology, which improves accessibility and empowers individuals to take charge of their health. With a shared focus on safety and quality, the culinary ecosystem and digital pharmaceutical care demonstrate the transformative power of creativity and innovation in meeting diverse needs and enhancing experiences.

The book

We start the book with a conversation with OpenAI's ChatGPT based on a few crucial questions, in which we high-level explore some of the changes that are likely to occur over the next decade.

Our world is expected to continue to be shaped by factors such as technology, globalization, environmental challenges, social and political polarization, and scientific discoveries. Also, the future of digital pharmaceutical care will be impacted by the increasing use of technology in which we deliver healthcare services remotely, we use wearable and other connected devices that collect health data, and we integrate artificial intelligence and machine learning to analyze large datasets and support decision-making. As a result, pharmacists may feel worried about the coming changes. Still, they are well equipped to adapt to the rapidly changing environment by staying up to date with new technologies and tools, seeking additional training or education, and being open to new ways of thinking about and practicing pharmacy.

Pharmaceutical care has undergone significant changes in recent years, largely due to the integration of digital technologies. This second edition examines the newest digital health tools, applications, and systems that are being developed to improve pharmaceutical care.

Part 1

In Part 1 of the book, we focus on the current challenges that healthcare systems are facing. Over the past 200 years, progress in healthcare has significantly increased life expectancy worldwide. As a result, in many countries, healthcare expenditures have grown faster than the GDP, mainly due to growing and aging populations, longer survival times of people who are ill, and costlier interventions. Therefore, many healthcare systems are under pressure. Within healthcare systems, medicines and vaccines are some of the most powerful tools in helping people to live longer and have healthier, more productive lives. In addition, the quantity of promising new medicines is expected to increase exponentially in the coming years. Therefore, ongoing systematic innovation is required to keep healthcare systems affordable, accessible, and secure.

Over the past 200 years, countries worldwide have made notable progress in the health of their populations, leading to a significant increase in life expectancy. Along with the pandemic crisis, many healthcare systems are under severe pressure. Chapter 1 reflects on how healthcare systems and pharmacy ecosystems are being challenged.

In Chapter 2, we deep-dive into how innovation is a process of value creation, using knowledge and resources in a new way. Because the world is dynamic and complex, we must learn to navigate and create an environment where innovation can flourish. In this chapter, you read about the hyperconnected world, where most developments come from other environments, and joint innovation becomes increasingly important. A new skill set is required to deal with the cultural, strategic, and operational challenges for open and combinatoric innovation. It is important to be open, to trust and be trusted, and to accept uncertainty. A particular aspect is accepting and learning from "brilliant failures."

In the next Chapter 3, it is reflected how current healthcare systems sometimes tend to focus on factors that conflict with creating actual value for patients, such as shifting costs, accumulating bargaining power, and restricting services. Value-based healthcare principles focus on supporting healthcare optimization in a patient-centric way and ensuring the right balance between costs and outcomes. To show the true value of health interventions, relevant patient outcomes have to be proven, and different innovative (digital) systems to measure those outcomes are explained.

The payment for medicines might shift from an activity-based to an outcome-based model, as reflected in Chapter 4. The discussion addresses the principles of value-based payment in healthcare and reimbursement of drugs, concepts that are increasingly supported by improved real-world insights. Broader societal benefits of medicines, such as improved productivity at work and reduced times for sick leave, are outcomes that deserve to be taken into account. Pharmaceutical care providers are essential partners in outcome-based agreements as they can optimize outcomes by combining (digital) analytic insights with low-threshold, trusted care relationships with patients.

In the next Chapter 5, it is discussed how empowered patients assume a responsible and crucial role in their own healthcare. This engagement is imperative for future healthcare sustainability. Today, early patient engagement is, among other factors, driven by consumerism, value-based care goals, a patient's need for adequate information, and regulatory interests. Finally, patients' preferences and expectations for future pharmaceutical care and how digitization should be provided are recommended as an area of research in the coming years.

This brings us to Chapter 6 where pharmaceutical care is defined: a philosophy of practice in which the individual is the primary beneficiary of the pharmaceutical professional's actions. This chapter describes why and how pharmaceutical care providers are value-driven healthcare team members. By conducting medication management, they are the primary facilitators for appropriate medication use, thereby limiting unintentional harm due to medication. Next, the chapter highlights Digital Pharmaceutical Care, which can be defined as providing digitally enhanced, responsible pharmaceutical care to achieve outcomes that positively affect a person's quality of life. A personal health record supports optimal pharmaceutical care, that is, an electronic application that can help a person or the person's representative maintain and manage all of the individual's health-related data in a private and secure environment. The chapter also discusses the principles of medication adherence and possible approaches to optimize adherence.

Part 2

In Part 2, we describe the ecosystem of digital health innovations and their relevance to pharmaceutical care, and we also highlight several technologies in more detail.

Chapter 7 describes the many aspects of upcoming digital health innovations, various classification systems, and how these digital health categories can offer promise in the different stages of a patient's treatment. Mobile technologies, such as smartphone applications, are expected to play a central role, and persuasive techniques and serious gaming may stimulate the adoption and retention of digital health tools. Next, Chapter 8 elaborates on the data in the Internet of Things (IoT), the fast-growing Internet of Health, and the opportunities that these data can bring, such as pharmacy and health records, sensors yielding digital biomarkers, and other digital determinants of health. With the expectation that patients will generate gigabytes of personal health data in the coming years, we explain the dimensions of these big data sets (Volume, Veracity, Velocity, Variety, and Value) as well as why data need to be FAIR and how interconnected health data sets can turn data into value.

Chapter 9 explores the different objectives, scopes, and functionalities of health apps, particularly those relevant to the pharmaceutical care ecosystem. Thoughts are offered on finding the right pairing of app and patient via these pharmaceutical care providers, navigating the changing landscape of app review platforms, staying cognizant of certification requirements related to reimbursements, and how to determine the efficacy of future health apps.

In the following Chapter 10, you read about wearables and insideables (the latter being the phase after external wearables), which contain sensors that collect data on human vital signs and activities. The "quantified self" becomes a reality with the digital biomarker data that these devices track. Integrating these data into patient profiles can further develop the concept of the Digital Twin, where individuals can monitor themselves by analyzing the digital version.

In Chapter 11, artificial intelligence (AI) technology is explained, which can offer pharmaceutical care providers smart support systems, given that it can access complete, adequate, and holistic health data sets. AI can support trend analysis and decision-making that augment pharmaceutical care expertise. This is what we may call "apothecary intelligence." With AI-driven pharmacy-as-a-service platforms, pharmaceutical care providers can spend more time working on what they do best: using human judgment, empathy, and consideration to provide good patient care.

In the next Chapter 12, we deep-dive into conversational AI. This technology has undergone huge evolution in the last decades, as chatbots were augmented with improved AI, text-to-speech, and visual empathic features. Nowadays, Virtual Personal (healthcare) Assistants (VPAs) are quickly finding their way into healthcare to support healthcare systems and triage, diagnostic, and disease management applications. In the pharmaceutical arena, these VPAs can support blended pharmaceutical care as an augmentation of human care, for example, by providing drug information, adherence support, or consulting for adequate, rational drug use.

Conversational AI can be combined with the opportunities that virtual, augmented, and mixed reality (VR-AR-MR) applications can bring to medical and pharmaceutical care. This is elaborated upon in Chapter 13. The VR-AR-MR examples included here act as concrete treatments for diseases, reducing the need for medication or removing the fear of medical intervention. Visualization, combined with computer-simulated environments, can enhance pharmaceutical care concepts and improve understanding and literacy among those who use medication.

The basis of all information and communication technology in pharmacies, the Pharmacy Information Systems (PIS), is broadly described in Chapter 14. The PIS can impact, positively and negatively, pharmaceutical care. The chapter offers a historical overview of the technology and its evolution. Next, we explore the nature of information systems and how a PIS relates to other healthcare information systems. In particular, we examine how PIS can support care and how they have influenced core responsibilities in the delivery of pharmaceutical care.

From the PIS, we evolve the fourth generation medicine: digital therapeutics. Chapter 15 discusses digital therapeutics (DTx) solutions, a fast-growing treatment group that uses technology to provide evidence-based software to treat, manage, and prevent medical conditions. DTx can be standalone apps or combined with medication or another piece of technology such as wearables, AI, or virtual reality. DTx utilizes health technology to treat medical and psychological conditions by digitally engaging patients, which can lead to clinically relevant outcomes. Clinical evaluated DTx products have undergone rigorous clinical testing through randomized clinical trials and real-world pilot projects to demonstrate safety and efficacy. In addition, some DTxs claim to be able to reduce, augment, or replace the need for medications and thus can be considered as a synergistic combinatory package with some drugs.

We finalize Part 2 in Chapter 16 by providing an outlook on four currently used technologies that are expected to be developed toward maturity in 2028 and will change healthcare paradigms in that process: Specifically, precision medicine, the opportunities afforded by 3D printing of medicines, the availability of social robots, and blockchain technology. Having these technologies in every home are innovations that will significantly affect how we provide pharmaceutical care. The overview provided in this chapter is not meant to be all-conclusive but is meant as an inspiring view of what lies ahead.

Part 3

In Part 3, the essential conditions for enhancing pharmaceutical care through the use of digital innovation are described. In addition, experts in their field describe the crucial governance and compliance required for digital pharmaceutical care, the ethical considerations necessary when implementing advanced digital tools, and the continuous educational framework required.

In Chapter 17, you will learn about contributing aspects to a safe and effective digital health solution: risk management, data protection principles, quality requirements and information security supplemented by organizational rules. A compliance-by-design approach is suggested by integrating various management systems to implement these requirements.

Compliance does not make sense once it is not embedded in the right ethical framework. Thus, in Chapter 18, you will read about how the core values of pharmaceutical care professionals are the fundament of providing care that patients consider good and meaningful. These values act as guiding beacons in the open-ended journey of complex ethical decision-making in the daily practice of pharmacists in the digital era. We delve into why the appropriate use of data and sound scientific research supports integrity and ethical framing, what is considered a meaningful life, and why human rights may become more pivotal in the digital age. Healthcare providers should be facilitated, rewarded and granted time to solve ethical dilemmas that come with the digital revolution.

Knowledge building of all the chapters above can only be done once awareness exists that we are entering a new era of pharmaceutical care. Therefore, Chapter 19 discusses the development of the digitally enabled pharmaceutical workforce through education in light of the new digital environment for pharmaceutical care. Digital health education is essential and must be part of undergraduate education and continuing professional development. The authors propose the characteristics of professional practice, knowledge, skills, and competencies that will be required for the new roles in the digital era. They strongly believe that pharmaceutical care providers will not be taken over by machines any time soon but will evolve and adapt to their adjusted and new role descriptions. The fundamental competencies relevant to pharmaceutical care and digital health, including literacy, are discussed. Examples of newly developed digital health courses and pharmacy informatics to educate and train the future pharmaceutical workforce to embrace the impact of the technological revolution can be found in this chapter.

Part 4

Part 4 describes inspirational concepts, visions, and thoughts on developing innovative digital pharmaceutical care pathways in daily practice. We also give advice on creating an organizational culture that can help ensure an effective transition into the digital epoch.

In Chapter 20, the concept of Digital by Design (DbD) is explained. DbD is a structured framework that can be used as a guide to effectively set up, execute, analyze and optimize digital innovation projects. DbD is accomplished in several phases, which address the domains why, who, what, and how, followed by the do (execution) and sustain phases.

Chapter 21 outlines how to build a high-performance culture in digital pharmaceutical care. You will never get the new results that you want from the existing behaviors that you like. This chapter provides an actionable blueprint consisting of six keys describing how digital pharmaceutical care providers can immediately start role-modeling the behaviors to build a high-performance organizational culture focused on the future. The six keys are creating clarity around goals; practical ways to measure progress; a mindset of playing to win; an attitude of falling in love with patients; using the power laws of time, place, and knowledge; and understanding how to let go in order to reach out.

We finalize the book by examining the progress made in digital health between the first and second editions of this book, as well as discussing the over-promising of some technologies. We also look back at this book's foreword and reflect on the four questions we asked at the start. Finally, we conclude on how a balanced approach to digital opportunities can help pharmacists use blended pharmaceutical care to improve the lives of their patients and themselves.

Introduction

It's funny how day by day nothing changes, but when you look back, everything is different.

C. S. Lewis

Imagine health-tracking wearables measuring every detail of our lives and giving us continuous feedback on how to stay in *optima forma,* algorithms and artificial intelligence techniques persuading us to follow healthier lifestyles and be more thoughtful about medication use, and voice-and-bot technologies residing in our homes, giving us advice we want (and potentially do not want) on all aspects of pharmaceutical care. In this world, we no longer need to visit physical pharmacies for care; instead, we have a menu of digital channels to use in our homecare environments.

Welcome to the epoch of health digitization and a special welcome to the ecosystem of the second edition of *Pharmaceutical Care in Digital Revolution.*

This book has a significant objective, that is, to elicit thoughts on how to provide blended pharmaceutical care so that our healthcare systems and the medicines we take help us live better and longer lives. Blended pharmaceutical care is defined as providing digital pharmaceutical care where possible and human pharmaceutical care where required. Digital pharmaceutical care is defined as *the provision of digitally enhanced, responsible pharmaceutical care to achieve outcomes that positively affect a person's quality of life* (see Chapter 6).

Ideally, blended care is organized as a regenerative system in which medications, tools, knowledge, and services are provided in closed loops or cycles, with the goal of continuously optimizing patient outcomes, reducing waste, and avoiding harm due to the use of medications. This approach is in contrast to a linear pharmaceutical care model, which is a "take-make-dispose" concept and is less focused on the ongoing integration of innovations based on new insights in healthcare. Instead, circular, blended pharmaceutical care ensures sustainability, supports improved patient experiences, and prepares us for the "day after tomorrow."

The WHY

Due to challenges inherent in pharmaceutical ecosystems, patient access to (innovative) medication is increasingly under pressure in many countries. This is a hard fact to accept, and we, along with every pharmaceutical care stakeholder we encountered, believe that steps to address this issue should be a priority of all of us. In light of the booming digital revolution, the healthcare professionals that populated this book believe that the primary challenge is knowing how to adequately select and use digitization to optimize pharmaceutical care processes and patient outcomes.

This book is written by an impressive group of international key opinion leaders who gained together hundreds of years of experience in epidemiology, pharmaceutical care, innovation, performance, compliance, and education. These colleagues share the expectation that digital tools will make the delivery of pharmaceutical care more efficient and, at the same time, significantly improve the outcome of patient treatments and the patient's quality of life while also reducing the monetary cost for such care as well as the harm derived from inappropriate drug use.

Purpose of book

The pharmaceutical pathway has always been driven by technology. The discovery, development, manufacturing, administration, and service of drugs all rely on sophisticated hardware and software applications that facilitate the innovation, accessibility, and usability of the drugs.

This book is best positioned as a so-called semiscientific educational and inspirational must-have for pharmaceutical care providers who wish to be optimally prepared for the future.

The primary purposes of this book are to create general awareness about impending digital health opportunities, inspire pharmaceutical care stakeholders to envision their profession's potential future and help frontrunners in the pharmaceutical landscape take an informed, balanced, patient-centric, and structured approach to blended pharmaceutical care.

This book is not intended to be a scientific reference but as an inspirational, thought-provoking work that supports the facets shown in the following figure:

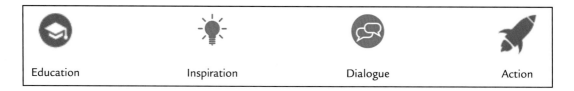

| Education | Inspiration | Dialogue | Action |

Culinary analogy

This book uses culinary metaphors. The innovative culinary ecosystem can serve as an excellent metaphor for the evolution of digital pharmaceutical care due to the many parallels that exist between the two fields. Both realms have experienced significant advancements and transformations over time, driven by creativity, technology, and a desire to meet the diverse needs of their respective audiences. Let us zoom in on a couple of the relevant metaphoric aspects.

- Variety and personalization: Just as the culinary ecosystem has evolved to offer a wide range of cuisines, flavors, and dietary preferences, digital pharmaceutical care is increasingly catering to individual patient needs. This shift is evident through the development of personalized medicine, tailored blended care treatment plans, and targeted therapies considering patients' unique geno- and phenotypical profiles, life-styles, and health conditions.
- Collaboration and interdisciplinary approach: The culinary world thrives on collaboration, with chefs and food experts blending their expertise to create innovative dishes and techniques. Similarly, digital pharmaceutical care benefits from cross-disciplinary collaboration, as medical professionals, pharmacists, data scientists, and software engineers work together to develop integrated solutions that improve patient outcomes and streamline healthcare delivery.
- Technological advancements: In the culinary realm, new technologies have revolutionized cooking techniques, food production, and delivery systems. Likewise, innovations such as telemedicine, electronic health records, artificial intelligence, and wearable devices have transformed digital pharmaceutical care. These technologies enable pharmaceutical professionals to monitor patients remotely, predict potential health risks, and optimize treatment plans for better results.
- Access and education: The culinary ecosystem has become more accessible and inclusive due to the proliferation of cooking shows, online tutorials, and food delivery services. Similarly, digital pharmaceutical care is making healthcare more accessible and patient-friendly by leveraging telehealth platforms, mobile apps, and patient portals that empower individuals to take charge of their health.
- Quality and safety: In the culinary world, there is a strong emphasis on food safety, hygiene, and quality control to ensure that consumers receive a high-quality, safe dining experience. In the same vein, digital pharmaceutical care prioritizes the safety and quality of patient care by implementing rigorous standards, data security measures, and regulatory compliance.

It is a delicate balance of mixing traditional and innovative ingredients and techniques that motivates the use of the culinary ecosystem as a metaphor in this book.

Humankind definitely needs optimization of our pharmaceutical care realm because, as we will explain thoroughly in this book, our healthcare systems are becoming exhausted under the pressures they face today.

However, without balanced implementation, digitization can result in a toxic side dish that will jeopardize the sustainable future of our care systems rather than fuel them.

In other words, this book—like the first edition of the book—is about balance: the balance between using technology and using human care, the balance between digitally augmenting the professional expert and securing the personal touch, and the balance between enhancing the impact of drugs based on (digital) data and securing the privacy of patients. We also need the knowledge that will enable us to define the proper balance in future pharmaceutical care, that is, between digital services where possible and human services where needed.

That said, the core values of pharmaceutical care providers are the compass for substantiating the principles of good care. The skills needed to authenticate these values cannot be robotized, and factors that cannot be automated are expected to remain highly valuable.

Scope of book

As indicated, this book is meant to introduce, educate, inspire, and prepare professionals for the dynamic future of pharmaceutical healthcare services. However, due to the space allowed, we limited the book's scope as defined in the following sections.

Audience scope

This book targets professionals who are responsible for providing pharmaceutical care. We frequently write from the stance that the pharmaceutical care provider, which is often a pharmacist, is the central player in this sector. While this may seem logical, and we had to start somewhere, pharmaceutical care is not only provided by pharmacists. Therefore, we propose that this book is also relevant for other stakeholders who drive pharmaceutical care, such as physicians, pharmacy chains' employees, payers, regulatory affairs associates, governmental entities, and patients.

Additionally, the book may attract those who want to transform pharmaceutical care by successfully implementing smart technology. You do not need to be a digital expert to understand the content of this book. In the domain of pharmaceutical care providers, the core knowledge areas are related to understanding drugs and how they work in the human body and effectively coaching people on how to use them. Even if you have reservations about the value of such technology and some mistrust about sharing data, this book can still offer you a fundamental, "helicopter" view of technology's future role in the industry.

In all cases, enabling an informed point of view is what this book is about.

Geographical scope

In the interest of brevity, this book focuses to a large extent on the pharmaceutical care situation in Western-oriented countries and their healthcare systems.

Some of the earliest digital concepts described in this book may not be integrated into all countries yet and, in such countries, may represent innovative, cutting-edge healthcare situations. However, the authors trust that disseminating these concepts will drive cross-fertilization in different regions, cultures, and systems.

Time scope

This book primarily focuses on developments over the next 5 years, largely because making predictions in the digital sector's fast-paced environment is rather tricky. Moreover, because of this speed, some of the book's content may already be slightly outdated at the time of publishing. In light of this fact, the authors provided links to dynamic QR codes and animations and attempted to present a book that will retain its value for readers over time.

Content scope

The book starts with a broad view of the challenges healthcare systems face and how pharmaceutical care will be affected, followed by a more focused discussion on how several digital health technologies can be used to address these challenges. Finally, the book describes the conditions and steps needed to initiate blended pharmaceutical care. Thus, the book is ideal for innovation-minded generalists who want to understand the bigger picture first and then perhaps study more deeply specific areas relative to the topic.

The authors hope that after reading this book, pharmaceutical care providers, and related stakeholders, will feel engaged and enabled to move from a general understanding of the digital revolution to taking concrete steps to implement digital innovations in daily practice.

This book will never be complete or one hundred percent accurate. But, first, it is meant as a holistic and inspirational insight into future digital opportunities and only hits the outer circle of knowledge about a number of key technologies.

Second, as addressed before, completeness is a challenge due to the speed of the digital revolution. Thus, some concepts may be obsolete in years to come, and some examples mentioned in the book may cease to exist. Others may go faster or be completely different than expected, and information in the book may become outdated sooner rather than later.

Third, as this book looks into the future, interpretations of digital opportunities may change due to ongoing insights. Initially, what was considered a promising development in 2019 was overhauled in 2020 with the start of the COVID-19 pandemic. Now in 2023, the future will tell us what is to be expected.

Readers are cordially invited to send comments, additions, and notation of errors or ideas to the editor so that together we can make the second edition of this book even better.

How this book is organized

In Part 1 of this book, we zoom in on the current challenges that healthcare systems are facing.

Without exception, in both developed and low- and middle-income countries, healthcare costs are rising due to a growing and aging population, the availability of increasingly more expensive technology, higher survival rates in chronic diseases, and inefficient healthcare systems. This part describes how healthcare systems are facing pressure, gives options for structural solutions, explains how the role of patients in those systems is changing, and defines what the global definition and context of pharmaceutical care might be in this respect.

In Part 2, Chapters 7 and 8 describe in general the ecosystem of technological health innovation and its relevance to pharmaceutical care, whereas Chapters 9−16 provide more detail on individual digital solutions and their relationship to supporting efficiency, personalization, and self-management in pharmaceutical care.

Promising digital technologies are described in Chapters 9−16 in a fixed format of four key items:

- Explanation of the individual digital technology
- Impact on the five core responsibilities in pharmaceutical care, as described in Chapter 6
- Implementation in daily practice
- Considerations for the use of the technology

Part 3 of the book describes the essential conditions for enhancing pharmaceutical care through digital innovation. Experts in their field have laid out the crucial governance and compliance required for digital pharmaceutical care, the ethical considerations necessary when implementing advanced digital tools, and the (continuous) educational framework required.

Finally, in Part 4, practical tips and tricks are provided on implementing technology in daily practice and transforming your way of working into a ready culture for the future.

Every chapter of this book ends with a summary of the most important priorities for creating a circular pharmaceutical pathway.

A number of QR codes are included in this book. Simply hover over the code with the QR reader on your smartphone or tablet, and you will be linked to inspiring materials, such as websites and videos, that support the topic you are reading about. If you are reading this book as an e-book, you have got it easy; just click the link and you will be directed to the web page.

Most important, you do not need to read the book from beginning to the end. You can instead just turn to the subjects you are interested in and read the individual chapters in any order you like.

Assumptions made

To help ensure that readers derive the full potential of this book, the authors made a few assumptions about a reader:

- You are interested in focusing on how pharmaceutical care providers can use upcoming technology to improve drug use and balance healthcare costs.
- You are aware that digitalization, among other fields, is changing drug development, clinical trial execution, pharmaceutical regulation, and more, although a detailed discussion of these fields is beyond the scope of this book.
- You know the basics on how healthcare systems and pharmaceutical care pathways are organized.
- You have access to and know how to use a computer, tablet, or smartphone with an internet connection.
- You are open to learning about new technologies that go beyond your area of competency and are willing to invest time in identifying its opportunities.

Icons used in this interactive book

Tip: Marks tips and shortcuts that you can use to integrate digital knowledge and tools in daily practice

Remember: Marks information that is especially important for pharmaceutical care practice and that bears repeating

Examples: Includes general trend updates, best practices, company information, digital-pharma collaborations, partnerships, and synergies

Warning: Signals where things could go wrong. This may be in terms of privacy, regulations, and governmental or other barriers related to going digital

Ethical Consideration: Gives a recommendation on when to make a balanced decision to protect the well-being of the patient

QR code: Refers to an illustrated website or video or other online information relevant to the topic of the respective paragraph. To be read with a QR code reader

Beyond the book

The book *Pharmaceutical Care in Digital Revolution* stands as a testament to the importance of interdisciplinary collaboration in the advancement of digital healthcare. Authored by over 15 international key opinion leaders, this groundbreaking second edition brings together diverse perspectives and expertise from various fields, including pharmacy, medicine, education, compliance, data science, and technology. The collective insights of the thought leaders provide a comprehensive understanding of the current state and future direction of digital pharmaceutical care.

PART 1

Why: global healthcare systems under pressure

CHAPTER 1

Pharmacists in need of sustenance*

Claudia Rijcken
Pharmi, Maastricht, The Netherlands

Under pressure everything becomes fluid

Unknown

We live in an epoch where humanity itself determines our earth's future, which is why some call this era the Anthropocene. The Anthropocene (although no formal epoch nomenclature yet) is considered the period of time during which human activities have impacted the environment in such a way as to constitute a distinct geological change. The technological revolution and the rapid incline of our population exhaust our living environment, whereas our globe is constantly in need of nourishment to bloom in its beauty. It means our globe needs elements necessary for growth, health, and keeping in good condition.

Our healthcare systems in general and our pharmacists in particular need such a sustenance as well, definitely in an era where life expectancy has increased significantly in recent decades.

Over the last two centuries, humanity's average life expectancy has increased from 40 years in the 1800s to 71 years in 2021. This increase in life expectancy can be attributed to improvements in healthcare, sanitation, and global medical practices [1]. However, there are still some gaps. For example, across the sexes, women live 5.4 years on average longer than men. And in certain parts of the world, this gap is even wider. The gap is caused by a mix of biological (e.g., hormonal and genetic) and societal (e.g., dietary, infrastructural) influences, which differ per region globally [1].

The share of the global population aged 65 years or above is projected to rise from 10% in 2022 to 16% in 2050 [2]. This trend provides a set of challenges for modern healthcare

---

*In this chapter, you will read about the impressive progress in global healthcare systems, the pressure they are experiencing, the value of medicine in these systems, and the global ambition and perceived urgency to innovate to warrant healthcare access.

Pharmaceutical Care in Digital Revolution. https://doi.org/10.1016/B978-0-443-13360-2.00012-5

3

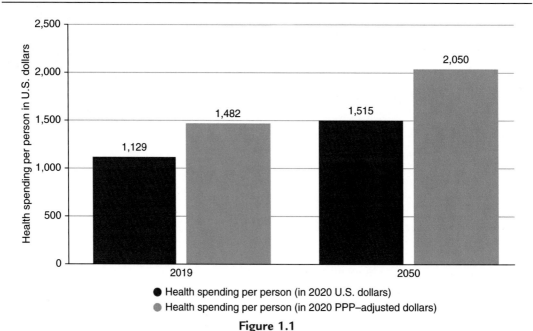

Figure 1.1

View on average health spending per capita in 2019 and in 2050. *Source: https://www.statista.com/ statistics/856380/per-person-health-spending-globally/.*

systems, as growing demand for care and changing age ratios have dramatically increased financial expectations of health budgets.

Health expenditures include the consumption of health goods, services, public health programs, insurance, and government spending. Globally, those health expenditures are on the rise.

Among all countries, the average per capita health expenditure is projected to nearly double from the 2017 totals by the year 2050. Total health spending per person globally in 2019 averaged to some 1129 US dollars annually and is estimated to increase to 1515 US dollars annually by 2050; see Fig. 1.1 [3].

According to the World Bank, the United States had one of the highest percentages of gross domestic product (GDP) spent on healthcare in 2022. The United States spent nearly 17% of its GDP on healthcare services. Canada, Germany, and France followed the United States with distinctly smaller percentages. The United States had significantly higher private and public health spending than other developed countries [4].

In most developed countries, healthcare expenses have grown faster than the GDP for decades, mainly due to increased population and improved therapeutic interventions. Should this trend continue, total health expenditures may more than double as a share of GDP, rising to an average of about 14% of GDP among the Organisation for Economic Co-operation and Development (OECD) member countries in 2060, resulting in percentages above 20% in high-income countries (QR Code 1.1).

Most policymakers and citizens do not consider this ratio sustainable; thus, system transformations are required to warrant sustainable access to healthcare.

QR Code 1.1
OECD health statistics.

Sustainability focus

Healthcare ecosystems worldwide were tested in ways that have never been imagined possible due to the COVID-19 pandemic. Overall, healthcare systems so far showed resilience, and the majority of people had the same as, or even better access than before the pandemic—while a third reported worsening of access [5].

Assuring sustainability in pressured systems is a delicate task: changes to healthcare systems are ultimately complex in terms of policy and are politically sensitive everywhere on the globe. Moreover, transforming current care forms in order to achieve global equality and affordable and accessible healthcare systems requires a unified approach within developed as well as low- and middle-income countries.

The sustainability challenge stresses the need for creative, innovative, and progressive solutions to warrant access to care in optimized future-proof systems. It also emphasizes the push for patients, providers, governments, and payers to share the responsibility for innovating healthcare, as will be explained in more detail in this book.

Given the complexity of healthcare's social and economic impact and the strong links between health, workability, employment, and social care (including people's individual preferences), a broad range of disciplines, sectors, and ministries must collaborate closely to ensure that policies and practices are consistent, strategically aligned, and focused on future needs of individuals and the population as a whole. Effective cross-sectorial collaboration is required to minimize resource waste while maximizing outcomes for patients, workforces, and societies.

Patients are in general positive, but expect better

Although it is difficult to generalize globally, patients, on average, are demanding a better experience, friendlier treatment, and assured outcomes in return for their substantial personal investment, as well as data sharing in healthcare. See Chapter 5 for further discussion.

Moreover, more focus on generational differences may be needed. For example, research among 12,000 healthcare consumers in 14 countries revealed that a great healthcare experience for people from Gen X or older seems to depend more on clear explanations and advice from medical providers. In contrast, millennials and younger people are more open to providers who use innovative digital technologies and information from other sources [5].

As a healthcare experience domain, patient centricity is a key concept, which means care to be convenient, transparent, and personalized. Consuming patients expect to be treated as whole people with individualized needs, not merely as problems to be solved. Therefore, they wish to consume care in their personalized environment as much as possible, preferably in blended care models: using digital technology if possible and allowing human care once needed.

In a recent McKinsey report, at least 60% of consumers expect to be able to change or schedule a healthcare appointment, check medical records and test results, and renew a medication online [6]. Consumers expect that healthcare information should be available at their fingertips. This expectation has grown with the ubiquity of mobile phones and was exponentially affected by the pandemic with increasing telehealth and virtual care services [6].

System change required as nourishment for healthcare system sustainability

Given the global ambition to prevent healthcare systems from collapsing under the weight of their success, that is, the provision of better treatment and extension of longevity, there is a strong need to bring increased healthcare expenditures more in line with the rate of economic growth, or even below that rate. For years, healthcare systems promised transformations, and in many cases, the pandemic was a catalyst for fulfilling those promises.

These healthcare systems used innovative nourishment to promote prevention and healthier lifestyles (broad determinants of health), reduce waiting times for care, restructure the delivery of care to make it more efficient, and implement cost containment measurements.

Since 2010, in some countries, health-related spending has declined for the first time since 1973, healthcare budgets and spending today are still a mysterious black box, and there is, in general, a lot of waste in all global healthcare systems.

Safe waste management services for healthcare waste are lacking globally, especially in the least developed countries. The latest data (from 2019) indicate that one in three healthcare facilities globally does not safely manage healthcare waste. The COVID-19 pandemic has led to large increases in healthcare waste, straining underresourced healthcare facilities and exacerbating environmental impacts from solid waste [7].

Therefore, policymakers increasingly agree that we need to move toward a model where every dollar spent goes toward producing optimal outcomes, e.g., return on investment. For decades, systems generally kept the incentive systems for care interventions firmly planted in fee-for-service models, also called activity-based costing. Not until the past decade did charges reach beyond the horizon. The proposed approach is called value-based healthcare, perhaps better stated as value-driven healthcare; the principles are explained in Chapter 3.

The benefits and budgets of medication in healthcare systems

Medicines and vaccines are some of the most powerful tools in helping people live longer, healthier, and more productive lives. For example, since the 1980s, we have seen death rates from human immunodeficiency virus fall by over 80%. Since the 1990s, cancer deaths have fallen by 20%, and recent pharmaceutical innovations mean that 90% of people living with Hepatitis C can be cured through a 12-week course of medicines [8] (QR Code 1.2).

QR Code 1.2
EFPIA data center.

After years consumed by vaccines and treatments for COVID-19, innovation in the pharmaceutical industry has evolved. At one stage, research focused on the mechanisms at work in existing drugs, but it has now shifted to refocusing on diseases that have had burdensome treatments or, worse, no treatment.

Medication innovation means, for example, drugs made from living cells, targeting a specific genetic makeup, or focusing on immunotherapy that harnesses the body's immune system to fight diseases. Also, using techniques to change genetic materials to treat diseases, such as chimeric antigen receptor T-cell therapy or clustered regularly interspaced short palindromic repeats to edit genomes, is expected to disruptively change the prognosis for several disorders in the coming years.

At the same time, companies are beginning to redefine what it means to be medicine. Software is starting to treat physical ailments just like pills, as reflected in Chapter 15. Treatments blend different care forms into caring and curing models delivered increasingly in the patient's home environment.

Value for medication money

Over recent decades, the average per capita retail pharmaceutical expenditure (prescribed and over-the-counter medicines) in OECD countries has increased from 308 US dollars in

2000 to 554 US dollars in 2018. The growth rate of pharmaceutical expenditures in hospitals for a selection of OECD countries reporting this information is greater than that of retail pharmaceuticals. Consequently, it is increasingly important to consider pharmaceutical expenditure in hospitals when analyzing total pharmaceutical expenditures since this accounts, on average, for an additional 20% on top of retail spending [9].

Most innovative drugs that determine the budget have been able to reduce other costs, such as avoiding clinical and surgical interventions, shorter hospital stays, less need for caregivers, or improved working productivity (referred to as broader societal benefits, as explained in Chapter 4).

Global spending on medicine continues to grow. In 2021, approximately 1.42 trillion US dollars had been spent on medicines, up from just 887 billion US dollars in 2010. That number is expected to increase to nearly 1.8 trillion by 2026. Spending on medicines has increased everywhere globally [10]. This figure excludes the significant list-price reductions rebated back to payers, governments, and other stakeholders in many countries, comprising as much as one-third of a medication's price.

Although the absolute budget spent on medicines is increasing, we also saw a reduction in the growth rate of drug budgets, which is driven by many mechanisms. First, the introduction of generics and biosimilars has led to an 85% switch from branded medicines during the past 15 years. This switching has led to significant price drops, as generics are only a fraction of the cost of branded medicines, and biosimilars are also less costly.

Also, companies that develop drugs are modernizing drug discovery and development processes to optimize and hasten developmental and regulatory approval timelines, which can be reflected in the price of innovative drugs. Moreover, new access models driven by value-based healthcare principles (see Chapter 3) and innovative payment models based on data-driven outcomes (see Chapter 4) are codeveloped by governments, physicians, patients, and manufacturers to ensure that future healthcare systems pay as much as possible for optimal patient outcomes, rather than purely for product delivery.

However, such approaches do not and would not happen spontaneously. They require a joint effort among all parties involved in the care process. When parties join forces and live up to the principles of—later in this book explained—value-based healthcare, the value for money spent on medication will increase, and access may be warranted, as such principles are meant to ensure that medication reaches the right patients, at the right time, in the right way.

This collaboration, focused on sustainability, innovation and payability, will be the new nourishing concept that healthcare systems require from the pharmaceutical ecosystem.

Principles on anchoring innovation in existing systems are discussed in Chapter 2.

This means for blended pharmaceutical care:

- Healthcare systems are under serious pressure due to aging populations, longer survival rates from illnesses, and more costly innovative treatment options.
- Ongoing system innovation is required to keep healthcare systems affordable, accessible, and unified.
- Medicines and vaccines are some of the most powerful tools in helping people to live longer, be healthier, and have more productive lives.
- The coming years will introduce a wealth of innovative measures that will make medicines again the cornerstone for changing the prognosis of many serious conditions.
- Generic introductions and innovative approaches in access models, like value-driven payment models, are concepts that support the sustainability of healthcare systems.

References

[1] Alvarez P. Animation: global life expectancy (1950-2021). 2022 [cited 2022 28/12/2022]; Available from, https://www.weforum.org/agenda/2022/11/global-life-expectancy-male-female-world.

[2] Economic, U.N.D.o. and P.D. Social Affairs, World population prospects 2022: summary of results. UN DESA/POP/2022/TR/NO. 3. 2022.

[3] IHME. Global health spending per capita in 2019 and projection for 2050 (in U.S. dollars) [Graph]. Statista; 2021. Available from, https://www.statista.com.statistics/856380/per-person-health-spending-globally/.

[4] World Bank. Current health expenditure (% of GDP). In: World health organization global health expenditure database. The World Bank; 2022. Available from, https://data.worldbank.org/indicator/SH.XPD.CHEX.GD.ZS.

[5] Accenture. The ultimate healthcare experience: what people want. In: 2021 Accenture health and life sciences experience survey—global report. Accenture; 2021.

[6] Singhal S, Vinjamoori N, Radha M. The next frontier of healthcare delivery. In: Healthcare practice. McKinsey & Company; 2022.

[7] World Health Organization. Global analysis of healthcare waste in the context of COVID-19: status, impacts and recommendations. 2022.

[8] EFPIA. Value of medicines. 2022 [cited 2022 28/12/2022]; Available from, https://www.efpia.eu/about-medicines/use-of-medicines/value-of-medicines/.

[9] García-Goñi M. Rationalizing pharmaceutical spending. IMF Working Papers 2022;2022(190).

[10] IQVIA. Global spending on medicines in 2010, 2021, and a forecast for 2026 (in billion U.S. dollars). Statista; 2021. Available from, https://www.statista.com/statistics/280572/medicine-spending-worldwide/.

CHAPTER 2

Experimental digital: innovation required*

Paul Louis Iske

Institute of Brilliant Failures, the Personalised Healthcare Catalyst Foundation, Maastricht University, Maastricht, The Netherlands

The alchemists in their search for gold discovered many other things of greater value.

Arthur Schopenhauer

Innovation is a much-discussed and written-about subject that always seems to be at the forefront of everyone's mind. This is not surprising: the world is changing rapidly. As addressed in the previous chapter, the pharmaceutical care ecosystem needs nourishment to move to a new, sustainable, balanced future.

Experimental cooking can be interpreted as trying new ingredients, techniques, and combinations to create unique and delicious dishes. Also, in the context of the required innovation, experimentation and creativity are crucial for coming up with new and unique ideas to drive innovation. Additionally, just like an experimental cook, an innovator should be willing to take risks and try new things, even if they may not work out as planned. For example, an experimental cook may create a dish that does not turn out well, but they can learn from their mistakes and try again. Similarly, an innovator may come up with the idea that does not work, but they can learn from their failures and try again.

Historically, system transitions take about 30 years. We do not have that time. What is needed to realize the ambitions is a collaborative approach aimed at ensuring that existing and future healthcare solutions quickly reach daily practice and can be deployed. With the current technological possibilities, it should also be possible to do this faster, as long as there is a sufficient sense of urgency and focus on innovation. There are many different definitions of innovation in the literature, and based on experiences in many different

---

*In this chapter, you will read about the principles of innovation and how to implement them effectively, what combinatoric innovation between pharmaceutical and digital technology providers is, and why the concept of brilliant failures is essential to drive digital transformation.

Pharmaceutical Care in Digital Revolution. https://doi.org/10.1016/B978-0-443-13360-2.00023-X

companies in various industries, the following general description of innovation seems suitable for the purpose of this book:

"Innovation is a process in which ideas and knowledge are applied to achieve new ways of value creation."

 Several words in this definition are relevant to this book:

1. **Innovation**: Innovation always has something to do with "new." This becomes clear when we look at the meaning of the Latin word "innovare," which means "to renew" or "to change."
2. **Process**: Innovation is a process in the sense that there is input (ideas, experiences, resources), activities (R&D, technical implementation, product launch, etc.), and output (product, service, new business model, etc.). This process usually consists of identifiable steps.
3. **Ideas and Knowledge**: During the innovation process, input is converted to output. The input often consists largely of ideas, information, and insights; these are the constituents of knowledge. Knowledge might be found within an organization, but it might also be (partly) brought in from the outside. It might even come from another industry. Of course, no matter which organization one works for, there will always be considerably more knowledge on the outside than on the inside (unless one works for an organization with 7.9 billion colleagues). But innovation can also be driven by the (re-)use of new and/or existing resources, including technology.
4. **Value**: Innovation is not just something new but involves a development with a certain value to those involved. This value is not necessarily financial; it can also be related to happiness, health, convenience, a better society, a cleaner environment, expansion of knowledge, new relationships, and so on. This is the reason that we often talk about *value* cases rather than *business* cases.

 ## *From innovation to value*

Innovation is not just about new products and services. Each new implementation within and around an organization that has value for its stakeholders can be considered an innovation. For example, new revenue models, new partnership models, developments in staff management, (social) innovation, and so on are just as much innovations as innovations resulting from hard-value propositions (products and services). Thus in healthcare, new medications (or administration forms) and new ways to interact with patients or different working processes in hospitals are considered innovations as long as they create additional value.

Technological developments can greatly accelerate the pace of innovation, but more is needed to maximize value creation. In several editions of the Erasmus Innovation Monitor, it was found that technological innovation contributes less than half to the realization of disruptive innovations; the remaining, bigger part is contributed by "social innovation," that is, innovative ways of managing, organizing, working, and collaborating.

In spite of the opportunities for social innovation, organizations frequently invest in technological innovation and subsequently make little to no changes in communication, adapting work processes, or driving cultural transformation to working with this new technology (as described in Chapter 21). Sometimes this is even the case when new technologies are introduced to customers.

In these cases, the well-known formula $NT + OO = EOO$ applies. It says: New Technology in an Old Organization results in an Expensive Old Organization [1]. Obviously, this is not the most optimal way for integrating innovative concepts, as one of our healthcare systems' big ambitions is to make them financially sustainable.

To determine the essence and value of innovation, it may be helpful to map the innovation against the value blocks of an organization via the Business Model Canvas (BMC; see Fig. 2.1), a framework that captures the essential building blocks of an organization, including health institutes [2].

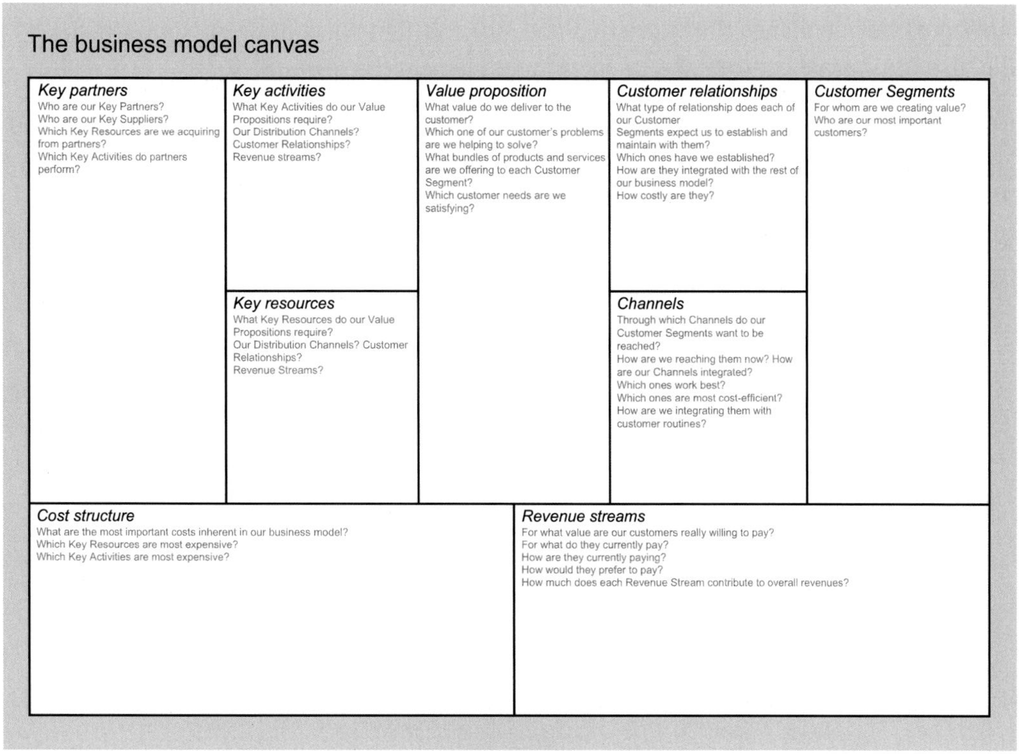

The business model canvas

Key partners	Key activities	Value proposition	Customer relationships	Customer Segments
Who are our Key Partners? Who are our Key Suppliers? Which Key Resources are we acquiring from partners? Which Key Activities do partners perform?	What Key Activities do our Value Propositions require? Our Distribution Channels? Customer Relationships? Revenue streams?	What value do we deliver to the customer? Which one of our customer's problems are we helping to solve? What bundles of products and services are we offering to each Customer Segment? Which customer needs are we satisfying?	What type of relationship does each of our Customer Segments expect us to establish and maintain with them? Which ones have we established? How are they integrated with the rest of our business model? How costly are they?	For whom are we creating value? Who are our most important customers?

Key resources
What Key Resources do our Value Propositions require? Our Distribution Channels? Customer Relationships? Revenue Streams?

Channels
Through which Channels do our Customer Segments want to be reached? How are we reaching them now? How are our Channels integrated? Which ones work best? Which ones are most cost-efficient? How are we integrating them with customer routines?

Cost structure
What are the most important costs inherent in our business model? Which Key Resources are most expensive? Which Key Activities are most expensive?

Revenue streams
For what value are our customers really willing to pay? For what do they currently pay? How are they currently paying? How would they prefer to pay? How much does each Revenue Stream contribute to overall revenues?

Figure 2.1
Business Model Canvas [2].

The BMC is a great tool for communicating with and among stakeholders and addressing the most important aspects of business development. For readers of this book, all building blocks are relevant, especially the ones referring to value proposition, channel, customer relationship, revenue model, and key activities. It goes beyond the scope of this book to explain the different compartments of this grid, as they need to be worked out in more detail; however, for those interested in systematically introducing value-adding innovations, the instructions on how to use this grid (which can be found on the internet or in books about the BMC) may be considered as valuable.

As stated before, the concept of business cases is being extended to value cases, in which positive/negative value creation (financial, social, intellectual capital) is considered. Furthermore, since in the healthcare system usually many stakeholders play a role, we speak about a 'collective value case,' again demonstrating the need to see the anticipated innovation from many perspectives (patient, caretaker, management, finance, payer, technology, government).

General principles of successful innovation

Successful innovators spot opportunities for industry revolution just a bit faster than the rest of the pack. They apparently seem to visualize how new practices will fundamentally change customer expectations and behaviors or break long-established industry paradigms. Simply put, they challenge the status quo and strive to find ways of doing things better while also having the competency to actually implement the changes.

An interesting book for those who aim to become top-notch innovators is *The Four Lenses of Innovation* by Rowan Gibson [3]. The book identifies four key business perspectives that enable readers to discover groundbreaking opportunities as the keys to successful innovation.

As a reader, one has probably already started using the first and second lenses from the left, shown in Fig. 2.2, in order to challenge the current pharmaceutical care dogmas.

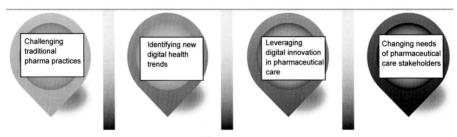

Figure 2.2

The four lenses of innovation in pharmaceutical care. *Adapted from Gibson R. The four lenses of innovation: a power tool for creative thinking. John Wiley & Sons; 2015.*

Therefore, picking up this book to understand what's going on is an important step. After reading it and understanding the trends changing the healthcare landscape, you will be halfway to innovation leadership.

One of the outcomes of reading this book or individual chapters may be that new ideas will inspire pharmaceutical care providers (PCPs) to build new concepts for reorganizing patient care. This would lead to the blue lens of innovation, meaning getting followers of the new ideas and resources to put new concepts into practice. But first, the ideas must be validated thoroughly to ensure that they truly meet the targeted audience's needs (last lens) and have the potential to "disruptively" change and direct pharmaceutical care toward improvement and sustainability.

About disruptive innovation

 In general, if we look at the current understanding of what real disruptive innovation is, we see that it consists of three basic elements [4]:

1. **Technological enabler**: Typically, this refers to sophisticated technology whose purpose is to simplify; it routinizes the solution to problems that previously required unstructured processes of intuitive experimentation.
2. **Business model innovation**: This model can deliver simplified solutions to customers in ways that make the innovations affordable and easily accessible.
3. **Value network**: This model is most often a commercial infrastructure in which constituent organizations have consistently disruptive, mutually reinforcing socioeconomic models.

Complexity and paradigm shifts are especially, but not exclusively, found in these transformative innovations. Clayton Christensen's *The Innovator's Dilemma* [5] provides a good description as well as many examples of disruptive innovations with a large impact on established companies and even on entire industries. For decades almost every field has seen disruptive innovations that led to dramatic increases in the quality of knowledge, resulting in a high level of expertise and high-quality knowledge centers, networks, and institutions.

Developments in such systems lead to emergent phenomena, that is, disruptive developments that cannot be controlled but instead require "navigation" skills such as agility and learning capacity; the impact of these new skills have on the pharmaceutical care are described in Chapters 19 and 21.

Disruptive changes usually do not come from within an industry but from the outside. The taxi industry was not disrupted by a taxi company but by the Uber IT platform. Airbnb introduced a new hotel model without owning any hotels. Banks no longer look to each other but to tech companies such as Google, FinTech startups, and crowd-funding platforms. Former IT companies now produce phones. The oil industry is about to share the playing field with sustainable energy sources, and street retailers are competing with internet parties. In short, it turns out that the world is bigger and more complex than just the limited environment in which we have always operated and competed.

⚠ We are familiar with the term "kodakized," a verb reflecting the fact that the photo company Kodak did not adjust fast enough to the upcoming digitalization of the photo world and completely lost its market leadership to new entrants in the digital picture arena. Societies' big challenge is determining whether healthcare systems in general and pharmaceutical care processes, in particular, are deemed to be kodakized under the pressure of sustainability and by new entrants that adjust faster to innovation than the traditional systems can.

The innovation funnel

In general, the innovation process consists of several stages (see Fig. 2.3): ideation (generation of ideas), concept (developed idea), quick scan (validated concept), business case (substantive reporting, including planning for development and implementation), prototype (development of products and services to the point where those involved have a representative image and are able to give feedback), and last but not least the launch (market introduction).

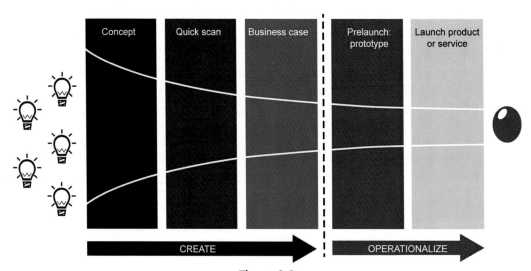

Figure 2.3
The funnel approach to the innovation process [1].

Organizing processes in an agile (flexible, adaptive) way is becoming increasingly more common, allowing for adjustments during and especially between the stages. This requires a type of decision-making that does not determine all goals and milestones in advance but allows decisions to be made and resources to be allocated based on intermediate results and trial and error.

That said, innovation always starts with a promising idea. How to get to that idea is the question.

 ## *Open innovation*

The idea of using knowledge and inspiration from outside an organization is not new. Organizations already know that it is often more effective not to develop all required knowledge themselves but to search for external parties that already have complementary knowledge or are more capable of developing it. This is known as "open innovation." This type of innovation is logically positioned on the opposite side of the more traditional "closed innovation" model, which involves parties developing and marketing their own internal ideas and knowledge.

An essential aspect of open innovation is that it requires the ability to use one's own knowledge internally as well as find it externally and expand the relevant knowledge elsewhere. For pharmaceutical care, this means that PCPs must develop a number of additional skills, including

- the ability to find knowledge outside the organization;
- the ability to assess that knowledge;
- the ability to integrate external knowledge into the existing knowledge;
- the ability to connect to other parties; and
- the ability to determine how the combination can successfully market the results.

An organization must therefore have minimal knowledge of other parties and be prepared to share its success, in line with the phrase, "A small piece of a large pie is better than a large piece of a small pie." In short, existing knowledge is joined with another ability: interface management (see Fig. 2.4).

Therefore, it is crucial to the success of open innovation that organizations and professionals have the alliance skills (as explained later in this book) needed to bridge the digital and pharmaceutical sectors, but also between the various stakeholders in the healthcare system (professionals, patients, managers, payers, government, industry, science). These skills are crucial to finding a fit between the potential partners in the innovation alliance.

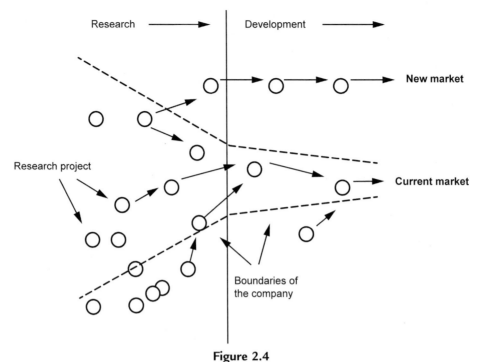

Figure 2.4
Open innovation requires looking into other industries [6].

Three areas are essential for establishing a fruitful collaborative climate: a cultural fit, a strategic fit, and an operational fit.

1. **Cultural fit**: It is important to acknowledge and work with stakeholders' different backgrounds, needs, and viewpoints in an innovation network. Collaboration and joint innovation may be very problematic if parties cannot agree on the basic, most important paradigms.

2. **Strategic fit**: The parties work on a joint goal in an alliance. However, most often, they will also have to deal with individual ambitions and targets, and if these do not match well, the alliance will probably suffer, making it difficult to achieve a sustained commitment.

3. **Operational fit**: Even when parties have the ambition and will to cooperate and jointly develop new propositions, practical issues may create challenges. These issues include availability, communication (between people, but possibly also between systems that use different data models), finance, and so on.

Examples of open innovation are everywhere. For example, the business world collaborates with knowledge institutions (e.g., pharmaceutical companies collaborate with academia), larger organizations collaborate with smaller, specialized companies (e.g., pharmaceutical chains collaborate with specialized digital companies), and some companies leverage the knowledge of their suppliers and partners.

The challenge in this open innovation setting is to bring together unfamiliar parties (e.g., the pharmaceutical sector and digital health providers) that are able to create synergy in their business propositions.

Combinatoric innovation

Combinatoric innovation is a methodological approach to multidisciplinary value creation. It emphasizes diversity and presupposes that it is worthwhile to bring together parties with diverse skills, backgrounds, ideas, customers, and interests in order to let them explore and discover how they can create value together in an innovative way.

Combinatoric innovation is also a creative process that combines trial and error, learning, and renewal. It is, by definition, nonlinear and, to a certain extent, unpredictable. It often cannot be captured in quick, short-term outcomes that positively influence profit and loss margins.

Moreover, a combinatoric innovation process can unveil new forms of value creation by combining and applying previously unrelated intellectual capital. This discovery process can result in serendipity, which is the skill of finding something important by coincidence. It, indeed, is a skill to create an environment of trust, understanding, and ambition in which parties, together, are motivated to find new opportunities for value creation for themselves and others.

Combinatoric innovation is in large part, a social innovation, as it is often about a new way of organizing, collaborating, and innovating.

Creating the best environment for combinatoric innovation

The dynamics of successfully innovating together can, to a certain extent, be compared to managing successful alliances.

In addition to cultural, operational, and strategic fits, for an organization to be innovative and thrive, a number of environments are essential:

- Social space
- Process and organization space
- Virtual and digital space
- Physical and real space

In this book, we do not delve into the details of optimizing these four environments, but for a more detailed description of their characteristics, refer to the book *Combinatoric Innovation* [1]. The point we want to make is that although we cannot always manage or control the process of (open, combinatoric) innovation, we can manage interventions in the environment that support it.

 An interesting healthcare example of combinatoric innovation testing can be found in the United Kingdom's National Health Service (NHS). The NHS's Five Year Forward View, published in October 2014, described the NHS's intention to develop a small number of "test bed" sites. These projects will serve as real-world sites for evaluating "combinatorial" innovations that integrate new technologies and other novel approaches that offer the prospect for better care and better patient experiences at the same or lower overall cost. Upon opening QR Code 2.1, you will find an explanation about how innovators can express interest, as well as the process the NHS followed to set up this initiative.

QR Code 2.1

Example of combinatoric innovation in healthcare.

Ideas ready to survive in a complex world: "the last mile"

"Without implementation, there is no innovation." Many innovative developments fail (brilliantly) because they cannot survive in a complex world. Research shows that the 'innovation paradox' is persistent, meaning that many promising innovations are ultimately never (fully) implemented. The success of an innovation is only 25% determined by the innovation itself. The other 75% is determined by social innovation: the system innovations and/or changes that are needed to implement innovation in daily practice. In business development terms, one might say that a successful startup will not automatically be successful in the next (scaled-up) phase. There are essentially three phases:

- Proof of concept
- Proof of business
- Proof of success

Where in general, a lot of attention and resources are available for innovation ('Proof of Concept'), this is much less the case for the implementation of the next and most difficult phase of the innovation process ('Proof of Business'). And while using the implemented innovation, we will discover whether we can enjoy sustainable value creation ('Proof of Success').

Lack of implementation, and therefore value creation, creates growing frustration, making innovation less and less popular. Therefore, we need to look for the factors, the barriers, that stand in the way of (rapid) implementation. An important cause for the difficult implementation of healthcare innovation is the fact that a new medical model also requires adjustment or readjustment of a large part of the healthcare system. The current healthcare system is complex, rigid, conservative, and responds too slowly to innovations. We are missing out on health gains as a result. What is needed is a resilient, flexible, experimenting and learning (together an evolving) system in which optimal use is made of all available (new) data, tools and knowledge, and applications. In such a system, optimal learning occurs from successful and unsuccessful projects. It is especially important to look at developments that face implementation barriers and therefore struggle with the 'Last Mile' or fail to complete it (die before the finish line). That is, something that works in a limited environment may be confronted with new circumstances and demands in a broader environment and may fail (Fig. 2.5).

At the point of transition between phases, it is important to consider certain aspects that might change or need to change. These include the team's skills (which could lead to changes in the team itself, as described in Chapters 19 and 21), the type of customers, and the model of financing and governance. Several brilliant failures stem from the inability to keep a concept alive in an increasingly complex context. The characteristics of each phase can be found in the book *Combinatoric Innovation* [1]. An overview of challenges in the last mile in healthcare innovation can be found in a report about implementation barriers for PHC (personalized healthcare) [7].

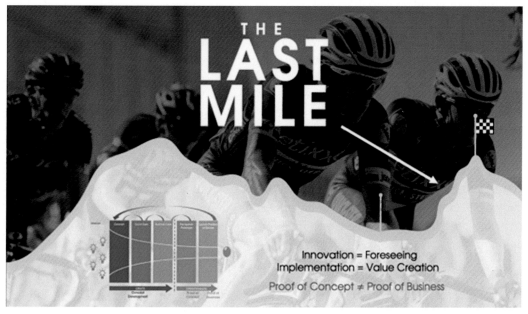

Figure 2.5
The last mile.

When executing the goal of integrating new digital technology with pharmaceutical pathways, it is important to take these steps into account in order to develop a valuable product or service.

Risks for failure

Research has also been into the factors that cause combinatoric alliances to fail. The most frequent reasons are changes in management, changes in priorities, slow or no results, cultural differences, weak commitment to the alliance, poor alliance management, poor communication, and changes in the business environment.

Also, many people are comfortable in their current situation, which can result in a tendency to discourage innovation rather than encourage it. Just by making critical, energy-draining remarks, a person can negatively impact the enthusiasm of people and organizations for innovation. There are many such innovation-killer remarks [1], and interestingly many of them suggest a fear of the unknown and of failure.

For example, "Can you guarantee that this will work?" is a perfect example of a question that should not be asked where innovation is concerned. As Einstein said, "If we knew what we are doing, we wouldn't call it research!" The word research in Einstein's statement could easily be replaced by the word innovation.

Other innovation killers related to fear of failure include "That is impossible," "We have never tried this before," "You can never make this happen," "We will make a fool out of ourselves," "In our organization, this will never work," "We have always managed without it," "You will never find a customer for this," and "We are too small for this."

Learning from brilliant failures

The importance of experimenting and daring to take risks to innovate, especially in these turbulent socioeconomic times, should not be underestimated. Progress and innovation go hand in hand with experimenting and taking risks, as Columbus discovered long ago. It cost Dom Perignon thousands of exploded bottles before he was able to bottle his champagne. And Viagra would never have been discovered if its manufacturer, Pfizer, had not persisted in looking for a new medicine for a completely different problem, that is, angina pectoris.

Healthcare systems may sometimes suffer from what can be called "corporate anorexia nervosa" and may create an unfavorable climate for enterprising people who want to explore the unknown, taking a chance that the result might not meet expectations.

However, in complex environments, progress cannot be forced or predicted. For sure, combinatoric innovation is, per its definition, not an efficient process, in the sense that many of the meetings set up would not produce immediate results. Thus, a failure-and-risk-accepting culture toward innovation is essential for motivating employees to explore the unknown and initiate disruptive ideas. Additionally, learning from failures should be encouraged.

Mediocrity, which is directly linked to fear of failure, just does not cut it. Michael Eisner, the former CEO of the Walt Disney Company, is convinced that punishing failures always leads to mediocrity because "mediocrity is what fearful people will always settle for." In other words, it is becoming increasingly important to have an open attitude to taking risks, experimenting, daring to fail, and learning from them.

The Institute of Brilliant Failures, which was founded in the Netherlands (QR Code 2.2), reinforces the culture of creating a failure-and-risk-accepting attitude toward innovation. The institute aims to reduce the fear in two ways: by increasing the appreciation of entrepreneurial activities and by stimulating learning from failed attempts. This is particularly relevant to combinatoric innovation, as the outcome of this process is by nature uncertain.

QR Code 2.2
Institute of brilliant failures.

The institute has seen the result of many failures. However, often universal lessons are found within such failures: patterns or learned lessons that exceed a specific experience that can be applied in many other innovation projects. Based on these patterns, the Institute of Brilliant Failures has developed 16 archetypes that help people identify and learn from failures (Fig. 2.6).

The archetypes also function to classify. Failure can happen at (a combination of) four levels: system failure, organizational failure, team failure, and individual failure.

Based on analysis of a few hundred cases, the most frequently observed failure patterns in healthcare are as follows:

- 'Empty spot at the table': this refers to innovations in which not all relevant stakeholder groups are involved in the design and development stages. Consequently, it is more difficult to get their commitment and support during the implementation phase.
- 'Canyon': this archetype refers to the many worn-in patterns in the healthcare system that block renewal. These could be procedures, protocols, laws, guidelines, best practices, etc., but also personal factors, such as habits, resistance to change, existing power, lack of knowledge, and politics.
- 'General without an Army': Shortage of resources, including employees, time, and money, can increasingly be observed throughout the healthcare system. Because of this, great ideas cannot be realized because especially in the last mile, there are not sufficient resources.

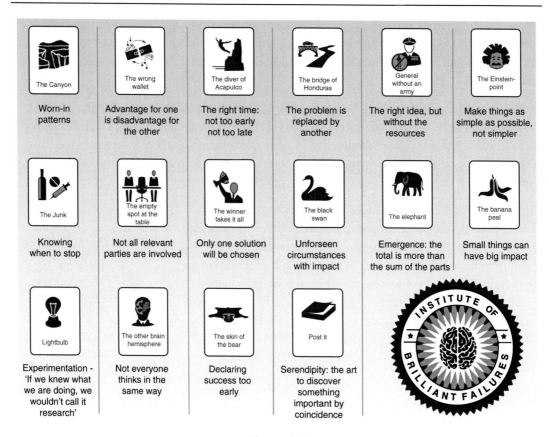

Figure 2.6
16 basic patterns (archetypes) of failure [8].

Chapter 3 discusses why proofing value-based innovation is important for the sustainability of future healthcare systems.

 This means for blended pharmaceutical care:

- PCPs should be equipped with the principles of innovation to prepare for upcoming disruptive innovations in the pharmaceutical care chain.
- Adhering to combinatoric innovation principles between current healthcare systems and (new) digital health providers will enhance the likelihood of successful innovation pathways toward circular pharmaceutical care.
- Vital conditions in which innovation can thrive need to be consciously facilitated in order to increase the likelihood of success and sustainability of digital innovation in pharmaceutical care.
- A failure-and-risk-accepting culture is crucial to stimulate innovation and learn from brilliant failures.

References

[1] Iske PL. Combinatoric innovation: Navigating a complex world. KnocoM; 2017. Available from: http://www.chairedelimmateriel.universite-paris-saclay.fr/wp-content/uploads/2012/06/3-IC8_Iske.pdf.

[2] Osterwalder A, Pigneur Y. Business model generation: a handbook for visionaries, game changers, and challengers, vol. 1. John Wiley & Sons; 2010.

[3] Gibson R. The four lenses of innovation: a power tool for creative thinking. John Wiley & Sons; 2015.

[4] Christensen CM, Grossman JH, Hwang J. The innovator's prescription: a disruptive solution for health care. McGraw Hill; 2010.

[5] Christensen CM. The innovator's dilemma: when new technologies cause great firms to fail. Boston: Harvard Business Review Press; 2013.

[6] Chesbrough HW. Open innovation: the new imperative for creating and profiting from technology. Harvard Business Press; 2003.

[7] van Schaik JGM, Iske PL. Implementation barriers for PHC in The Netherlands. 2021. Available from, https://www.phc-catalyst.nl/wp-content/uploads/2021/12/PHC-Catalyst-Report-Implementation-barriers-for-PHC-in-the-Netherlands.pdf.

[8] Iske PL, Bovelander M. Institute of brilliant failures: make room to experiment, innovate, and learn. 2019.

Healthcare's nutritional value*

Claudia Rijcken[1], Michel van Agthoven[2]
[1]*Pharmi, Maastricht, The Netherlands;* [2]*J&J Campus, The Netherlands*

Price is what you pay. Value is what you get.

Warren Buffet

Nutritional value refers to the amount and types of nutrients (such as proteins, fats, carbohydrates, vitamins, and minerals) that food contains. It is a crucial element for maintaining good health and preventing chronic diseases. Therefore, a balanced diet with a variety of nutrient-dense foods is essential for maintaining good health. Similarly, a well-rounded and sustainable healthcare system should include various services and treatments that guarantee the highest value to maintain a solid and reliable care system.

On the other hand, a diet high in processed foods and low in nutrients can lead to chronic health problems. Similarly, a healthcare system heavily focused on treating symptoms and insufficiently measuring the value added of services and products rather than addressing underlying issues and promoting preventative care can be costly and inefficient in the long run.

How to quantify a balanced approach to healthcare, in which the quality of future care, the financial well-being of all stakeholders in the healthcare system, and the stability of government budgets are addressed, is a crucial question nowadays (see as well Chapter 1).

Current healthcare systems sometimes tend to focus on competing issues such as shifting costs, accumulating bargaining power, and restricting services rather than creating true value for patients. This competition occurs more at the level of health plans, networks, and hospitals and, unfortunately, less where it matters most: in the diagnosis, treatment, and prevention of specific health conditions.

As Michael Porter indicated in 2006, the solution for keeping healthcare sustainable may be found in implementing value-based competition on outcomes [1].

---

*In this chapter, you will read about the principles of a value-based healthcare concept, how to quantify the value of pharmaceutical interventions, and how this relates to the core values of the pharmaceutical care provider.

Pharmaceutical Care in Digital Revolution. https://doi.org/10.1016/B978-0-443-13360-2.00022-8

In the value-based healthcare paradigm, healthcare providers are encouraged to prove the value of their interventions, as Porter described in this formula:

$$\text{Patient value} = \frac{\Delta\text{Health Outcomes}}{\Delta\text{Costs of Services}}$$

Any intervention that leads to a cost increase without better patient outcomes moves a system into an unsustainable, nonbeneficial situation and thus requires adjustment. Porter and Lee, in 2013, defined six steps to transform healthcare organizations into value-driven ways of working; among these six steps, they considered a rigorous measurement of value (outcomes and costs) as perhaps the single most important step to optimizing healthcare. When systematic measurement of results in healthcare took place, they found an improvement in the treatment results [2].

Value-driven healthcare systems are characterized by the following measures:

- Focus on value for patients, not just on lowering costs.
- Drive for high-quality care that is most cost-effective.
- Focus on measuring value in the total patient pathway and beyond (broader societal value).
- Reduce variation by learning from failures and extrapolating best practices.
- Reward innovation that increases outcomes and value.
- Use technology as an enabler for the preceding characteristics.

Concerning the latter point, value-enhancing IT platforms are expected to be centered on patients, use common data definitions, and acquire holistic patient data accessible to all parties involved in care. These platforms will include expert systems for each professional attribution and allow quick and easy data analysis and extraction [2].

Measuring outcomes

The World Health Organization defines an outcome measure as a "change in the health of an individual, group of people, or population that is attributable to an intervention or series of interventions." Outcome measures (i.e., disease progression, mortality, readmission, patient experience) are the quality and cost targets healthcare organizations are trying to improve. A value-based healthcare approach will:

QR Code 3.1
WEF global coalition for value in healthcare.

1. Improve access to appropriate care,
2. Spur innovations in treatment and care delivery, and
3. Provide new business opportunities for the public and private sectors (for more detailed information, see QR Code 3.1).

In addition to measuring differences in clinical parameters, outcomes can be measured using, for example, the International Consortium for Health Outcomes Measurement, which offers standardization of outcomes for many individual diseases [3].

Furthermore, the quality of life of health processes can be measured, for example, by Patient Reported Outcome Measures (PROMs) and Patient Reported Experience Measures (PREMs). PROMs measure a patient's health status or health-related quality of life at a single point in time. PREMs are focused on measuring a patient's experience with healthcare processes. Both data can be tracked by surveys or by digital applications.

In addition to the standardized approaches to measuring patient outcomes, pharmaceutical care stakeholders can survey patients not only on direct outcomes but also on other determinants of health from a physical, mental, and societal perspective—for example, "what matters to patients" rather than "what is the matter with your disease?"

What people value is different for everybody

Take, for example, an active hypertension patient who is prescribed a beta-blocker. Although the treatment choice may be according to clinical evidence and prevailing guidelines, the patient may decide not to take the pill. This is because the adverse events of a beta-blocker may be such that the patient feels hampered in active daily life. Thus, the overall quality of life experience has deteriorated from the patient's perspective. That negatively impacts therapeutic adherence and the outcome of a treatment.

In order to determine what patients value, a personalized holistic approach, potentially supported by digital data on lifestyle and living preferences, is recommended. In addition, validated instruments like the global attainment scale can be used to monitor progress.

In the example case, an antihypertensive without fatigue adverse events could have been a better fit for treating this "specific" patient.

Taking this individual approach is essential once aiming for a holistic value approach, where health status is just one parameter within a broader spectrum of aspects that determine positive health [4,5].

Investing in medicine can bring significant societal benefits, including improved health and longevity, reduced healthcare costs, and increased productivity. For every dollar invested in medicine, there can be a return in terms of reduced healthcare costs due to the prevention and treatment of diseases, as well as improved quality of life and increased productivity for individuals who can maintain their health. Additionally, medical research can lead to new treatments and technologies that can positively impact society as a whole.

The WHO calculated that every dollar invested in drugs has an approximate fourfold return in broader societal benefits; thus, pharmaceutical care providers are recommended to put these broader determinants of health into the equation when moving to value-driven pharmaceutical care [6].

Quadruple aim and proving value of medicine

Quadruple Aim is the expansion of the established Triple Aim concept, which says that any innovation and/or activity needs to either enhance patient experience and/or improve population health and/or reduce costs.

A decade of working with the Triple Aim, has learnt that the Triple Aim is not achievable without attention to healthcare personel experience and, in the next step, without focus on maintaining equity in access to the healthcare system. Many who have resisted prioritizing the well-being of healthcare workers as a fourth aim has found that it is demonstrably impossible to fully achieve the Triple Aim without seriously addressing workforce safety and satisfaction [7]. And, as our understanding of what it will take to create a better health-creating system for all evolves, it becomes increasingly clear that the explicit pursuit of health equity is fundamental to all other aims.

Thus, an additional fourth goal of improving the work life of healthcare providers has been added to the Triple Aim. Organizations view this expansion in different ways, but the Institute for Healthcare Improvement (IHI) calls this new aim "Joy in Work."

Many healthcare organizations have adopted the framework of the Triple Aim, but the stressful work life of clinicians and staff has proven to play a large role in the ability to achieve and maintain the three aims. In primary care, adopting the Triple Aim has enhanced the patient experience, but resources are lacking to help providers and staff maintain these overarching goals. Professional burnout and reduced job satisfaction have hindered the ability of providers and staff to provide quality care. Therefore, a fourth aim focusing on improving the work life of clinicians and staff has been proposed to create a more symbiotic relationship between patients and healthcare providers [8].

In order to work according to the Quadruple Aim, the IHI recommends a process that includes the identification of target populations, definition of system aims and measures, development of a portfolio of project work that is sufficiently strong to move system-level results, and rapid testing and scale-up that is adapted to local needs and conditions [9]. The IHI even goes beyond this "quadruple aim" (addressing clinician burnout) to add a "quintuple aim" that includes advancing health equity as well in the equation. Although this is a relatively new parameter, there is a growing belief that the explicit pursuit of health equity is fundamental to all other aims. Making equity the fifth aim may radically accelerate improvement in population health, enhanced care experience, cost reduction, and improved workforce safety and well-being. The excess in morbidity and mortality, poor patient experience, and unmet need is concentrated among marginalized, underresourced, disenfranchised, and historically oppressed populations. Many of the failure modes associated with the Triple Aim and the Quadruple Aim (when equity is left out) concentrate where inequities are steepest [7].

Health technology assessment agencies all over the world are working on how to adequately define, analyze, and position the value of medical interventions (see QR Code 3.2), the value of a life year, and how to regulate healthcare costs in a solidary way. Precision medicine tests, technologies, and therapeutics (as described in Chapter 16) are increasingly being adopted into clinical practice, and prescription as evidence of their effectiveness grows. However, justification of their actual budget impact and true added value requires adequate measurement of outcomes and a growing need for regulatory reform to safeguard equitable access [10].

QR Code 3.2
The value of medicines.

A potential dilemma of the Quadruple and the Quintuple Aim concept for pharmaceutical care professionals is reflected by the example that a proposed intervention may positively influence one of the three pillars but cause friction in another. For example, clinical guidelines may conflict with economic arguments (depending on the viewpoint taken in the economic analysis), and there might be a conflict with improving a patient's quality of life. The professional standards that pharmaceutical care providers adhere are to require a balanced judgment of the patient's well-being versus societal, economic arguments, which sometimes creates complex dilemmas (more information in Chapter 18).

The quantified self to measure outcomes

The technologies mentioned in Part 2 of this book increase the possibilities for collecting remote patient data on outcomes, analyzing and visualizing results, and creating holistic pictures of patients and populations - under the conditions that the right privacy measures and conditions are in place.

The movement toward gathering these kinds of personalized data and using them in big data analysis is generally referred to as "the quantified me" or "the quantified self" also known as "lifelogging" In brief, quantified self delivers self-knowledge through self-tracking via technology.

The movement incorporates technology into the acquisition of data from a person's daily inputs (e.g., food consumption, quality of surrounding air), states (e.g., mood, arousal, blood oxygen levels), and health status (mental, physical, and social).

Other examples of outcomes that can nowadays be continuously tracked (obviously taking into account the appropriate privacy and compliance restrictions) are:

- self-monitoring and self-sensing devices that combine wearable sensors (e.g., EEG, ECG, and echography) and wearable computing;
- biometrics and biomarkers, which are, for example, insulin, cholesterol, glucose and cortisol levels, DNA sequencing, microbiome testing, pharmacogenetic testing, and so on;
- semantic data, for example, data on interactions with virtual personal assistants; and
- quality of life and other social and/or mental digital assessment scales.

This quantification approach makes it possible to measure an intervention's outcomes, or ultimately, value, in a very holistic and longitudinal way. Although debates about healthcare costs are often focused on the short term, longer-term goals will become more interesting as prospective studies to prove the effects of major reforms with better data are more feasible than ever.

Driving value as a pharmaceutical care provider

With the aim to create as much health value as possible for patients, the world's pharmacy profession is moving from a product-oriented practice to a patient-centered practice.

In this respect, the primary contribution of the pharmaceutical care provider—beyond filling, dispensing, and counseling patients on how to take prescriptions—is a service best known as medication management, which is explained in depth in Chapter 6.

Pharmacists can play a vital role in improving clinical outcomes by providing medication management services. It involves, for example, reviewing a patient's medication regimen, identifying potential problems or interactions, and making recommendations to the patient's healthcare provider.

One example of the positive value of pharmacist interventions on clinical outcomes is in the area of diabetes management. In many countries, pharmacist-led medication therapy management (MTM) services for patients with diabetes have been shown to lead to improved blood sugar control and reductions in hospitalization rates and healthcare costs [11].

Another example is the case of hypertension management, where studies have shown that pharmacist-led interventions can lead to improved blood pressure control and a reduction in the number of medications required to achieve blood pressure control. In addition, such interventions can also lead to an improvement in patient adherence and satisfaction with their medications [12].

These examples indicate that pharmacist interventions can lead to improved clinical outcomes and can also help to reduce healthcare costs by preventing hospitalization and other complications.

As indicated in Chapter 1, in many countries, recent reforms in payment indicate a shift to holding providers more responsible for outcomes and quality and for coordinated care to reduce variation and fill the gaps when patients move from one part of the system to another.

This shift offers opportunities for partnerships between, for example, general practitioners and pharmaceutical care providers, who, on the one hand, have access to a broad set of patient data and, on the other hand, can harvest the advantage of a trusted, low-threshold, close relationship with patients, and thus are able to influence outcomes through both data and empathy.

This synergy is known to bring the highest value to healthcare systems and makes pharmaceutical care providers the optimal providers for maintaining a sustainable nutritional balance in bringing innovations with the highest outcomes in drug intervention programs.

In Chapter 4, there will be a description how new models for reimbursing these outcome-based activities look.

 This means for blended pharmaceutical care:

- Value-based or value-driven healthcare principles support sustainable systems that embrace the Triple Aim concept: more prevention, better treatment, and an improved evidence base for the relationship between outcomes and costs.
- Value-based healthcare also focuses on "what matters to patients" rather than "what is the matter with the disease"?
- In order to prove value, outcomes must be measured, preferably in a standardized way.
- Outcomes can relate to clinical results, disease measurement scales, quality of life, and to broader societal benefits.
- Balancing economic versus patient-related outcomes is a unique competency by which pharmaceutical care professionals can drive patient and, therefore, societal value.

References

[1] Porter ME, Teisberg EO. Redefining health care: creating value-based competition on results. Harvard business press; 2006.

[2] Lee T, Porter M. The strategy that will fix healthcare. Harvard Business Review Boston; 2013.

[3] ICHOM. International consortium for health outcomes measurement 2023 [cited 2023 25/01/2023]; Available from: https://www.ichom.org.

[4] Christensen CM. The innovation health care really needs: help people manage their own health. 2017.

[5] IPH. Institute for positive health. 2023 [cited 2023 25/01/2023]; Available from: https://www.iph.nl/en/.

[6] Nurse J, et al. The case for investing in public health: a public health summary report for EPHO 8. 2014.

[7] Nundy S, Cooper LA, Mate KS. The quintuple aim for health care improvement: a new imperative to advance health equity. JAMA 2022;327(6):521−2. https://doi.org/10.1001/jama.2021.25181.

[8] Huntsberry A, Wettergreen S. Quadruple aim. Learn the lingo: key terms for navigating the value based care world. 2023 [cited 2023 23/01/2023]; Available from: https://www.pharmacist.com/Practice/Practice-Resources/Learn-the-Lingo/quadruple-aim.

[9] IHI. The IHI Triple aim. 2023 [cited 2023 25/01/2023]; Available from: https://www.ihi.org/Engage/Initiatives/TripleAim/Pages/default.aspx.

[10] Gronde TVD, Uyl-de Groot CA, Pieters T. Addressing the challenge of high-priced prescription drugs in the era of precision medicine: a systematic review of drug life cycles, therapeutic drug markets and regulatory frameworks. PLoS One 2017;12(8):e0182613.

[11] Erku DA, Ayele AA, Mekuria AB, Belachew SA, Hailemeskel B, Tegegn HG. The impact of pharmacist-led medication therapy management on medication adherence in patients with type 2 diabetes mellitus: a randomized controlled study. Pharm Pract (Granada) 2017;15(3):1026. https://doi.org/10.18549/PharmPract.2017.03.1026. PMID: 28943985. PMCID: PMC5597801.

[12] Alshehri AA, Jalal Z, Cheema E, Haque MS, Jenkins D, Yahyouche A. Impact of the pharmacist-led intervention on the control of medical cardiovascular risk factors for the primary prevention of cardiovascular disease in general practice: a systematic review and meta-analysis of randomised controlled trials. Br J Clin Pharmacol 2020;86(1):29−38. https://doi.org/10.1111/bcp.14164. PMID: 31777082. PMCID: PMC6983518.

CHAPTER 4

Platters of paying for outcomes*

Claudia Rijcken
Pharmi, Maastricht, The Netherlands

> *Obstacles are those frightful things you see, when you take your eyes off your goal.*
>
> **Henry Ford**

Preparing a good but cost-effective platter of food in a sustainable way is complex in a world where resources and personnel are increasingly more expensive. It is all about balancing volume, quality, timing, and managing expectations. It is the customer who, with the tipping, decides whether expectations have been met or even exceeded.

Similar to this evolution in the cooking world, a healthcare revolution focused on sustainability may create winners and losers in the health provider space.

From activity-based to outcome-based financing

Healthcare stakeholders ultimately have the same goal: finding sustainable solutions that warrant accessibility to future (drug) innovations for the sake of improving patients' health. Moreover, they all tend to agree that the majority of innovative, specialty drugs referred to in Chapter 1 are not at all discretionary and cannot be dismissed as mere lifestyle improvement drugs, as many of these drugs represent significant medical innovations in their clinical realms. Thus, among other interventions, innovation in payment access schemes is the next step toward establishing future sustainable models and optimizing societal impact.

---

*In this chapter, you will read about the potential innovation of reimbursement schemes for pharmaceuticals, why outcome-based financing is considered a potential panacea, and how health digitization can augment the role of pharmaceutical care providers to drive these outcome-based agreements.

Pharmaceutical Care in Digital Revolution. https://doi.org/10.1016/B978-0-443-13360-2.00015-0

Philips: from products to solutions

Traditionally, Philips was a company selling light bulbs.

For many years, the company's sales model was based on selling as many bulbs as possible. However, as the bulbs' quality improved and were eventually replaced by long-lasting LED lights, the business model had to change.

Philips had much more lighting expertise than just producing the bulb; thus, their new business model is much more focused on integrated light solutions.

Now when clients contract with Philips for a light-solution plan, the company is reimbursed for providing the clients with a customized, adjustable, continuous light solution. Philips is paid for the solution rather than for only the product [1].

To optimize the cost-effective use of drugs and reward outcomes (refer to Chapter 3), payers are increasingly thinking toward "value-based" reimbursements. Value-based refers to if a drug does not perform as it is supposed to (i.e., according to outcomes in clinical trials), it will not be fully reimbursed. By extension, this is what we call performance-based or outcome-based financing (OBF).

An outcome-based or performance-based model takes a radically different approach to the structure of a health system by not funding the system with resources (i.e., personnel, budget, real estate). Instead, this model gives organizational units the right to make decisions about their resources (i.e., autonomy) to reach set, predefined performance levels. In this new paradigm, health systems may no longer be rewarded for providing patient interventions (i.e., activity-based interventions and delivery of drugs). Instead, they will be rewarded for providing effective solutions based on the outcomes explained in Chapter 3. This outcome-based approach also happens in other industries, as shown in the Philips example.

The performance-based model is particularly marked in relation to highly innovative and recently introduced drugs. Because societal risks are considered higher as real-world experience is less available, the outcomes are harder to predict (whether they resemble trial results). The budget impact is often significant compared to existing therapeutic options.

An important prerequisite for driving performance-based models is the availability of outcome data, as shown in Chapter 3. This is one of the biggest assets of the digital revolution; as in the days of the quantified self, much more health data are available. For example, medical records are digitized, interventions are digitally tracked, and real-time sensors record all kinds of patient data. These data could potentially give healthcare stakeholders better insight into which treatments and interventions worked and which did not. Additionally, while connecting the different data sets and linking them with artificial intelligence (AI) software, all stakeholders are expected to predict upfront better what the outcome of treatments will be (also see Chapter 11).

To meet payers' performance-based requirements, physicians, manufacturers, and pharmaceutical care providers (PCPs) are requested, or even expected, to install mechanisms with patients that prove the actual outcomes of drug and care interventions (QR Code 4.1).

QR Code 4.1
HIB: a form of social impact bond.

Changing models for spending control on drugs

In order to be ready to move into outcome-based payment models, providers' business models are changing significantly.

For example, in the pharmaceutical industry, whereas in the past, development, marketing, and sales of a specific product were the core activities, today the optimal outcome for individual patients is becoming the core strategy, as shown in Table 4.1.

Many countries seek to control overall spending on drugs either directly or indirectly by controlling the reimbursement and access to specific drugs. Direct controls include spending or growth caps and payback schemes, not a drug's immediate performance. An example of indirect control is assigning separate dedicated budgets for, say, hepatitis or oncology. Other indirect controls focus on evidence-based assessment of the value of medicines, which then influences either reimbursement or patient access to the medicines or both.

Table 4.2 provides an overview of different payment schemes as they are currently implemented in different payer—provider relationships.

Globally, innovative models are sometimes codeveloped by the pharmaceutical industry and other relevant stakeholders, such as physicians and patient associations. Fig. 4.1 shows

Table 4.1: Toward proving clinical outcomes.

Past	Future
Treating signs and symptoms	**Proving relevant clinical outcomes**
For example, lowering cholesterol, opening up airways	Fewer cardiovascular incidents, fewer *chronic obstructive pulmonary disease* (COPD) exacerbations
Offering products	**Offering solutions**
Drugs	Reduction of COPD via smart inhaler, drugs, and behavioral therapy
Negotiating price	**Partnering for better health**
Transactional collaboration based on volume	Collaboration based on best health outcomes

Table 4.2: Overview of payment schemes.

	More Outcomes/Performance Focus →	
Financial-based contracts	Intermediate outcomes	Final Outcomes/Outcome-Based financing (OBF)
Price-volume (no. of units)	Intermediate patient outcome, which are a marker for disease state, e.g., LDL, CRP	Actual patient outcome, e.g., cancer survival or multiple sclerosis relapse
Capitation	No payment for nonresponders	System usage outcomes, e.g., avoided hospitalization/emergency room visits
Financial risk share	Reimbursement only with evidence development in real life	Experience of healthcare treatment, e.g., QoL improvement
Volume-based discount		Broader societal benefits, e.g., less sick days at work
Payment per channel Free/discount treatment initiation		Integrated societal impact

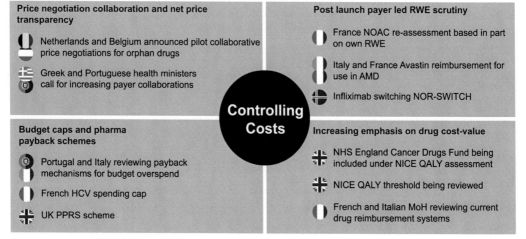

Figure 4.1

Changes in EU drug spending control mechanisms. *Reproduced from Aitken M. Outlook for Global Medicines through 2021. Quintiles IMS, Parsippany; 2016. https://www.iqvia.com/-/media/iqvia/pdfs/institute-reports/global-outlook-for-medicines-through-2021.pdf.*

an overview of recent changes in European spending control mechanisms; this overview indicates significant development of creative, innovative ideas for keeping access to drugs affordable and sustainable while optimizing societal outcomes and costs.

Real-world evidence

As OBF schemes are becoming increasingly popular in many healthcare systems, there is a growing need to provide real-world evidence of the outcome of drugs. Real-world evidence (RWE) is defined as data collected outside the clinical trial setting, including electronic health records, social media, and digital health devices.

Over the past decade, many countries with outcome-based healthcare systems initiated registries to analyze the real-world experiences of people using medications. A registry collects information about individuals, usually focused on a specific diagnosis or condition. For example, many registries collect information about people who have a specific disease or condition. In contrast, others seek participants with varying health statuses who are willing to participate in research about a particular disease. People provide information about themselves to these registries voluntarily. A governmental agency, a nonprofit organization, a healthcare facility, or a private company can sponsor registries.

Registries may make use of primary care data, hospital data, claims data, patient-reported outcomes, and, increasingly, data from digital health devices. The most time-consuming work in these large databases is combining, formatting, cleaning, and processing data to prepare the data for analysis.

Advanced analytics techniques, with statistical methods or AI algorithms (as explained in Chapter 11), can be applied to the collected registry data to help organizations analyze much broader data sets compared to past data. For example, upfront segmentation of patients based on RWE behavioral patterns and correlated risks of inadequate drug use can be considered, which in turn can help to develop better, more customized, and earlier intervention strategies.

Real-world evidence can be directly related to measuring a patient's disease status or general health and may also look at benefits outside the direct healthcare environment. For example, spending on drugs may not only improve the patient's health status but also decrease the need for care and improve work productivity.

There is a growing realization that registries seem to be too archaic. Today, the focus is moving toward federated data networks, which leave source data where they belong. These networks make use of the source data and, via complex algorithms, enable the anonymous use of the collective data. Federated data networks also give account to an often heard complaint on registries, e.g., that they do not (always) require additional data collection work by healthcare workers, which is a great advantage of federated data networks.

Unfortunately, in many countries, healthcare department and socioeconomic department budgets are yet completely separated, as profit-and-loss structures are organized in separate balances. Once the budget spent in healthcare benefits work productivity, this real-world benefit should also be considered when determining the real-world value of medicines.

In their reimbursement assessment procedures, many European health technology authorities consider these broader societal benefits (BSBs) of drugs. Nevertheless, due to broad differences in the cost of living among different countries, it is rather complex to compare BSBs between countries and come to joint conclusions on a more holistic assessment of the economic value of drugs.

Broader societal benefits and health impact bonds

In a value-based healthcare system, we need to look at the direct advantages of medications on the health of an individual or a population and the impact that drugs can have on people's ability to work or contribute to the economy and society.

There is a global trend in which employers are increasingly investing in the prevention of disease and the well-being of employees. For example, with careful plan design, employers can improve health outcomes. In a randomized clinical trial whose results were published in *The New England Journal of Medicine* and *Health Affairs*, patients from racial and ethnic minoritized groups whose employers covered all the costs of their preventive medications after they had suffered heart attacks had 35% fewer major complications than patients with copayments, and 70% lower total health care costs.

Employees' health, productivity, and diversity are key to an organization's success. The pandemic has magnified the wide inequities in health that prevent certain employees from achieving their optimal health. By using a health equity lens and proven strategies to eliminate disparities, employers can improve business outcomes, create a better employee experience, and advance health for all [2].

Although the figures are lower in Europe, the movement has started, and promoting high standards in working conditions, including in the area of health and well-being at work, is a key priority for the European Union [3].

Pharmaceutical care providers as drug outcome optimizers

The outcome-based payment schemes, as previously described, provide many opportunities for pharmaceutical care stakeholders. While the traditional activity-based model was focused on delivering products and care, evolving models are increasingly focused on incentivizing positive healthcare outcomes.

In this book, you will see how digital health technology can augment the role of PCPs to deliver health solutions and patient outcomes instead of predominantly providing products. By thoroughly understanding the opportunities of this digital arena, having access to broader health data sets, and using analytics, we may have the setup we need to make performance-based risk-sharing arrangements (PBRSAs) in pharmaceutical care a reality.

 PCPs need to be highly involved in setting up these PBRSAs (which are often initiated by payers and pharmaceutical industries), as PCPs have the holistic insight of the individual patient and may positively influence drug outcomes by combining analytic insights with a human, low-threshold, and trusted approach.

As the earlier Philips example indicates (where Philips moved from selling light bulbs to warranting light solutions), we can anticipate that in future healthcare systems, the hunting grounds of drug budgets will be better balanced by PCPs being paid based on providing circular pharmaceutical care outcomes rather than on the number of prescriptions delivered.

In the next Chapter 5, we will take patients' perspectives on these developments.

This means for blended pharmaceutical care:

- Payment models in healthcare are shifting from activity-based to outcome-based schemes.
- Outcome-based reimbursement of drugs is increasingly possible due to better real-world insights.
- In addition to the value of medicines on health status, BSBs of drugs need to be considered as well when determining value and driving circular pharmaceutical care.
- PCPs are essential partners in outcome-based payment models, as these providers can drive outcomes through strong, insightful analytics combined with low-threshold, trusted care relationships with patients.
- PCPs can be paid based on the provision of circular pharmaceutical care outcomes rather than the number of prescriptions delivered.

References

[1] Signify Holding. Signify. 2023 [cited 2023 25/01/2023]; Available from: https://www.signify.com/en-gb.
[2] Nundy S, Cooper LA, Kelsay E. Employers can do more to advance health equity. Harv Bus Rev 2023;1. Available from: https://hbr.org/2023/01/employers-can-do-more-to-advance-health-equity.
[3] Eurofound. Health and well-being at work. 2023. 17/01/2023 [cited 2023 25/01/2023]; Available from: https://www.eurofound.europa.eu/topic/health-and-well-being-at-work.

CHAPTER 5

#Including the consuming patient*

Lucien Engelen[1,2], Claudia Rijcken[3]

[1]Transform Health, LLC, Baltimore, MD, United States; [2]Strategist Health(care) Innovation for Deloitte C4E, Vodafone Group, Laurentius Medical Center, Roermond, The Netherlands; [3]Pharmi, Maastricht, The Netherlands

> *Diversity is the art of thinking independently together.*
>
> **Malcom Forbes**

Consuming healthcare is like eating a nutritious meal. Just as a healthy diet is essential for maintaining a strong and healthy body, regular healthcare check-ups and screenings are crucial for keeping our physical and mental well-being in check.

As we need to be mindful of the foods we put in our bodies, we also need to be mindful of the healthcare we consume, making sure to choose the right treatments and providers to nourish our overall health and well-being. Therefore, we as healthcare providers need to involve the consumer and the patient in our decisions, system setup, and future wishes.

A growing number of patients are researching, networking, and talking about health-related topics in the virtual world every day. They are accessing medical information that is freely available and shared. Increasingly, patients find themselves in the center of care.

The patient is increasingly becoming the expert in managing their own disease, as information comes online, research becomes open access, communities online are created, and user-generated data are becoming mainstream.

Patient centricity

Early patient engagement is essential in disease management, and patient centricity is a core element of the development of medicines and value-driven healthcare. In Chapters 3 and 4, we noted that health outcomes are highly dependent on active patient engagement

---

*In this chapter, you will read about the emerging engagement of patients in healthcare system optimization, the principles of good care, the competencies for shared care partnerships, and the expectations for future pharmaceutical care.

and that there is a clear need for healthcare system providers to partner with patients in optimizing the adequate use of medicines, among other activities, to bring about better outcomes.

Patient centricity is not an activity 'on the side,' but, similar to quality control and product development, it should be covered at the management level in healthcare systems. An example is the initiation of the #patientsincluded charter [1], which stimulated a chain of development for including patients in core business and development processes. An interesting example is also the "patient and public partnership" [2], where the British Medical Journal guidelines for authors require mandatory disclosure of patient involvement in the paper's design, operation, and results.

Although many definitions are being used, recent research suggests that patient centricity is defined as "putting the patient first in an open and sustained engagement of the patient to respectfully and compassionately achieve the best experience and outcome for that person and their family" [3].

This definition encompasses five clear themes: (1) achieving inclusiveness, (2) sharing goals that are patient- and family-centered, (3) empowering patients to take control of their own health, (4) working in a way that shows respect, compassion, and openness, and (5) working in partnership [3].

At first glance, the concept of patient centricity may seem easy to grasp; however, in today's society, this concept cannot be taken for granted universally. So let us take a look in more detail.

Why healthcare systems promote active patient participation

Of the many forces that drive the goal of healthcare systems to engage with patients and consumers actively, we pick four to elaborate on as they seem the most relevant ones for the upcoming years.

- Consumerism/retailization of healthcare to take autonomy on own healthcare
- Targeted information supply at individual literacy levels
- Care systems move from volume to value
- Regulatory interest in patient perspectives

Consumerism to take autonomy for own healthcare

As we indicate in Chapter 1, in many countries, there exists dissatisfaction with current forms of healthcare systems, and more patients than ever are criticizing the healthcare industry's once-paternalistic approach. Therefore patients are increasingly taking charge of their own care and proactively communicating their needs, desires, and concerns to healthcare institutions.

 Dissatisfaction and distrust of patients in current healthcare systems is also one of the pivotal reasons why retailers (e.g., Amazon, Apple, and Google) have become relevant players in the healthcare industry. These companies have created a consumer-centric, personalized, and intuitive buying experience and a growing number of people now expect to interact with a healthcare system in the same way. Thus, when patients are offered affordable healthcare options—that truly solve their daily problems—from providers with whom they are already familiar, patients readily tend to consider these stakeholders as trusted parties and are more open to adopting the new services offered [4].

Therefore, financially accountable, digital-savvy consumers increasingly avail themselves to a wide range of digital health services from both traditional providers and new entrants in the healthcare industry. Many consumers want to create their own health management ecosystems, act as stewards of their own care, and control not just where they access the care but also what, how, and from whom they acquire it, as well as the price they have to pay.

Society is largely anticipating consumerism's evolution through initiatives that disclose health information directly to patients. For example, institutions like myTomorrows aim to disclose information that will ensure that patients with rare diseases and their physicians do not miss out on available treatment options. There are institutions like the Patient-Centered Outcomes Research Institute, which aims to improve the quality and relevance of the evidence available to help patients, caregivers, clinicians, employers, insurers, and policymakers make better-informed health decisions. Finally, there are places like Ask a Patient (see QR Code 5.1), which is an environment that gathers and discloses experiences of drug users, thus empowering other patients to take control of their health by being better informed through peers.

QR Code 5.1
Askapatient.

Targeted information supply at individual literacy levels

Access to tailored, understandable, and executable information to make informed decisions is essential in the movement to take charge of own health. However, this is not as straightforward as it sounds; for example, having access to laboratory results is one thing, but interpreting the results as a layman and knowing how to adjust lifestyle or treatment accordingly is a different matter.

Offering optimal patient value is about supporting patients' holistic experiences and everything that goes into making those experiences as good as possible, including providing health information at an individual (patient/professional and others) level of understanding [5]. Thus, many consumers and patients may not only look for how a medication works or what a certain disease comprises, but they also may want to make completely informed and empowered healthcare decisions to reduce the likelihood of an inaccurate or delayed diagnosis, to lower the risk of hospitalization, and to maximize their quality of life. By becoming self-educated and gaining health literacy, they expect to optimize their own treatment pathways [6]. On the other hand, using well-crafted UI (user interfaces) and interpretation by healthcare professionals at tech corporates creates a piece of new information channeling, creating a better understanding of user-generated data (from smartwatches and wearables) and aggregating them info advice and suggestion.

Herein lies a huge opportunity for pharmaceutical care providers. Digital pathways offer a variety of mediums that give patients access to health information in a personalized manner. Providing individualized written, visual, and digital information communication is possible nowadays and can be aligned with patients' personal preferences. Part 2 of this book offers an extensive discussion about the different digital pathways that can deliver information at the level consumers seek.

Before developing these information gateways, it is essential to involve patient associations and individual patients. Thus, together, they can determine the highest priority areas for solving existing problems and where the most value can be created by implementing individualized support. All diseases are different, and preferences may be linked to the mobility of patient populations, the prognosis of a disease, age variations, treatment options, or the disease phase. Involving patients as equal partners from the start, as opposed to near the end or at the point of the process redesign, should be at the top of every health professional's mind and should be considered "the new normal"[7].

Care systems from volume to value

As discussed in Chapter 3, precision medicine has been described as disruptive in its ability to drive down healthcare costs without compromising quality or outcomes, thus supporting the move from volume-driven to value-driven healthcare [8].

Personalized medicine, in this respect, refers to an approach in which patients consider their genetic makeup with a focus on their preferences, beliefs, attitudes, knowledge, and social context. Conversely, *precision medicine* describes a model for healthcare delivery that relies heavily on data, analytics, and information. Precision medicine is an emerging model that aims to customize therapy to subpopulations of patients, categorized by shared molecular and cellular biomarkers, to improve patient outcomes. This model goes beyond genomics and has vast implications for a nation's research agenda and its implementation and adoption into healthcare. To succeed, precision medicine—and the ecosystem that supports it—must embrace patient-centeredness and engagement, digital health, genomics and other molecular technologies, data sharing, and data science [9].

The power of precision medicine is that it enables healthcare providers to choose the most effective treatment for an individual. However, precision forecasting (e.g., which drug might provide the highest patient value) currently is not yet common practice. It cannot be easily drawn from only the results of clinical trials. Moreover, real-world outcomes may differ from those in clinical trial settings, mainly because populations in the real world are much more heterogenous as compared with populations in which medicines have been tested. Nevertheless, the current real-world health data offer a wealth of new opportunities once the data are synergized by combining clinical development data, patient experiences, and real-life digital health biomarkers.

As a result, using multicriteria decision formulas that consider a broad set of data, third-party value assessment groups—such as the Institute for Clinical and Economic Review, the American Society for Clinical Oncology, and the European Cardiology Society, as well as many national disease-specific scientific associations—increasingly publish in a structured approach their own balanced decisions about drug value.

Those insights, preferably created with patients included in the guideline setup, empower both providers and patients to make better-informed decisions on treatments that best fit individual cases, thus fueling the goal of precision medicine within a circular care model.

Regulatory interest in patient perspectives

The move from a volume model to a value model requires that regulatory authorities and health technology assessment bodies use a proactive patient-inclusive approach. For example, when pharmaceutical companies aim to market drugs for diseases of low prevalence (called orphan indications), costs to develop these drugs are often higher, as the risk of development failure may be increased and the return of investment distributed among a lower group of patients. Therefore, to increase the likelihood of development and reimbursement success, both pharmaceutical companies and regulators strive toward better and earlier integration of the experiences of people who endure low-frequency, but often very serious, illnesses.

As part of the Food and Drug Administration Safety and Innovation Act of 2012, the Food and Drug Administration (FDA) set up a Patient-Focused Drug Development program to better engage with patients. As of 2018, the FDA had held 21 disease-specific meetings in the United States, asking patients for perspectives on their diseases, treatments, willingness to participate in clinical research, tolerance for risk, and digitalization perspectives on healthcare.

The European Medicines Agency (EMA) has a structured approach to patient interaction. The framework for engagement between EMA and patients, consumers, and their organizations outlines the basis for involving patients and consumers in Agency activities.

In 2022, the EMA's Management Board endorsed an updated framework [10]:

- supporting access to patients' real-life experiences of living with a condition, its management, and the current use of medicines complementing the scientific evidence provided during the evaluation process;
- promoting the generation, collection, and use of evidence-based patient experience data for benefit-risk decision-making;
- enhancing patients and consumers understanding of medicines regulation and their role in the process;
- contributing to efficient and targeted communication to patients and consumers to support their role in the safe and rational use of medicines and to foster trust in the EU Medicines Regulatory Network.

What do patients consider as good healthcare?

The importance of timely determination of whether expected outcomes of innovative treatments will meet patient expectations of good, and preferably easy, care has been explained. But what should we consider as the definition of good care? First, start with defining what is good health. Apart from many definitions and the one from the WHO, an often-used framework comes from the Institute for Positive Health [11] by Machteld Huber and colleagues [12]. It defines that Positive Health is a broader view of health (not only the absence of disease), and it is elaborated in six dimensions. This broader approach contributes to people's ability to deal with physical, emotional, and social challenges in life—and to be in charge of their own affairs, whenever possible. Health can only be achieved once these domains are in balance. Depending on how the patient perceives and defines priorities in life, the balance may differ and choices need to be adapted.

Whereas there is considerable literature on this topic, here we want to focus on the findings within a 2018 project. One of the world's largest personalized health networks, PatientsLikeMe, fielded a six-question online poll to a sample of its members, asking them what they consider as being "good care." A total of 2559 patients completed the poll, which asked a number of original multiple-choice questions with a section for additional written responses [13].

While opinions about care and provider performance varied across different disease conditions, in general, patient groups agreed on the top factors that constitute "good" care:

- Active patient role in care
- Effective treatment selection
- Effective care delivery
- Focus on outcomes
- Doctor or provider competence
- Individualized and empathic care
- Collaborative care
- Effective staff communication
- Care accessibility and cost
- Office management of the respective care institute

The findings in this survey were pretty much in line with other research published in this field. Also, as in previous studies, the "offer support in using digital health data and technology" has not been a dedicated item addressed.

Some of the 10 reflected topics can only be achieved by adequate use of available digital tools. Thus, one could state that adequate use of digital technology enables different perceptions of what is good care.

Definitions of good care in the digital revolution may not differ from those in the analog period because digital technology is seen as a way to serve patients well, just as human interactions do. Good care is the best possible outcome, and digital technology can be a vehicle for achieving that goal.

It is also crucial to realize that the more trust we place in future technology to deliver good care and support clinical decisions, the more studies and research we will need to validate such technology. Therefore, we must continue to evaluate whether technology goals remain aligned with our human goals and whether they are consistent with the previously mentioned definitions of good care. For example, when one measures their blood pressure, they may notice that it is within the correct range. However, when we look at blood pressure over time, we may notice an increase in levels signaling a decline in health. Thus, evaluating a single point in time is insufficient for proper assessment but should be based on a cumulation of activities based on real-world data.

Shared responsibility

To establish an environment where good care can thrive, many healthcare organizations have developed transparent communications on the shared responsibility of care providers and patients.

The way institutions provide healthcare can be found in their mission, vision, value, and process statements. Also, for many diseases, there are openly published regional, national, and international treatment guidelines (although not always at an appropriate literacy level). Additionally, institutional ambitions on private and secure data sharing, financial coverage, attitude, and expected professional behavior of providers are openly published in many healthcare environments. Thus, patients are informed on what to expect from the healthcare provider and the healthcare process, and if a patient does not feel well-informed, a proactive attitude and hand-raising are expected in many healthcare systems.

Some healthcare institutions publish what they expect from a patient, which can be regarded as a *psychological contract* between the healthcare system and the patient. An inspirational example is the UCLA hospital in Los Angeles, which transparently publishes its expectations to patients in a public environment as [14]:

- To report to your physician and other healthcare professionals caring for you accurate and complete information to the best of your knowledge about present complaints, past illnesses, hospitalizations, medications, unexpected changes in condition, and other matters relating to your health to be filed in your medical record, if applicable.
- To seek information about your health and what you are expected to do. Your healthcare provider may not know when you are confused or uncertain or just want more information. If you do not understand the medical words they use, ask for a simpler explanation.
- The most effective plan is the one to which all participants agree, and that is carried out exactly. It is your responsibility to tell your healthcare provider whether or not you can and want to follow the treatment plan recommended for you.
- To ask your healthcare provider for information about your health and healthcare. This includes following the instructions of other health team members, including nurses and physical therapists linked to this care plan. The organization makes every effort to adapt a plan specific to your needs and limitations.
- To continue your care after you leave UCLA Health, including knowing when and where to get further treatment and what you need to do at home to help with your care.
- To accept the consequences of your own decisions and actions if you choose to refuse treatment or not to comply with the care, treatment, and service plan offered by your healthcare provider.

Interestingly, many of the publicly available responsibility statements from hospitals and other healthcare providers do not yet make specific statements about the responsibility to transfer relevant quantified-self data (although this may be included in "sharing all knowledge about your health available"). Patients are not obliged to share these digital data, however, as data may be crucial for adequate treatment, actively reminding patients about this asset may help produce a favorable outcome of the proposed care.

Therefore, adding a statement about the potential use of such data, specifying that they may contain important health information required to optimize the outcome of the chosen treatment, might be considered, such as the following:

- *To discuss with your healthcare provider the option to transfer relevant digital health data* (e.g., *mobile apps, wearables, home robotics*), *as they may contain important information for your treatment plan.*

Patients getting acquainted with digital health technology

The global adoption rate of digital health technology largely relates to a population's health and technology literacy. In situations where there is no awareness of why a healthy lifestyle is important, technology will not be the primary answer to stimulating consciousness on the necessity of maintaining fitness and well-being. And if health literacy exists but interest in or access to technology is limited, the adoption rate of digital health tools is still at risk.

Health technology industries anticipate these factors by increasing the integration of health monitoring tools with low-threshold devices like watches and other wearable devices that do not need to be actively operated. For example, in a global study comprising 160 patient groups, Deloitte showed that 65% of the respondents used smartphones, of which 70% used their phone to manage their disease, and about 50% did so regularly [15]. Chapter 7 provides more information on factors that impact the adoption of digital health technologies.

In a 2015 study, the patient engagement rate with digital health technologies increased by 60% or more when physicians used apps and online portals to facilitate ongoing patient communication. Thus, the expanding digital environment is opening avenues for providers to improve communication with patients and remotely monitor disease status. Therefore, technology has the potential to bridge the still-existing gap between patients and the healthcare ecosystem [16].

A survey of 2301 US health consumers also suggests that consumers become more accepting of machines—ranging from artificial intelligence (AI), to virtual clinicians and home-based diagnostics—and those machines have a significantly greater role in their overall medical care. For example, one in five respondents (19%) said they have already used AI-powered healthcare services, and most said they are likely to use AI-enabled clinical services, such as home-based diagnostics, virtual health assistants, and virtual nurses, that monitor health conditions, medications, and vital signs at home [17].

Due to the COVID crisis, virtual care services saw a surge as in-person visits were put on hold. Digital healthcare quickly became a part of the clinical routine as both patients and providers adapted quickly. Despite the growth of digital healthcare, it was found that the challenges faced before the pandemic still persist, such as cumbersome digital experiences, concerns over privacy and security, and difficulties integrating new tools into daily clinical work. To make these digital healthcare advancements permanent, providers, payers, and consumers can take advantage of the forced adoption and tackle the preexisting barriers to digital health adoption. This can include increasing trust in virtual services by incorporating new tools, addressing privacy and security concerns, and improving technology access for all consumers, especially as nonmedical players become more involved in healthcare [18].

We cannot include all the available information on patients' adoption of digital healthcare in this book, but one commonality is obvious: it is the focus on simplifying and solving basic patient needs that drives adoption in healthcare, not the novelty or degree of innovation of the tools. Based on the fact that in 2018 there were about one billion chronically ill patients worldwide, it is clear that digital innovations are or are expected to become vital tools enabling patients to play an informed role in their healthcare, which is one of the strongest prerequisites for making value-driven healthcare systems work.

Some examples where patients are making a (digital) difference

An interesting example of where patients are voluntarily sharing health data that can be used to improve the health of specific populations is DigitalMe. The goal of this platform is to stretch the limits of breakthrough technologies to find new answers to existing and upcoming healthcare questions.

QR Code 5.2
DigitalMe.

It is an initiative of the platform PatientsLikeMe (a health data sharing platform), which combines multiple sources of patient health data, pulling together experiential, environmental, biological, and medical information to create a digital version of the participating patient. The platform has a business model of selling data to pharmaceutical companies and others, which contributors to the platform agree to upfront (QR Code 5.2).

Based on the patient's disease-specific data, what the platform is seeing across conditions, and what the platform learns from the data, it will choose from the most advanced scientific resources available, such as machine learning to examine RNA and DNA, proteins, antibodies, microbiome, and metabolites.

 Ultimately, the platform aims to make it possible for a patient to try an intervention first in the digital version of himself (called an avatar or digital twin) and see how it works before deciding with a healthcare provider to continue the treatment. Needless to say, adverse events and contraindications will be much better modeled upfront than is done in current practices.

ORCHA and www.myhealthappsblog.com are other examples of where patients can contribute their own or find the health experience and knowledge of others.

The site www.myhealthappsblog.com brings together information about healthcare apps that patients have tried and tested. Each app is reviewed by healthcare communities worldwide, including empowered consumers, patients, care providers, patient groups, charities, and other not-for-profit organizations. It is a community-based platform that endeavors to disclose information in a more user-friendly way than general app stores do, and that adds experiences that contributors had when they used a particular app (QR Code 5.3).

QR Code 5.3
MyHealthAppsblog.

The website gives consumers, patients, and care providers a quick-and-easy way to find trusted apps that can make a difference in a patient's health or that can support caregivers. Although the platform is not fully matured yet, it provides a good example of how patients can take power into their own hands and build a knowledge base worldwide (see also Chapter 9).

ORCHA is a leading provider of health-and-care app reviews and of the assessment of digital activation solutions. ORCHA is part of the NHS England National Innovation Accelerator program and supports many NHS (National Health Service) and local government organizations to drive the uptake of digital health among their populations. ORCHA's aim is to help remove the barriers that currently inhibit the true potential of digital health solutions and prevent the widespread adoption of great products and services by patients, health and care professionals, and health and care systems. ORCHA also drives the development of the first ISO certification for health apps (ISO 82304) [19].

What patients can expect from pharmaceutical care

Pharmacists in many countries around the world are praised for their professional service and their accessibility. However, next to being trusted advisors, the waiting time for pharmaceutical services pales compared to the waiting time many patients experience in a doctor's office. Although many doctors are praised for their good services, there is a growing demand for care. Suppose patients cannot get a timely appointment with their doctor and their condition deteriorates. In that case, they often turn to more expensive care providers such as emergency rooms or other hospital facilities. Often, pharmaceutical care is regarded as the highly educated, professional intermediary that may prevent emergency care and provide support for disease-related questions.

Also, for example, research has shown that US patients perceive their pharmacists as one of the most trusted care providers. The pharmacists' high rating is due mainly to the fact that they are regarded as clinically trained medication experts who—at a low threshold—adequately and quickly answer patients' questions and offer solid advice about their drug profile as well as their disease [20].

Pharmaceutical care providers strive to understand how patients think about their health and illnesses. Patients' personal perceptions of their health tell something about their ideas, feelings, and expectations about illnesses and their motives for why and how they see medication as a value in impacting their health. By talking with patients, pharmaceutical care providers often know the patients as well as their doctors, especially in rural areas. Thus, pharmacists know what matters most to patients and can align advice about treatment with the personalized situation a patient may be in.

In this matter, determining the channel or location of providing care is increasingly becoming important. Separating logistics from care, may be an option, as some logistical activities can be allocated to companies that are specialized in logistical operations.

Care needs to be provided by professional institutions, broader than the traditional brick-and-mortar locations, as it can be situated near the patient's activities like supermarkets or malls, or in digital channels where the patient is already active.

Unfortunately, pharmaceutical care is still a relatively untapped resource in many countries. Once pharmacists have access to key individual health information (preferably specific data from both first- and second-line care), they, together with physicians, are able to offer quick support to patients who need urgent advice, or need unplanned care, or even need help when their doctor's office is closed or busy.

To valorize this asset, in addition to linking primary and secondary care data, another option is to have an integrated patient record application that gives a patient's healthcare provider access to key health data. Those data may be originally stored in physician or hospital databases but can also be part of an online or mobile personal health dossier. If local regulations allow, patients (or their representatives) may grant pharmaceutical care providers access to certain medical data. With the upcoming European Health Data Space [21], the empowerment of citizens and patients will get a boost, whereas they gain the right to own and have full access and authority over their own (medical) data [22]. Conversely, physicians should have access to pharmaceutical care data, for instance, on adherence, adverse events, or other drug-related facts such as those acquired from digital health devices that a patient is using (you can find more on the topic of Personal Health Applications in Part 2 of this book).

Patients' level of trust in sharing their health data with pharmaceutical care providers will grow as the providers continue to adapt positively to the changing nature of healthcare delivery. These changes include, for example, setting up more coordinated care with other healthcare providers, analyzing and using shared health data, and ensuring an understanding of the data with the aim of driving better health outcomes.

Not just a shop or department

Although there is great variability among regions and countries, sometimes hospital pharmacies are criticized as being invisible in direct patient care. Community pharmacies are often seen as just a shop, with drugs dispensed at the back of the facility and employees focusing on earning money by selling over-the-counter medications. In those settings, it seems difficult for many people to position the pharmacist as the healthcare professional, with a five- to six-year postgraduate education who can drive the highest patient value and outcome.

Also, in the digital epoch, we are approaching, new logistic entrants are claiming to be better capable of the pure drug "distribution and shopping" concept than traditional pharmacy models. Cost Plus [23] of multientrepreneur Mark Cuban is a recent example [24] trying to disrupt the market of generics.

As much as this may be true in some situations, such as the delivery of over-the-counter medications or the relatively straightforward care for hay fever or contraception use, the professional human competency to deliver adequate and good care should not be overlooked. In addition, a physical presence in the community or hospital offers professionals the ability to meet patients at a low-threshold level of healthcare and to use technology to turn pharmacies into little mini-clinics that can consult on all kinds of health and wellness concerns [25].

Additionally, in the digital epoch where blended care approaches will thrive, certain pharmaceutical interventions will require a trusted face-to-face interaction or a direct drug delivery within minutes to hours. Examples from daily practice that continue to require human support include accompanying patients with complex polypharmacy interaction profiles; dealing with difficult innovative drug administration schemes in hospitals (e.g., in oncological situations); consulting with patients on ethical questions, for instance, euthanasia; or urgent recall situations with polluted drugs like the valsartan recall in 2018 [26].

In some of the patient surveys done in past years, overall outcomes have revealed that those patients living longer with multiple morbidities prefer to see pharmaceutical care providers especially visible, actively promoting tools around health promotion and screening, supporting efficient medication management of long-term conditions, enabling easy and accessible drug monitoring, educating the public about timely and innovative (digital) tools that are easy to integrate into patients' daily lives.

However, more extensive client satisfaction surveys are required to gain a deeper understanding about patients, and can be optimally nurtured in the future pharmaceutical.

In Chapter 6, we discuss how pharmaceutical care providers view their role and responsibilities in this endeavor.

 This means for blended pharmaceutical care:

- A growing number of patients play a responsible role in their own health, which is a strong prerequisite for making value-driven healthcare systems work.
- Many forces drive increasing engagement of patients in healthcare system optimization, with some of the important drivers being consumerism, information supply, value-driven healthcare, and regulatory patient interests.
- A number of factors determine the experience of "good care" delivery, in which a dedicated description of the impact of digital health data sharing.
- Actively depicting both institutional responsibilities and patient responsibilities in a healthcare environment can help to ensure that the patient's voice is really heard.
- Patients' preferences about the format (digital) of future pharmaceutical care need to be further researched.
- Real-world and real-time data become a nonneglectable source to be included in decision-making and research.

References

[1] Richards T. Is your conference "patients included?". BMJ 2015. Available from, https://blogs.bmj.com/bmj/2015/04/17/tessa-richards-is-your-conference-patients-included/.

[2] BMJ. Patient and public partnership. 2023 [cited 2023 29/01/2023]; Available from, https://authors.bmj.com/policies/patient-public-partnership/.

[3] Yeoman G, et al. Defining patient centricity with patients for patients and caregivers: a collaborative endeavour. BMJ innovations 2017;3(2).

[4] Atluri V, et al. How tech-enabled consumers are reordering the healthcare landscape. McKinsey & Company; 2016.

[5] Sittig DF, Singh H. A new sociotechnical model for studying health information technology in complex adaptive healthcare systems. Qual Saf Heal Care 2010;19(Suppl. 3):i68−74. https://doi.org/10.1136/qshc.2010.042085.

[6] COUCH Medical Communications. Study finds almost half of patients skip medication. 2018 [cited 2023 26/01/2023]; Available from, https://www.prnewswire.com/news-releases/study-finds-almost-half-of-patients-skip-medication-300647249.html.

[7] Engelen L. Patients included. 2023 [cited 2023 26/01/2023]; Available from, https://patientsincluded.org/.

[8] Christensen CM, Grossman JH, Hwang J. The innovator's prescription: a disruptive solution for health care. McGraw Hill; 2010.

[9] Ginsburg GS, Phillips KA. Precision medicine: from science to value. Health Aff 2018;37(5):694−701. https://doi.org/10.1377/hlthaff.2017.1624.

[10] European Medicines Agency. Engagement Framework: EMA and patients, consumers and their organisations. 2022. Amsterdam. Available from, https://www.ema.europa.eu/en/documents/other/engagement-framework-european-medicines-agency-patients-consumers-their-organisations_en.pdf.

[11] IPH. Institute for positive health. 2023 [cited 2023 25/01/2023]; Available from, https://www.iph.nl/en/.

[12] Huber M, et al. How should we define health? BMJ 2011;343(jul26 2). https://doi.org/10.1136/bmj.d4163. d4163-d416.

[13] Delogne MC. New PatientsLikeMe studies reveal how patients Experience and define "good" health care. 2018. Available from, https://www.businesswire.com/news/home/20180328005084/en/New-PatientsLikeMe-Studies-Reveal-How-Patients-Experience-and-Define-%E2%80%9CGood%E2%80%9D-Health-Care.

[14] UCLA Health. Patient rights and responsibilities. 2023 [cited 2023 27/01/2023]; Available from, https://www.uclahealth.org/patients-families/support-information/patient-experience/patient-rights-and-responsibilities.

[15] Taylor K, Ronte H, Haughey J. Pharma and the connected patient−how digital technology is enabling patient centricity. 2017. Available at, www2.deloitte.com/uk/en/pages/life-sciencesand-healthcare/articles/pharma-and-the-connected-patient.html. [Accessed 11 November 2018].

[16] Wicklund E. Using the survey as a patient engagement tool. 2015 [cited 2023 27/01/2023]; Available from, http://mobihealthnews.com/news/using-survey-patient-engagement-tool.

[17] Accenture. 2018 consumer survey on digital health - US results. 2018. Available from, https://www.accenture.com/t20180306T103559Z__w__/us-en/_acnmedia/PDF-71/accenture-health-2018-consumer-survey-digital-health.pdf.

[18] Safavi K, Kalis B. How can leaders make recent digital health gains last. Re-examining the Accenture; 2020. Available from, https://www.accenture.com/content/dam/accenture/final/a-com-migration/pdf/pdf-130/accenture-2020-digital-health-consumer-survey-us.pdf.

[19] ORCHA. Orcha. 2023 [cited 2023 29/01/2023]; Available from, https://orchahealth.com/.

[20] Norman J. Americans rate healthcare providers high on honesty, ethics. Washington, DC: Gallup; 2016.

[21] European Commission. European health data space. 2023 [cited 2023 27/01/2023]; Available from, https://health.ec.europa.eu/ehealth-digital-health-and-care/european-health-data-space_en.

[22] European Commission. European health data space - factsheet. 2023 [cited 2023 27/01/2023]; Available from, https://ec.europa.eu/commission/presscorner/api/files/attachment/872447/Factsheet%20-%20EHDS. pdf.pdf.

[23] Mark Cuban Cost Plus Drug Company. Mark cuban cost plus drug company. 2023. Available from, https://costplusdrugs.com/.

[24] Cohen J. Mark cuban's cost plus drug company continues to revolutionize generic drug pricing, in Forbes. Forbes 2023. Available from, https://www.forbes.com/sites/joshuacohen/2023/01/01/mark-cubans-cost-plus-drug-company-continues-to-revolutionize-generic-drug-pricing/?sh=6054f98b7919.

[25] Engelen L. Augmented health(care). 1st ed. UK: Lightning Source; 2018.

[26] European Medicines Agency. EMA reviewing medicines containing valsartan from Zhejiang Huahai following detection of an impurity. 2018. Available from, https://www.ema.europa.eu/en/documents/press-release/ema-reviewing-medicines-containing-valsartan-zhejiang-huahai-following-detection-impurity_en. pdf.

CHAPTER 6

The pharmaceutical care buffet*

Carl R. Schneider

School of Pharmacy, Faculty of Medicine and Health, The University of Sydney, Australia

Variety's the very spice of life, that gives it all its flavour.

William Cowper

When you visit a buffet, you are exposed to several dishes simultaneously. From these dishes, we will find some dishes we have not had before. Trying some of these new dishes can expose you to new directions. As one experiences life, one should be open to new and enriching experiences. The digital revolution has afforded us the opportunity to integrate technology to a greater or less extent across the vast span of human endeavor. From technology-aided physical tasks, we now have the capability to use technology to enhance cognitive activities. We are even exploring the use of technology to improve one's affective condition.

Similarly, pharmaceutical care can be a rich and gratifying experience, as it can help improve an individual's health and quality of life. To benefit from the options in our metaphorical buffet of drug treatments, we must place importance on the judicious application of digital pharmaceutical care (DPC), in order to provide a wholesome repast.

Pharmaceutical care (PC) is a philosophy of practice in which the person is the primary beneficiary of the pharmacist's actions.

Pharmaceutical care

Pharmaceutical care may be defined as "Any professional activity by which the pharmacist is linked to the person (and/or caregiver) and other healthcare professionals, to attend to the individual according to their needs, setting out strategies to align and achieve the short- and medium-/long-term objectives of pharmacotherapy and incorporating new technologies and the means available to continuously interact with

---

*In this chapter, you will read about the principles of pharmaceutical care and medication management, the concepts and causes of inadequate drug use and nonadherence, and the personalized opportunities that digital pharmaceutical care provides to optimize the value of drugs.

Pharmaceutical Care in Digital Revolution. https://doi.org/10.1016/B978-0-443-13360-2.00019-8

people in order to improve their health outcomes" [1]. Pharmaceutical care has also been described as the pharmacist's contribution to the care of individuals in order to optimize medicines use and improve health outcomes [2,3]. Pharmaceutical care aims to optimize an individual's health-related quality of life and achieve positive clinical outcomes, within realistic economic costs [4].

The practice was developed to meet the standards of and be consistent with the professional practices of medicine, nursing, dentistry, and veterinary medicine. As a professional practice, pharmaceutical care is guided by a philosophy, a purpose, and values in its resolution of specific problems. This mandates a strong commitment to using the profession's knowledge for the good and well-being of others, which implies a clear ethical component (turn to Chapter 18 for more on this topic).

Pharmaceutical care providers (PCPs) are professionals, as they become competent in their role through solid academic training; they maintain their skills through continuing professional development and commit to behaving ethically to protect the interests of the individual in the context of societal needs.

Pharmaceutical care focuses on the functions, knowledge, responsibilities, and skills as well as the attitudes, behaviors, commitments, concerns, and ethics that a pharmacist is required to fulfill, as previously defined. Above all, the provision of person-centered drug therapy has the goal of driving optimal outcomes toward individuals' health and quality of life.

To understand what drives the individual, it is necessary to understand what people value most (refer also to Chapter 5). Clinical intervention is more than the competent application of pharmaceutical knowledge to the resolution of health problems. It is also the value-laden context in which the provider deals with the process of decision-making, judgment, and justification of choices made [5].

The pharmaceutical care process can take place in a hospital setting (hospital pharmacists), in the transition from hospital to home care (e.g., elderly wards), in an outpatient clinic, a pharmacy or primary care clinic, and homecare setting.

The clinical care process parallels the practice management activities conducted by pharmacists and ensures personnel support, document management, a supply chain, good distribution and manufacturing practices, and so on (Fig. 6.1).

Although not all have equal accountability for clinical programs, pharmacists with a pharmaceutical care focus can be found in clinics and hospitals, in community pharmacies, in the pharmaceutical industry, and in wholesale pharmaceutical companies. They may also work in policy-making organizations, health insurance companies, research

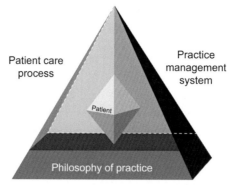

Figure 6.1
Components of person-centered pharmacy practice [5].

laboratories, and governmental agencies, and may be involved in academic and postacademic education and research.

Digital pharmaceutical care

An individual's medication experience can be described as the sum of all the events the person has in his/her/their lifetime that involve drug therapy. These combined experiences reveal how the individual values his/her/their health, how the person makes personal decisions about medications, and the person's beliefs and habits around adhering to proposed healthcare interventions.

Increasingly, components of those experiences are built by and recorded in digital ecosystems. The technologies discussed in Part 2 of this book, combined with data on social media and on geographic, demographic, and cultural environments, and so on, form an individual's medication footprint, which PCPs need to understand. To gather all the insight required to personalize care pathways, the healthcare provider must be part of that digital ecosystem.

Historically, pharmaceutical care was provided predominantly in a face-to-face manner; however, over time, it has gradually shifted toward a format that includes digital environments, which we discuss in detail in Part 2 of this book. Based on the situation, pharmaceutical care can (and will) be given remotely; it should also consider multiple sources of digital health data and be augmented by analytics more so than in the past.

Therefore, DPC can be defined as *the provision of digitally enhanced, responsible pharmaceutical care for the purpose of achieving outcomes that have a positive effect on a person's quality of life.*

In many cases, it is up to the professional whether pharmaceutical care can be provided fully digital or whether (additional) human interaction is required. A blended care approach may be feasible for most people: *digital if possible and human where required* for individual well-being.

Whereas the individual largely leads the professional through a process of shared decision-making, considerations like the complexity of dosage regimens, initial versus refill medication, and prior adherence experience may be taken into consideration when considering whether to provide care digitally or in person. Pharmaceutical care professionals have a responsibility to support adequate understanding about the use of medications (medication literacy) [6] and digital technology (digital literacy) [7], as we further elaborate on in the course of this book.

Independent of the mode in which it is provided, pharmaceutical care should consist of a number of activities to ensure a structured and solid approach, as discussed in the following section.

Five essential domains of pharmaceutical care: The role of pharmacists

The American Pharmacists Association defined five domains for PCPs, mainly pharmacists, which determine adequate pharmaceutical care [4]. These are presented below, adapted to use person-centered language:

 A. Establish and maintain professional relationship with individuals

 B. Maintain adequate collection and recording of health data

 C. Review health data and provide adequate PC proposal

 D. Ensure person alignment and facilitate execution of PC plan

 E. Ensure circular management of PC plan

Although the outcome of either digital or human provision of pharmaceutical care should be focused on achieving optimal person-centered outcomes, digitization of healthcare interventions will have an impact on the execution of those domains. In Chapters 9—15, we take these five domains through an iterative process to explain how each type of technology is expected to change the nature of these domains.

First, let us take a deep dive into the basic expectations of each of these five domains, where we focus primarily on the role of the pharmacist as the PCP while realizing that a number of other stakeholders support this process as well (e.g., pharmacy technicians and physicians) [4].

A *A professional relationship must be established and maintained*

Interaction between the pharmacist and the individual must occur to ensure that a relationship based upon caring, trust, open communication, cooperation, and mutual decision-making is established and maintained. In this relationship, as in the Hippocratic Oath, the pharmacist holds the individual's welfare as paramount, maintains an appropriate attitude of caring for the welfare of the individual, and uses all of their professional knowledge and skills on the person's behalf. As part of the relationship (as we note in Chapter 5), the person provides their consent to supply personal information and preferences and participates in the therapeutic planning process via shared decision-making. In addition, the pharmacist develops mechanisms to ensure that the individual has access to pharmaceutical care at all times.

B *Person-specific medical information must be collected, organized, recorded, and maintained*

Subjective and objective information should be collected regarding the individual's general health and activity status, past medical history, medication history, social history, diet and exercise history, history of present illness, and economic situation (financial and insured status). In general, this is done by the physician and the pharmacist, and ideally, a connective data set is shared across healthcare professionals.

Sources of information in addition to the person's perspective may include, but are not limited to, quantified self data, medical charts and reports, pharmacist-conducted health/physical assessment, the person's family or caregiver, the insurer, and other healthcare providers, including physicians, nurses, allied healthcare practitioners, and other pharmacists.

Since it will form the basis for decisions regarding the development and subsequent modification of the pharmaceutical care plan, the information must be timely, accurate, and complete, and it must be organized and recorded to ensure that it is easily retrievable and is updated as necessary and appropriate.

In addition to the preceding data sources, it is imperative to consider data regarding an individual's beliefs, concerns, and expectations (BCEs) for medication use, as they carry great weight in determining how people regard their medication intervention. Also, discussing and recording what matters most to people in other domains that determine a "good life" should be taken into account in order to develop a plan that is as personalized as possible. Two concepts that propagate the idea that a holistic approach to individual values is needed to improve health are the Positive Health approach and the Whole-Person approach. They are relatively new concepts within healthcare that consider six domains of what determines good life: physical functioning, mental well-being, meaningfulness, quality of life, participation, and daily functioning [8].

These approaches focus on supporting people in defining how to live a truly meaningful life, more than on recovering from a disease (which is not always possible). Taking data from an Institute of Positive Health measurement tool into account will enable PCPs to make a more holistic treatment plan with a higher likelihood of acceptance and adherence by the individual.

Clinical information must be collected and maintained in a confidential and privacy-compliant manner (one can find more information on this topic in Chapters 17 and 18).

C *Person-specific medical information must be evaluated, and a pharmaceutical care plan developed mutually with the individual*

Based on a thorough understanding of a person's beliefs and his/her/their condition or disease and its treatment, the pharmacist must, with the individual and with relevant other healthcare providers as necessary, develop a value-driven, outcomes-oriented pharmaceutical care plan.

The plan may have various components that address each of a person's diseases or conditions. In designing the plan, the pharmacist must carefully consider the psychosocial aspects of the disease as well as the potential relationship between the cost and complexity of therapy and medication adherence.

As an advocate, the pharmacist assures the coordination of pharmaceutical care with other healthcare providers and the individual. In addition, the pharmacist strives to address medication literacy by providing explanations at the level of the person's understanding of the various pros and cons of the options relative to drug therapy and instances where one option may be preferred, based on the pharmacist's professional judgment.

The pharmaceutical care plan must be documented in the individual's pharmacy record and communicated to the person's other healthcare providers as necessary.

D *The pharmacist assures that the person has all supplies, information, and knowledge necessary to carry out the pharmaceutical care plan*

The PCP must assume ultimate responsibility for assuring that the individual has been able to obtain, and is appropriately using, any drugs and related products or equipment called for in the pharmaceutical care plan.

The pharmacist also assures that the person understands the disease thoroughly and the therapy and medications prescribed in the plan.

 E   *The pharmacist reviews, monitors, and modifies the pharmaceutical care plan as necessary, in alignment with the physician and in close collaboration with the individual and healthcare team*

The PCP takes a circular approach toward the service provided, which means feeding information on response, tolerability, and beliefs via a medication monitoring process into a continuation or adaptation of the care plan, with a focus on achieving the best person-centered outcomes possible.

From hospital or community to home pharmaceutical care

Provided infrastructure and technology allows, an increasing number of people across countries are being treated with complex therapies in intermediate care facilities or in their own homes. For example, the Mercy Virtual Hospital is transforming healthcare by creating new care models fully supported by telehealth teams and technology. As a result, people no longer have to physically seek out care or entirely reorient their lives to gain access to specialists. Instead, virtual technology brings care to them [9]. This healthcare modality accelerated in use as a result of the COVID-19 pandemic [10].

There are several reasons for the shift toward homecare:

- Most people prefer to stay at home, if possible.
- The number of older adults in the population is overtaking the capacity of hospital beds.
- Hospital treatment timelines have reduced significantly in past years (e.g., about a hip replacement, which used to be a seven-to-ten day hospitalization and is almost an outpatient intervention).
- There are lower cost projections when treating people at home.

Consequently, PC provision is expected to increasingly extend beyond the traditional pharmacy establishments, which emphasizes the need for different types of pharmacists and other care providers to collaborate and exchange data in an integrated care environment to ensure the continuity of PC, optimize strategies, and reduce where possible harm from medication [11].

Integrated care

With a person's well-being at the center of decision-making, it is vital to have one environment where all data are accessible to relevant care providers. Ideally, this is an environment managed by the individual, where they authorize care providers to see, use, and review data as needed. This environment is referred to differently in various countries, for example, Personally Controlled Electronic Health Record, My Health Record, or a Personal Health Application (PHA), which we use in the remainder of this book. The PHA should always be accessible via a centralized cloud or a decentralized technology, as discussed in Chapter 8.

In general, information on the person is currently stored in an electronic health record.

In many countries, there is a major challenge to connect siloed healthcare applications with this electronic health dossier [12], as shown in Fig. 6.2.

Technology may be a strong driver toward this connectivity, but it is currently lagging, as many different healthcare applications exist but many of the systems are not (yet) compatible.

The Internet of Things will enable interoperability, machine-to-machine communication, information exchange, and data movement, making healthcare service delivery effective. A promising approach to secure interoperability is the use of blockchain technology [13]. One can find more information on establishing integrated data systems with standardization of interoperability in Chapter 8.

An important responsibility of PHA system owners is to establish a systematic approach to optimizing digital literacy, as medical and pharmaceutical transparency that is not understood may inadvertently create stress for people and their caregivers. When individuals have access to health data and cannot understand their relevance, questions

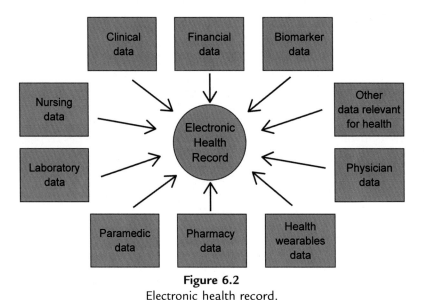

Figure 6.2
Electronic health record.

may arise, and an explanation should be given. Providing this transparency can be handled by making literacy a crucial part of the design phase (e.g., add explanatory text fields to the PHA) and offering a virtual personal assistant that explains to the person how to interpret data in the PHA, before concerns are raised, which would create more work for providers and more discomfort for the individual.

 Maintaining the balance between having as much transparency as possible while avoiding unnecessary worries and questions makes achieving PHA literacy a complex matter.

Preventing inadequate drug use

The objective of reducing avoidable harm due to medication and inadequate drug use has received global attention in recent years.

Avoidable harm due to medication

In March 2017, the World Health Organization (WHO) launched the third global safety challenge on the topic of 'Medication without Harm,' with the intention to reduce severe, avoidable medication-associated harm in all countries by 50% over the following 5 years [11].

Medication errors injure approximately 1.3 million people annually in the United States alone. Although low- and middle-income countries are estimated to have rates of medication-related adverse events similar to those in high-income countries, the impact is about twice as high in terms of the number of years of healthy life lost. Unfortunately, many countries lack good data, which are being gathered as part of the WHO initiative.

Globally, the costs associated with medication errors (not including indirect costs related to nonadherence) have been estimated at $42 billion annually or about 0.5% of total global health expenditure [11].

Inadequate drug use

In principle, inadequate drug use can be placed into four main categories [14]. Table 6.1 depicts a number of situations that lead to inadequate drug use.

Depending on a specific problem in the adequacy of drug use of an individual, digital health technology may offer solutions to limit the occurrence of situations described in Table 6.1. Those technologies are described in Part 2 of this book, and referrals will be made to the topics in the preceding table to address potential benefits to reduce avoidable harm.

Table 6.1: Categorization of inadequate drug use.

Indication	Effectiveness	Safety	Adherence
Drug therapy unnecessary: - No medical indication - Duplicated therapy - Nondrug therapy indicated - Treating avoidable ADR - Dose set too high in clinical trials - Unnecessary dose escalation or combinations	**Requires different drug product:** - More effective drug available - Condition refractory to drug - Dosage form inappropriate - Not effective for condition - Dosage too low	**Adverse drug reaction:** - Undesirable effect - Unsafe drug for individual - Dose changed too quickly - Allergic reaction - Contraindications present	**Drug not taken according to directions:** - Directions not understood - Individual prefers not to take - Person forgets to take - Drug product too expensive - Cannot swallow/ administer - Drug product not available - More reasons reflected below in text
Additional drug therapy required, but not provided: - Untreated condition - Preventative/ prophylactic - Synergistic/ potentiating	**Wrong dose:** - Frequency inappropriate - Duration inappropriate - Drug interaction - Dose set too high in clinical trials		

Adapted from Vrijens B, Heidbuchel H. Non-vitamin K antagonist oral anticoagulants: considerations on once- vs. twice-daily regimens and their potential impact on medication adherence. Europace 2015;17(4):514–23.

Adherence, its relevance and taxonomy

 Medication adherence is the process by which people take their medication in accordance with the mutually agreed upon care plan.

As the healthcare community adopts the concepts of person-centeredness and empowerment, it is moving away from the previously more frequently used term *compliance,* which affords a lack of agency in following the prescriber's recommendations.

Another term often heard in adherence is persistence, which refers to the length of time from initiation to discontinuation of therapy compared to the initial treatment goals.

Medication nonadherence is an important public health consideration, strongly affecting health outcomes and overall healthcare costs. It is widespread and varies by disease, person characteristics, and insurance coverage, with nonadherence rates ranging from 25% to 50% [15].

Chronic conditions such as diabetes, hypertension, and asthma can be effectively managed with low-cost medications. Unfortunately, around 50% of people taking pills for these conditions fall out of adherence [16]. And of that 50%, half will stop taking their pills within the first year.

Classification system for nonadherence using the theoretical domains framework

Successful interventions in medication adherence ideally target current modifiable determinants and are tailored to the unmodifiable determinants.

Potential interventions and individual determinants from published literature on medication adherence can be categorized in 11 domains according to the Theoretical Domains Framework [17]:

Knowledge	**Skills**	**Social/professional role and identity**
Beliefs about capabilities	Beliefs about consequences	Intentions
Memory, attention, and decision processes	Environmental context and resources	Social influences
Emotion	Behavioral regulation	

Those categories are useful to consider as both modifiable and unmodifiable determinants need to be assessed at the inclusion of intervention studies to identify people most in need of an adherence intervention [18].

Medication nonadherence places a significant financial burden on healthcare systems. Although some literature suggests that healthcare costs attributed to nonadherence are as much as $300 billion each year in the United States and about $125 billion each year in Europe (no global data are available), current research assessing the economic impact of medication nonadherence is limited and of varying quality, failing to provide transferable data sufficient to influence health policies. In addition, differences in methods make comparison among studies challenging, and an accurate estimation of the true magnitude of the cost is still impossible [19] (QR Code 6.1).

QR Code 6.1
An explanation of adherence.

Multiple studies and metaanalyses show that more than 700 different factors are associated with adherence, as reflected in Table 6.1 [20]. However, the predominant cause of nonadherence is socioeconomic rather than medication or disease-related factors [21].

Measuring adherence

A key process in managing adherence consists of monitoring and supporting an individual's adherence to proposed treatments and interventions.

Pharmaceutical care stakeholders have a key responsibility to drive adherence in a positive direction, as this is one of the primary elements of the joint pharmaceutical care plan.

Adherence patterns can be measured indirectly or directly. Table 6.2 gives an overview of the systematic calculation of adherence rates.

As reflected in Table 6.2, a frequently used indirect metric can be derived from prescription refill data, which most pharmacies now collect in automated systems called electronic pharmacy records. The refill rate divides the number of days pharmacy medication was picked up within a certain time period by the number of medications prescribed by the physician.

Table 6.2: Methods to measure adherence.

Methods	Data source	Definition
Indirect measurements used in research and administrative settings		
MPR[a]	Pharmacy claims = (total days supplied)/(number of days between the first and last refills)	
PDC[a]	Pharmacy claims = (total days supplied)/(number of days in refill interval)	
Indirect measurements used in clinical care settings		
Self-report	Person	Person recalls medications taken in response to care team query
Questionnaire	Provider	Use of validated tool for adherence markers
Pill counting	Provider	Staff member reviews medication supply for doses remaining
Dose counting device	Device	Device includes electronic or manual counter that tracks doses released
Electronic-prescribing	PBM interface	Reports transmitted from a pharmacy benefit manager to provider usually via EMR link
Direct measurement		
Direct observation	Provider	Individual receives and takes medication at health care facility
Drug levels and markers	Laboratory	Blood or urine sample tested

EMR, electronic medical records; MPR, medication possession ratio; PBM, pharmacy benefit manager; PDC, proportion of days covered.
[a]Generally not used in direct clinical care.
From McGuire M, Iuga A. Adherence and health care costs. In: Risk management and healthcare policy. 2014. p. 35.
Adapted from Anghel LA, Farcas AM, Oprean RN. An overview of the common methods used to measure treatment adherence. Med Pharm Rep 2019;92(2):117–22.

Other indirect adherence metrics, reflected in Table 6.2, that have been used for decades in pharmaceutical care research are the medication possession ratio (MPR) and the proportion of days covered, both referring to measuring continuous medication availability (CMA). A more recent way to measure CMA is found in the AdhereR example box.

AdhereR

AdhereR is an add-on package for the widely used free statistical software R developed for the estimation of adherence based on electronic healthcare data [22].

AdhereR implements a set of functions consistent with current adherence guidelines, definitions, and operationalizations. It is open source, runs on any platform on which R runs (including MS Windows, macOS, and various others), and its source code is openly available in a public GitHub repository.

Researchers and clinicians can use AdhereR to visualize medication histories and calculate medication availability and persistence in a flexible, transparent, and reproducible way. In addition, users can choose among different options depending on their needs, perform sensitivity analyses with alternative options, and share their analysis code.

Being written in R and hosted on GitHub, AdhereR allows independent development and testing of new functionalities by different teams, which will be incorporated regularly in new AdhereR releases.

An MPR of 80% is often used as the cutoff between adherence and nonadherence based on its ability to predict hospitalizations across selected high-prevalence chronic diseases; however, although it is frequently used, this percentage is not based on sound arguments.

Technology to support adherence

In past decades, many (digital) applications have been developed that help people remember to be more adherent and to adapt their lifestyle toward adequate use of drugs.

 For example, improving adherence can be achieved through:

- better understanding of a person's BCEs;
- better education;
- value-based insurance plans;
- use of individual incentives;
- adoption of medication adherence systems, including hardware-based medication adherence systems (e.g., smart pill bottles, smart caps, automated pill dispensers,

electronic trays, smart cabinets, smart medical watches, smart medical alarms, wearable health sensors, packaging systems, and robotics); and

- software applications (e.g., mobile apps, sensor-enabled software solutions, mobile medication management applications, patient portals, health programs, web portals, voice-user-interfaces, and others) [23].

To choose the technology that fits the needs of an individual, it is crucial to identify which measures are best suited based on their advantages and disadvantages, as shown in Table 6.3.

Once a method is selected, it is important to realize that a tool can create a certain bias, and this should be considered when analyzing the data. For instance, home sampling may be forgotten, individuals may be "white-coat" adherent or self-reporting may have a desirability and recall bias.

Some tools, such as SMS reminders and behavioral apps, have moved the needle to the positive side in certain settings [24,25], whereas others could not yet make a

Table 6.3: Overview of assessment methods of adherence.

	Examples	Advantages	Disadvantages
Direct measurement tools	Institutional sampling/ home sampling by digital devices	Accurate Objective, proving the ingestion of the drug	Costly Invasive Interindividual differences
Self-reporting	Survey/digital tools/ phone calls	Easy to use Inexpensive	Overestimate adherence Subjective, influenced by recall or reporting bias
Pill counts	Dispensing tools/digital counting	Simple Mostly used in clinical trials	No evidence of ingested medication
Prescription and refill databases	Link physicians with pharmacy database/ combined database analysis	Easy to use Inexpensive Noninvasive, people not aware that they are being monitored Especially specific to identify nonadherent individuals	Evidence of the drug being dispensed but not ingested
Electronic monitoring	Hardware and software solutions including initial support	Objective Additional information on the degree of adherence One of the most accurate methods	The person is aware of the evaluation No actual evidence that the medication is being ingested

significant difference [26]. A metaanalysis of mobile apps to support adherence suggests that there is an overall positive effect as an intervention to improve adherence [27].

Individualized goal setting

It is clear that the adherence landscape is full of choices when it comes to finding a vehicle that best meets an individual's expectations and delivers the lowest level of bias.

Please also refer to Chapters 3 and 4, where the importance of considering holistic individual life preferences regarding "what matters most" from a physical, mental, and societal perspective are described. Common sense tells us that individuals will engage most readily in adherence goals directed toward BCEs that are important to them. The consensus among experts in the adherence community is that successful interventions need to target individual reasons for nonadherence and require tailoring to individual characteristics. Thus only personalized, multifaceted interventions show positive effects at a population level.

Therefore, PCPs ideally understand, for example, how an individual rates being healthy, maintaining a social life, fulfilling all work environment obligations, and high-risk sports.

Through ongoing dialogue between the individual and the PCP, negotiations of shared goals that are not only realistic but also well aligned to the individual's priorities for drug adherence will lead to increased satisfaction with the overall outcome of the intervention.

Goal attainment scaling (GAS) is a technique that can be used, for example, as a supportive mathematical technique for quantifying the achievement of goals set. GAS outlines the process of setting goals appropriately so that the achievement of each goal can be measured on a 5-point scale ranging from -2 to $+2$ and then explains a method for quantifying the outcome in a single aggregated goal attainment score [28].

The GAS process can further facilitate pharmaceutical care by helping identify a person's priorities and providing a systematic method for measuring and achieving outcomes that are important to the individual.

As we move into the era of the longitudinal quantified self and an integrated PHA, it will become easier to understand and track individual health benefits obtained from adequate pharmaceutical care adherence interventions and then recalculate them in terms of cost benefits.

This transparency is crucial as it will reinforce the value of pharmaceutical care support and deliver a rationale for appropriately reimbursing adherence tools.

Return of investment of an adherence program

The majority of direct costs attributed to medication nonadherence result from avoidable hospitalization. Due to the progression of controllable diseases, additional direct costs are incurred through (1) increased use of services at physician offices, emergency rooms, and urgent care and treatment facilities such as nursing homes, hospice facilities, and dialysis centers, (2) avoidable pharmacy costs related to intensified therapy as comorbid conditions develop, and (3) diagnostic testing that could be avoided by controlling the primary illness [15].

Indirect costs include factors such as loss of the caregiver's productivity and loss of a person's autonomy.

Strategies to enhance drug adherence need to consider the impact on overall healthcare costs, weighing potentially increased drug expenditures against savings from improved outcomes and a better quality of life.

 Quantifying the benefits of investing in adequate drug use programs is rather complex, mainly for the following reasons:

- **Lack of standard approach:** this lack is due, for example, to different ways of reporting costs within and between countries.
- **Bias effect or "healthy-user" effect:** the type of people who voluntarily enroll in adherence studies may not be representative of the general population.
- **Time preference trade-off:** stakeholders may not be willing to trade short-term increases in medication costs and complementary goods or services for long-term savings or health gains.
- **Time to attain a return on investment (ROI) differs across stakeholders:** this is definitely an issue for pharmacists, who are often paid on a population-based level and will see benefits of adherence interventions only after a certain amount of time (less hospitalization, less deterioration). Individuals may even receive a later ROI (depending on the progression rate of a condition), as well as the payers, who may see lower healthcare costs only after a significant amount of time due to better treatment of people. This variability of return and the relative short-term focus of many systems may discourage healthcare system partners from making investments [29].

In conclusion, the pharmaceutical care buffet is one of many picturesque vistas, but the scenes from past decades will not be the same as the ones in the coming years. Part 2 describes the technologies that will restructure this scenery.

This means for blended pharmaceutical care:

- PCPs are value-driven healthcare team members and gatekeepers for reducing avoidable harm due to medication and optimizing medication outcomes.
- DPC can be defined as the responsible digital provision of pharmaceutical care to achieve definite outcomes that improve a person's quality of life.
- Optimal pharmaceutical care is facilitated once an individual's values, preferences and beliefs, as well as all clinical data, are collected in a PHA, a digital environment that puts all health-related data in one dossier that is owned and managed by the individual or a representative.
- PHAs should entail a system to facilitate literacy for individuals, as not understandable medical and pharmaceutical transparency may cause avoidable stress for individuals and caregivers.
- Depending on the specificity of individual adherence challenges, digital health technology may offer personalized solutions to optimize medication management.
- The choice of a particular digital health technology support tool for pharmaceutical care should depend on individual BCEs of the individual.
- In DPC, professionals have a responsibility to support the adequate use of medication as well as the use of digital technology.
- Strategies to enhance drug adherence should consider the impact on overall healthcare costs, weighing potentially increased drug expenditures against savings from improved outcomes and better quality of life.

References

[1] Morillo-Verdugo R, et al. A new definition and refocus of pharmaceutical care: the Barbate Document. Farm Hosp 2020;44(4):158−62.

[2] Allemann SS, et al. Pharmaceutical care: the PCNE definition 2013. Int J Clin Pharm 2014;36(3):544−55.

[3] Pharmaceutical Care Network Europe. Position paper on the definition of pharmaceutical care 2013. 2013.

[4] American Pharmacists Association. Principles of practice for pharmaceutical care. APhA: American Pharmacists Association; 2021.

[5] Cipolle RJ, Strand LM, Morley PC. Pharmaceutical care practice: the patient-centered approach to medication management. McGraw Hill Professional; 2012.

[6] Neiva Pantuzza LL, et al. Medication literacy: a conceptual model. Res Social Adm Pharm 2022;18(4):2675−82.

[7] Marinkovic V, et al. Person-centred care interventions in pharmaceutical care. In: Intelligent systems for sustainable person-centered healthcare. Cham: Springer International Publishing; 2022. p. 53−68.

[8] IPH. Institute for positive health. 2023. Available from: https://www.iph.nl/en/. [Accessed 25 January 2023].

[9] Mercy-Virtual. Mercy virtual hospital—about. 2018. Available from: http://www.mercyvirtual.net/about/. [Accessed 28 January 2023].

[10] Sitammagari K, et al. Insights from rapid deployment of a "virtual hospital" as standard care during the COVID-19 pandemic. Ann Intern Med 2021;174(2):192—9.

[11] World Health Organization. Medication without harm. Geneva: World Health Organization; 2017.

[12] Shull JG. Digital health and the state of interoperable electronic health records. JMIR Med Inf 2019;7(4):e12712.

[13] Jabbar R, et al. Blockchain technology for healthcare: enhancing shared electronic health record interoperability and integrity. IEEE; 2020.

[14] Cipolle RJ, Strand L, Morley PC. Pharmaceutical care practice: the clinician's guide: the clinician's guide. McGraw-Hill Medical; 2004.

[15] McGuire M, Iuga A. Adherence and health care costs. In: Risk management and healthcare policy; 2014. p. 35.

[16] Heldenbrand S, et al. Assessment of medication adherence app features, functionality, and health literacy level and the creation of a searchable web-based adherence app resource for health care professionals and patients. J Am Pharm Assoc 2016;56(3):293—302.

[17] Lawton R, et al. Using the theoretical domains framework (TDF) to understand adherence to multiple evidence-based indicators in primary care: a qualitative study. Implement Sci 2015;11(1).

[18] Allemann SS, et al. Matching adherence interventions to patient determinants using the theoretical domains framework. Front Pharmacol 2016;7:429.

[19] Cutler RL, et al. Economic impact of medication non-adherence by disease groups: a systematic review. BMJ Open 2018;8(1):e016982.

[20] Kardas P, Lewek P, Matyjaszczyk M. Determinants of patient adherence: a review of systematic reviews. Front Pharmacol 2013;4:91.

[21] Gast A, Mathes T. Medication adherence influencing factors—an (updated) overview of systematic reviews. Syst Rev 2019;8(1).

[22] Dima AL, Dediu D. Computation of adherence to medication and visualization of medication histories in R with AdhereR: towards transparent and reproducible use of electronic healthcare data. PLoS One 2017;12(4):e0174426.

[23] BCC Publishing. Medication adherence: systems, technologies and global markets. BCC Research; 2021.

[24] Mack H. Study: texting to improve medication adherence shows high engagement. In: MobiHealthNews. HIMSS Media; 2017.

[25] Vrijens B, Urquhart J, White D. Electronically monitored dosing histories can be used to develop a medication-taking habit and manage patient adherence. Expert Rev Clin Pharmacol 2014;7(5):633—44.

[26] Choudhry NK, et al. Effect of reminder devices on medication adherence. JAMA Intern Med 2017;177(5):624.

[27] Armitage LC, Kassavou A, Sutton S. Do mobile device apps designed to support medication adherence demonstrate efficacy? A systematic review of randomised controlled trials, with meta-analysis. BMJ Open 2020;10(1):e032045.

[28] Turner-Stokes L. Goal attainment scaling (GAS) in rehabilitation: a practical guide. Clin Rehabil 2009;23(4):362—70.

[29] Cognizant. Medication adherence in the real world. 2016. Available from: https://www.slideshare.net/cognizant/medication-adherence-in-the-real-world-63632949. [Accessed 28 January 2023].

[30] Vrijens B, Heidbuchel H. Non-vitamin K antagonist oral anticoagulants: considerations on once- vs. twice-daily regimens and their potential impact on medication adherence. Europace 2015;17(4):514—23.

[31] Anghel LA, Farcas AM, Oprean RN. An overview of the common methods used to measure treatment adherence. Med Pharm Rep 2019;92(2):117—22.

PART 2

What: digital advances to innovate pharmaceutical care journeys

CHAPTER 7

The digital health technology menu*

Jaime Acosta-Gomez[1,2]

[1]Technology Advisory Group, FIP, Madrid, Spain; [2]Farmacia Acosta, Madrid, Spain

Technology is neither good nor bad; nor is it neutral.

Melvin Kranzberg

The organization of a kitchen is critical in how the food is prepared. The organization of a kitchen has two main components: staff and equipment. Staff positions can highly vary according to the type of restaurant: executive chef, station chef, expediter, sauce station chef, pastry chef, purchasing manager, dishwasher, and porter, among others. Equipment is the gear used to cook and eat, such as pots and pans, utensils, electricals, cutlery, tableware, and drinkware. As is the case in healthcare, the restaurant industry is a dynamic, ever-changing business, and how the kitchen is organized directly correlates to the experience a guest receives. We can apply this perspective metaphorically to healthcare systems, with the staff being doctors, nurses, and pharmacists and the equipment being, for example, money, healthcare machines, medicines, and digital technology. The organization and management of these factors determine the success of both ecosystems.

Let us start with a hypothetical example of patient Jeanny, reflecting how digital health is changing treatment paradigms.

Jeanny had not been feeling well for the past several weeks, and she could not fully grasp what was happening. Although she used to be in top physical shape, she had been sweating while sleeping for days, she had been feeling very tired for weeks, and she had lost some weight, even though she had stopped dieting some time ago. Her daily job had been rather stressful for a number of months, and she did not have sufficient time to relax and do sports-related activities, but could that explain the decline in health she was experiencing?

---

*In this chapter, you will read about the classification of digital health, considerations for adoption, economic benefits, and potential hurdles. We also consider the impact of persuasive techniques and serious gaming on the uptake of digital health technology.

Pharmaceutical Care in Digital Revolution. https://doi.org/10.1016/B978-0-443-13360-2.00006-X

Furthermore, her smart health trackers and home equipment reflected issues. Her daily step count had decreased, her blood pressure tracker showed abnormal measurements, her sleep-tracking mattress was emitting stress signals, the microchip in the toilet was detecting elevated lab markers in her urine, the smart scale measured ongoing weight loss, and her digital mirror reflected an unhealthy pale look with large, dark circles under her eyes. Then suddenly, she received a digital invitation to run a triage chatbot conversation and see her doctor face to face. Probably this invitation was raised based on ongoing health data that some years ago Jeanny had decided to share with her healthcare team.

She thought her malaise might result from her stressful job and many side activities. Yet, according to the data collected by the sensors, the symptoms could also point to an underlying malignant process, which she and her doctor might now be able to catch in its earliest stage and thus prevent a further deteriorating illness that could have a lifelong effect. On the other hand, her condition might be such that it could be easily treated in a homecare situation, allowing her to receive the care she needed from her comfortable hammock.

This example is no longer the stuff of science fiction. It is fast becoming a "science fact." It is, to a certain extent, already possible and is expected to become a full reality in the upcoming years.

Technology is shifting power away from traditional healthcare providers and placing it increasingly in the hands of consumers (patients), payers, and emerging digital entrants. Moreover, when individuals integrate smart technology into their living environment, they can monitor their disease and detect it in an earlier stage and intervene more effectively.

People like Jeanny are now better informed, more connected, and increasingly engaged in keeping fit and healthy as long as possible (as we also note in Chapter 5). They prefer to receive their care at home as long as possible and avoid visiting their doctor's office or going to hospitals and other healthcare facilities.

As of 2022, mobile phones are a 1000 times more capable than they were only 10 years ago, and they will become at least a 1000 times more powerful over the next 10 years. Together with the sensors in their homes and on and within their bodies, Jeanny and many others will feel reassured that potential health issues will be identified in a timely way and that they will get the best outcomes from care and experience a better quality of life, even when ill.

Millennials are currently known to be the largest group to seek out alternative modes of healthcare delivery [1], and like Jeanny, they are the earliest adopters of a broad range of digital health innovations.

Digital health

When technology meets medicine, it is generally referred to as telehealth, telemedicine, e-health, or digital health.

The World Health Organization (WHO) describes telemedicine as follows: "The provision of healthcare services at a distance with communication conducted between healthcare providers seeking clinical guidance and support from other healthcare providers (provider-to-provider telemedicine); or conducted between remote healthcare users seeking health services and healthcare providers (client-to-provider telemedicine)." [2] QR code 7.1 visualizes the definition further.

QR Code 7.1
Consolidated telemedicine implementation guide.

Digital health has to a certain extent become, in the eyes of many, a panacea for the democratization of healthcare (bringing it into people's homes and environment). Digital health is also an opportunity to fight the challenges caused by an aging society, the epidemic of noncommunicable and chronic diseases, and the dramatically rising healthcare costs, as described in Chapter 1.

Booming digital health environment

Digital health is expected to grow significantly in many countries in the upcoming years.

Figure. 7.1 gives an overview of how digital technology has now been developed and applied to every aspect of health and health care. It groups the various digital health tools into a dozen application arenas, but the individual applications number in the thousands.

The global digital health market was valued at USD 145.57 billion in 2021 and is projected to surpass the valuation of USD 430.52 billion by 2028 at a compound annual growth rate (CAGR) of 16.9% during the forecast period 2022−28 [4]. Furthermore, the Europe digital health market size was valued at USD 39.3 billion in 2021 and is expected to expand at a CAGR of 27.1% from 2022 to 2030 [5].

Chapters 9−16 describe in detail the digital health technologies that the authors assume will impact future pharmaceutical care.

Digital health classification by type of data transfer

There are many classification systems for digital health. One involves the classification into two categories that are based on the type of data transmission [6]:

1. Store-and-forward technology, which involves the transmission of packages of data.
2. Real-time interactive services involve direct (virtual) interaction.

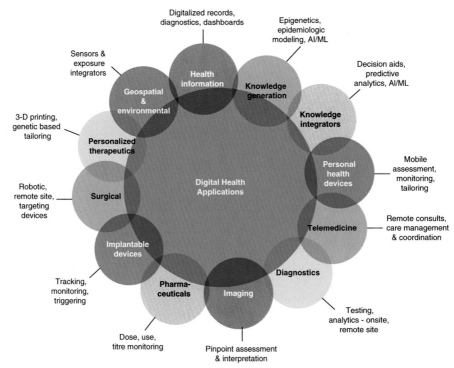

Figure 7.1

Evolving applications of digital technology in health and healthcare [3]. *Source: National Academy of Medicine. 2019. Digital Health Action Collaborative, NAM Leadership Consortium: Collaboration for a Value & Science-Driven Health System.*

Both categories are relevant for pharmaceutical care providers.

Concerning the first category, in many countries, electronic pharmacy records (EPRs) are already linked to laboratories that, for example, transfer renal or liver function data into EPRs. The same applies in some countries where genomic data on poor or fast metabolization of drugs are transmitted into EPRs, as essential information to better predict medication responses and adverse events.

The second category of real-time virtual interaction is being adopted gradually by pharmaceutical care stakeholders. For example, data from health trackers, virtual personal assistants, and digital therapeutics can be connected to electronic medical records (EMRs) and EPRs, allowing for a better understanding of responses to treatment and personalized follow-ups. However, interconnectivity and the possibilities for secure data transfer are potential hurdles to adopting these innovations, as we describe later in this part of the book.

WHO classification of digital health interventions

The WHO offers a classification of DHIs that categorizes the different ways digital and mobile technologies are used to support health system needs. Historically, the diverse communities working in digital health—including government stakeholders, technologists, clinicians, managers, implementers, network operators, researchers, and donors—have lacked a mutually understandable language to assess and articulate functionality. As a result, a shared and standardized vocabulary was recognized as necessary to identify gaps and duplication, evaluate effectiveness, and facilitate alignment across different digital health implementations. The classification framework aims to promote an accessible and bridging language for health program planners to articulate digital health implementations functionalities and facilitate the dialogue between public health practitioners and a technology-oriented audience [7].

 The WHO DHI categories are organized into the following overarching groupings based on the primarily targeted user:

- **Interventions for clients:** clients are members of the public who are potential or current users of health services, including health promotion activities. Caregivers of clients receiving health services are also included in this group.
- **Interventions for healthcare providers:** healthcare providers are members of the health workforce who deliver health services.
- **Interventions for a health system or resource managers:** health system and resource managers are involved in the administration and oversight of public health systems. Interventions within this category reflect managerial functions related to supply chain management, health financing, and human resource management.
- **Interventions for data services:** this consists of cross-cutting functionality to support a wide range of activities related to data collection, management, use, and exchange.

Details of the content of the classification can be found in QR Code 7.2.

QR Code 7.2
Digital health intervention classification.

Health technology at different stages of the patient pathway

Digital health technology can be used in different stages of a treatment pathway. From a patient's perspective (which may differ from a physician's point of view), an example of classification of tools within this pathway may look as shown in Fig. 7.2.

Patients' trust in digital health tools must be earned and maintained. Choosing a particular technology in the initial phase of a patient pathway can seriously impact treatment in a

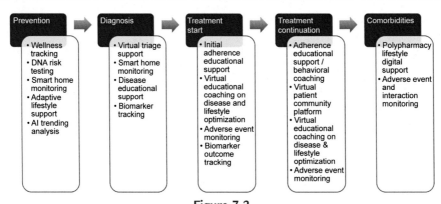

Figure 7.2
Examples of digital health in different patient pathway stages.

later stage. For example, suppose virtual triage or digital disease education is done in an inappropriate way or results in suboptimal care. In that case, that might also lower a patient's trust in supportive digital technology at a later stage, resulting in technology adversity or nonadherence later in the disease. Conversely, positive experiences in an early stage may result in better virtual expectations during the remainder of the treatment.

Additionally, once a certain technological platform or device is chosen to support the patient at the start of treatment and the patient becomes familiar with a certain platform and interconnectivity, switching to another platform or device may be increasingly complex and hard to achieve. The necessity of the Bring Your own Health Device strategy is explained in Chapter 10.

Health data are a potential treasure trove of information. So-called 'secondary use,' or reuse of patient data, whereby information collected for clinical care by health systems and hospitals is used for purposes other than medical record-keeping, offers myriad opportunities [8]. However, experts have been warning for some time now that ambiguity about managing data privacy laws could cause a crisis of public trust.

As pharmacists traditionally perform their role in close proximity to society and because pharmacy is one of the most trusted professions globally, it is considered a low-threshold environment for professional care; thus, a pharmaceutical care provider may take on additional responsibilities in future care systems since pharmacists are uniquely positioned to help drive the digital health wave into the future. Due to pharmacist accessibility, patients will seek out their local pharmacist for technology and data synchronization issues with devices, technology, and software. We need to be prepared to answer patients' questions and play an integral part in how patients incorporate digital health solutions into their health management [9]. A small fraction of practitioners have received digital health education or training, including continuous education, as pharmacists more frequently recognize the ability of digital health tools to save time compared with other benefits such as improved outcomes of medicines use [10].

Technology adoption

In general, the adoption rate of digital technology varies among countries, as shown in Fig. 7.3.

Healthcare, in general, has always been a technology-receptive area, embracing the development of diagnostic support tools such as X-rays, MRI, and ECG. In the pharmaceutical care environment, since the beginning of the third revolution (around 1969), drug development, production, and distribution have been increasingly infused by technological advances like genetic profiling, robotics, and EPRs.

For 2 decades, digital advances in patient interaction have been adopted by healthcare sectors. With the global digital developments around 2000, many healthcare providers became aware of the need to offer online information about their services via their own websites.

Around the same time, providers began to use social media to reach a greater number of customers and also offered support through interactive health services on Facebook and Twitter, for example.

Subsequently, providers' digital priorities changed again toward having their own health apps, which put the healthcare provider directly in the patient's pocket.

Since 2018 more healthcare providers have been considering using voice—user interfaces like chatbots, which take health and pharmacy records, clinical assessments, and other data to be processed by algorithms into supportive machines, thus helping both patients and providers. The behavioral data captured from these experiences will fuel the machine learning and cognitive capabilities required for more sophisticated conversations that integrate a given voice assistant's conversational knowledge from multiple sources and drive a dialogue [12]. In addition, when patients get very little time with a physician and leave the office and pharmacy with a handful of papers they may never read, voice assistants have the opportunity to bolster patient education and health literacy.

The promise of smartphones and access to the internet

In the digital revolution, the adoption of mobile technology has been extremely fast. In 2021, there were about 8.6 billion mobile device users [13], representing more than the global population (7.87 billion people) [14]. Mobile phones are being replaced by smartphones, which are mobile phones with a touchscreen and a connection to the internet that can perform a range of similar functions to a computer.

Digital Evolution:
State and Momentum

An analysis of the current level of digital development
and pace of digital growth of 90 global economies
divides those economies into four distinct zones:
Stall Out, Stand Out, Break Out, and Watch Out.

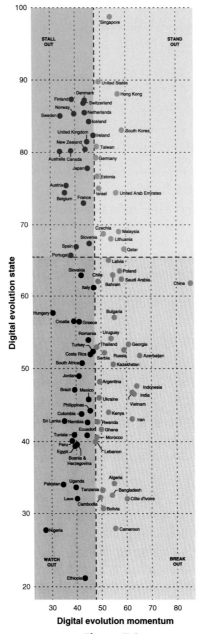

Figure 7.3
Which economies showed the most digital progress in 2020? [11]
Source: Digital planet. The Fletcher school at Tufts University: Mastercard.

The share of Americans that own a smartphone is now 85%, up from just 35% in Pew Research Center's first survey of smartphone ownership conducted in 2011 [15]. In 2025, that number will increase to 87% [16]. In 2021, 474 million people in Europe (86% of the population) subscribed to mobile services, which is expected to grow to 480 million by 2025 [17]. The services smartphones offer are improving, and recent studies confirm that the average teen now spends more than a third of the day online [18], while the average American spent nearly a month and a half (44 days) on their phones in 2022. At the same time, the pandemic has impacted knowledge workers. During one of the most transformational periods in history, employee expectations and attitudes around work evolved in the wake of the COVID-19 pandemic, leading to 73.1% of "knowledge workers" currently working remotely in some capacity. This is a significantly higher percentage of workers than before the pandemic—previously at just 18% [19].

Still, some 30% of adults in the United States say they often or sometimes experience problems connecting to the internet at home, including 9% who say such problems happen often. As Fig. 7.4 shows, while a growing share of Americans say they have a high-speed internet subscription at home, 23% do not. Financial barriers are among the more common reasons Americans do not subscribe to high-speed internet at home. Not having broadband could be tied to a number of disadvantages—including difficulties finding health information.

The frequent connectivity via the smartphone makes it the ideal device for monitoring, checking, coaching, guiding, and supporting health topics. In Chapter 8, we discuss how the smartphone can become the home of an entire personal health application. Also, many biosensors are now either integrated into or connected to smartphones, making the device suitable to track health parameters through, for example, ECGs, ultrasounds, and biomarkers. Applications like triage chatbots are increasingly "standard" on mobile phones, and are further explained in Chapter 12.

⚠ Even with these positive opportunities offered by mobile phones, many predict that the smartphone is only an intermediate vehicle and that within a decade, augmented reality (AR) via glasses, body-worn solutions, and implanted neural laces will be our future, thus creating a cyborg-like, human—machine fusion called "transhumans." That may be the end of machines that we carry with us passively and the beginning of something that fuses our bodies directly with digital information. Yet, this vision also raises a number of ethical questions, which are discussed in Chapter 18.

Health technology adoption

Digital transformation has recently been a hot topic in the healthcare industry. Spending on digital transformation surpassed $1.3 trillion worldwide, growing at a whopping 10.4% year on year [21]. Around 92% of healthcare professionals and institutes achieved better

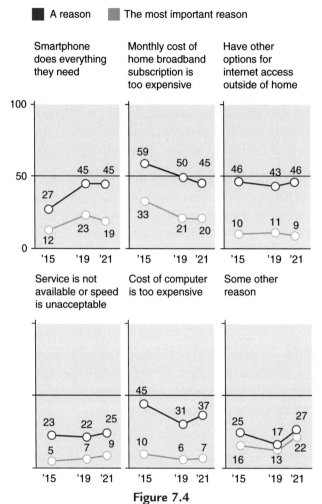

Smartphones, financial barriers and outside options for internet cited as reasons for not having home broadband

% of non-broadband users in the U.S. who say the following are ___ they do not have broadband at home

■ A reason   ■ The most important reason

Figure 7.4

Smartphones, financial barriers, and outside options for internet cited as reasons for not having broadband. *Reproduced from Pew Research Center (2021) Pew Research Center. https://www.pewresearch. org/internet/2021/06/03/mobile-technology-and-home-broadband-2021/. 2021 [cited 2023 02/02/2023]; Available from: https://www.pewresearch.org/internet/2021/06/03/mobile-technology-and-home-broadband-2021/; Note: Respondents who did not give an answer are not shown. Source: Survey of US adults conducted Jan. 25-Feb. 8, 2021. "Mobile technology and home broadband 2021."*

performance from digital transformation. The COVID-19 pandemic accelerated the convergence of several trends in the healthcare industry, particularly consumers prioritizing convenience and access to care. Leading health systems view digital transformation as a way to become more consumer-friendly while simultaneously changing their operations, culture, and use of technology [22].

- Health systems consider digital capabilities a path to transform their relationship with consumers. Designing processes and experiences from a consumer's perspective is a way to build their trust and loyalty—improving patient experience and building on newer forms of care delivery using digital technology.
- While the digital transformation journey is long, health systems are focusing on interim milestones to show value. Frequent checkpoints are needed to measure the value of the initiatives rather than waiting until the completion of the initiatives to measure returns on investments (ROIs).
- In addition to budget, talent, data, and setting key performance indicators are challenges to overcome.
- An executive champion is key to digital transformation success. Leadership and management of implementation (68%) are the key accelerators of digital transformation, and culture, communication ownership, and transparency are the key barriers. Organizational leadership is a crucial factor in the success of digital transformation efforts.

Although the adoption of digital health tools is definitely in an upward phase, the fast transformation of healthcare systems into one that uses predominantly digital pathways is not yet a reality in most countries.

 There may be a number of underlying reasons for this situation, such as the following:

- The principle of "**first do no harm**" is one of the primary precepts of bioethics, into which all healthcare practitioners are socialized both in training and in practice, and is a fundamental principle throughout the world. However, as long as digital innovation is in the early phases and its safety has not been proven sufficiently, healthcare professionals may regard its use as a risk for patients, which hinders adoption.
- The use of digital health, in general, will **require a different approach** to care delivery. Systems and cultures will have to adapt and engage informed patients while encouraging care providers to relinquish some control in exchange for useful real-time data.
- Those who market and develop new digital health technologies may yet underestimate the **distance between designing a wellness-like product** that appears to be associated with a healthy lifestyle and disease monitoring versus **a tool that also has the capacity to provide scientific evidence** to support underlying health claims.

- **Pharmacists, doctors, and patients are not always involved** in developing digital tools that are supposed to influence interventions set up by or for them. Thus, not involving key stakeholders may lead to innovations that (initially) do not adequately meet customer needs. A large proportion of pharmacy schools and faculties do not offer any digital health education. Expectations of practitioners around the clinical benefits of digital health in practice remain low. This might be because the implementation of digital health tools in clinical care is among the least likely concepts to be included in pharmacy education, based on academics' perspectives. Existing digital health education appears to be tailored more toward providing administrative and functional competencies for facilitating business processes and improving operational efficiency [10].
- Digital healthcare has posed a variety **of data validation, privacy, security, and reimbursement challenges,** as is explained in detail in the remainder of this book.
- **The connectivity** of different digital health solutions is yet suboptimal. Much of the data from wearables and apps available since 2018 have only limited ability to connect with existing electronic health software; thus, an integrated outlook for circular pharmaceutical care is not yet achievable.
- **Amara's law** may also be a potential rationale for slower adoption: people often overestimate the speed at which innovations will be implemented but underestimate how these innovations will ultimately significantly impact changes in long-term healthcare systems.
- The healthcare sector may also have **insufficiently focused on truly meaningful problems.** The question, "What healthcare or patient challenges need to be solved?" in some cases has become, "How can technology solve a healthcare problem?" This may sound like a subtle distinction, but the result is a glut of mobile technologies searching for a medical purpose and not meeting the future needs of healthcare systems.
- **Governmental priority** is variable among countries. A great European example in this respect is Estonia, where since 2008, the government has developed a strong digital (health) policy and has repeatedly focused on the right questions and prioritized the right solutions for enabling fast adoption and has modeled frameworks so that they are quickly integrated into systems.

In Estonia, doctors can access patients' electronic records, no matter where they are and can make better-informed treatment decisions. Each person in Estonia who has visited a doctor has an online e-health record, which contains his medical case notes, test results, digital prescriptions, X-rays, and a full log file tracking access to the data. Patients own their health data, and hospitals have made their data available online since 2008. Today over 95% of the data generated by hospitals and doctors have been digitized, and blockchain technology is used for assuring the integrity of stored EMRs as well as system access logs, while there is a detailed strategic plan for promoting the implementation of AI solutions in the public and private sectors.

Because of its focus on digitization in healthcare as well as in other sectors, Estonia has been referred to as the "most advanced digital society in the world" [23].

Despite all the challenges to adequately adopting digital health solutions, there is a strong, ongoing proliferation of applications. To stimulate adoption and retention, persuasive health technology techniques may be needed.

Persuasive health technology to drive adoption

Persuasive health technology is broadly defined as technology designed to change consumers' attitudes or behaviors through persuasion and social influence, but not through coercion.

Persuasive technologies have been exploited to tremendous effect with applications ranging from mobile healthcare, which persuades users to exercise more often and adopt a healthy lifestyle, to government programs encouraging civic engagement [24]. Examples of ways these technologies influence behavior include specific push messages, question-and-answer techniques, and guidance signals.

Gamification, understood as the use of game design elements in nongame contexts, is a research field integrating approaches from the human—computer interaction, psychology, and computer science fields. Gamification has increased popularity for designing software that covers enjoyment, immersion, and goal orientation, being a conventional approach for behavior change [25].

Gamification is primarily utilized in health and wellness applications dealing with disease prevention, self-management, medication adherence, and telehealth programs. The core of healthcare gamification is very patient-centric, as it aims to improve patient engagement by making their experience more personalized [26].

Patients can take part in different challenges and earn multiple badges as rewards. In some healthcare apps, they can compete with themselves by challenging personal goals, while in others, they can also compete against other patients. Competing in different challenges and achieving goals makes patients more motivated and involved in their healthcare activities [26]. As a useful tool for keeping users motivated, engaged and active, there is a wide interest in adopting gamification solutions for supporting and promoting positive behaviors and behavior change (e.g., smoking cessation, food choices, mental healthcare) [27].

Old habits die hard

Google is extremely dominant in the search market, with a market share of over 90%. Its position is largely due to its advanced search algorithms, which are able to provide relevant and accurate results to users. Other competitors, such as Bing and DuckDuckGo, may have advantages in areas such as privacy protection or offering a different interface. Now, thanks to ChatGPT, Microsoft Bing poses a real challenge to the Google search engine. However, they still have a long way to go in terms of catching up with Google in terms of market share. Although everyone does not like Google, it is used by an overwhelming majority.

Internet searches on Google occur so frequently that it has positioned itself as the only solution in many users' minds, making it very difficult for new platforms to enter the market successfully.

Google identifies users through tracking technology, automatically improving users' search results based on their past behavior to deliver more accurate and personalized experiences, thus reinforcing the users' preference for the search engine.

Nevertheless, in 2018, Google was penalized for "serious illegal behavior" in its attempt to secure the dominance of its search engine on mobile phones.

For new behaviors to really take hold, they must occur often. That is why technology uses the principle of creating hooks to stimulate the occurrence of new habits.

Persuasive "hooks" can be defined as experiences that connect a user's problems to a supplier's solution with enough frequency to form a habit. The more often users run through these hooks, the more likely they are to form habits, most often linked to the supplier behind a product.

The hook always begins with an internal or external trigger that motivates a person to find the technology. In this respect, the external trigger often raises the user's interest (the app sends a message, for example, on the risks of obesity and cardiovascular disease). In contrast, the action mostly follows only when the internal trigger is profound enough to drive activity (for example, can I use digital tools in my app to help me lose weight?).

The user then carries out a particular kind of activity (e.g., performs an exercise) and subsequently gets a reward, which can be tokens, applause, or perhaps even a reduction in health insurance fees. The next phase starts with discomfort when the exercise is not done, and no reward is received. For example, push messages are received with narratives about people who felt much more healthy at BMI 21 after successfully using the losing-weight app.

Such situations will motivate many people to perform the activity again, obtain a reward for positive behavior, and feel good. This is how the hook is created, and this is how the new habit is slowly formed after a number of reiterations.

In nonhealthcare environments, companies with habit-forming services usually link the services to users' daily routines and emotions. However, many marketing companies, large or startups, are now trying to change behavior profoundly by guiding users through a series of experiences, that is, through hooks, as previously described.

Some interesting fiction depicting what hooks can do to society can be found in the books *You've Been Played* by Adrian Hon (2022) and *The Circle* by Dave Eggers (2014), which has been transformed into a movie plot as well [28].

In terms of improving the adequate use of medication in general and medication adherence in particular, the principles behind creating appropriate digital persuasive hooks combined with human pharmaceutical support can be strongly augmented.

Creating hooks to improve adequate use of drugs

Being adherent to the use of a prescription drug is a fundamental habit, but one that for many is not easy to do (also refer to Chapter 6). Thus, pharmaceutical care providers have a clear professional responsibility to support the optimization of adherence behavior.

To change nonadherent behavior, the external trigger for adherence must be transformed into intrinsic motivation. This means that patients must be honestly convinced to use drugs to care for or cure their disease, or at least to alleviate the symptoms toward the best possible acceptable level. It is recommended that pharmaceutical care providers determine what a patient sees as personally relevant outcomes of treatment and consider a holistic perspective of determinants influencing health (see Chapter 3 for more information).

Once an intrinsic motivation has been sparked, persuasive technology may call for a personalized action to use the medication, which ideally should be rewarded by something that the individual finds relevant and that makes the adherence activity attractive enough to prompt future action. Interactive technologies such as virtual reality and AR are increasingly used in healthcare, especially inpatient education. Studies have demonstrated AR applications in multiple settings, including an app-based medication management plan and patient medication adherence [29]. This is where the Goal Attainment Scaling (GAS) score of Chapter 3 and the Institute for Positive Health (IPH) principles of Chapter 3 have relevance: when the pharmacist knows what matters most to the patient, the intrinsic motivation may be easier to spark. A blended care approach of digital as well as human coaching most often produces the greatest chance for success [30]. However, more research is needed to fully understand the benefits and limitations of blended care and determine when and how it should be used. Ultimately, the best approach will depend on individual patient needs and preferences and the availability of resources and technology.

Furthermore, all digital or blended programs that strive to change the habits of patients must at least have the principles of behavior change interventions (BCIs) integrated into them. Researchers have discovered that individuals go through a sequence of steps when it comes to changing behavior. Although the amount of time an individual can spend in each stage varies, the activities necessary to advance to the next stage do not. At each point, some concepts and change mechanisms work best to minimize opposition, promote growth, and avoid relapse [31]. Many frameworks of BCIs exist, but there is no gold standard yet. Therefore, before developing a digital tool that aims to change behavior, it makes sense to analyze which BCI framework could best support the tool's goal and thus further increase the likelihood of successful innovation.

Serious gaming to change habits

Gamification may also be considered as a suitable technique for achieving behavioral changes. This is because gamification triggers the brain's reward pathways and can be designed to promote positive action and reinforcement for the correct adherent behavior.

Serious gaming can be defined as the use of game principles for the purposes of learning, skill acquisition, and training. As reflected in QR Code 7.3, serious gaming has been shown in patient care to improve patients' cognitive abilities, rehabilitate disabled patients, promote healthy behavior, educate patients, enhance disease self-management, and attract participation in medical research.

QR Code 7.3
What is gamification?.

Serious games are expected to be increasingly prescribed as autonomous treatment regimens for patients. The company Akili Interactive (described in Chapter 15) received the Food and Drug Administration approval to market AKL-T01, a video game designed to treat pediatric ADHD. This is one of the first games to be considered a legitimate treatment option for pediatric ADHD [32].

One example of a serious gaming app in the cognition improvement area is Neurogrow which received a $7.5 million grant from the National Mental Health Institute to conduct clinical trials [33]. Another example is CogniFit, which is designed to measure, train, track, and monitor 22 cognitive skills. Based on AI and advanced adaptive algorithms, the system automatically adapts the training to the needs of each user. Based on the data acquired, the apps can signal improvement or deterioration and potentially underlying disease conditions.

Regulation at the EU level is complex, and there is a myriad of overlapping regulatory proposals, such as the AI Act, the Data Act, and the European Health Data Space. In parallel, given that health is a primary competence of Member States, it is imperative that national and European policies are aligned and harmonized, especially when it comes to data protection, as well as data access and reuse for multiple purposes, from care to research. And finally, we must not lose sight of international collaboration since health research is global—as the fast development of COVID vaccines made clear [34].

Economic benefits of digital health

The main benefits associated with digital health are often positioned as improved personalized access to healthcare, ameliorated health insights, and reduced healthcare-related costs.

Due to digital healthcare, patients may also experience a better quality of life, as they are treated in a more personalized and often geographically convenient way. In addition, with digital health's strong focus on prevention, people are protected as long as possible from deterioration or, perhaps, from getting sick.

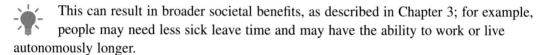 This can result in broader societal benefits, as described in Chapter 3; for example, people may need less sick leave time and may have the ability to work or live autonomously longer.

Digital health adoption as such will create additional benefits for healthcare systems as implementation may (or should) lead to more cost-efficient care, predominantly in home-situated environments. Thus, the need to maintain large, expensive hospitals and care institutions may also gradually decrease.

Additionally, the digital health epoch creates more opportunities for new entrants in the care arena, startups, and big corporations, who see the attractiveness of a suboptimal system that can benefit from digital optimization.

Research on digital health cost-effectiveness

Structured analysis of the costs, benefits, and added value of digital health innovations is needed to form the basis for developing new business models in healthcare and to facilitate payment systems to support the most promising services. In the absence of solid evidence, key decision makers in government and paying authorities may doubt the effectiveness of digital innovations, which, in turn, limits investment in and adoption of such models.

Fortunately, a significant amount of vital research is being done in this area. The scope of this book is too broad to provide a detailed discussion on this research; instead, here we look at a number of recent representative examples.

A systematic metaanalysis of peer-reviewed studies published in English from 2016 to 2020 examined the cost-effectiveness (or utility) of e-health technologies. Health technologies evaluated by these studies include video-monitoring service systems, text messaging interventions, web platforms and digital health portals, telephone support, mobile phone—based systems and applications, and technologies and innovations. Findings on the cost-effectiveness of digital interventions showed a growing body of evidence and suggested a generally favorable effect in terms of costs and health outcomes. However, due to the heterogeneity across study methods, comparing interventions remains difficult. Further research based on a standardized approach is needed in order to methodically analyze incremental cost-effectiveness ratios, costs, and health benefits [35].

Telehealth is becoming increasingly important for the management of patients with long COVID. Telehealth can help patients with the care and monitoring they need without having to leave the comfort of their homes. There are several ways patients may be able to receive care for long-term COVID-19 symptoms: Talking to their healthcare provider about telehealth options for follow-up care after leaving the hospital or their office; using remote patient monitoring devices so their healthcare provider can check on the patient at home; getting support for specialty care faster via telehealth than waiting to see a health care provider in person; discussing with a health care provider during a telehealth appointment the lab test results; asking their healthcare provider—especially pharmacists—about medications or treatments that can help manage their symptoms; and generally using telehealth as a bridge between in-person appointments [36].

The good times have been really good for digital health sellers over the last decade and increasingly so over the past few years. Even with recent pullbacks in 2022, digital health funding reached $6B in Q1 of this year (compared to $6.7B in Q1 of 2021), which is certainly nothing to sneeze at.

But with economic uncertainty comes increasing capital constraints, which stands to turn the longstanding burgeoning digital health market on its head in the years to come.

Gone are the days when digital health startups could sell based on stories and a promise. Now more than ever, digital health companies need to clearly demonstrate their value and prove a real financial ROI to the organizations they are selling to—showing the value to patients and healthcare system and the buyer's bottom line in both the short and long term [37].

Digital technologies often include innovative software solutions and algorithms that could be substantially cheaper than devices or drugs. In addition, these technologies tend to focus on solutions to the notoriously inefficient delivery systems of health care globally, as opposed to developing new treatments. Digital health will offer patients improved access to increased health services. We might embrace these technologies rapidly simply because of their convenience or reassurance. However, as evidence suggests, more is not always better in medicine, and careful evaluation of such interventions becomes ever more important. Otherwise, to paraphrase the remark made by the US economist Robert Solow, we will soon see digital health everywhere, but will it really bring health gains or cost reduction? [38].

This means for blended pharmaceutical care:

- Digital telehealth technologies will further mature toward 2024, offering possibilities for care in every stage of the patient pathway, whereas smartphones still seem to be the ideal devices to provide digital pharmaceutical care.
- The adoption of digital health tools by care providers still faces many rate-limiting hurdles.
- Persuasive technology and serious gaming are techniques that may positively stimulate the adoption and retention of digital health tools.
- To integrate digital health technology effectively into current healthcare systems, further systematic research on the (broader) economic benefits is crucial.

References

[1] Safavi K, Kalis B. *How can leaders make recent digital health gains last.* Re-examining the Accenture. 2020. Available from, https://www.accenture.com/content/dam/accenture/final/a-com-migration/pdf/pdf-130/accenture-2020-digital-health-consumer-survey-us.pdf.

[2] World Health Organization. WHO guideline: recommendations on digital interventions for health system strengthening: executive summary. World Health Organization; 2019. Available from, https://apps.who.int/iris/handle/10665/311941.

[3] Abernethy A, et al. The promise of digital health: then, now, and the future. NAM perspectives; 2022.

[4] Research VM. Digital health market size to reach valuation of $430.52 billion by 2028 | telehealth generates 38% market revenue | VMR. 2022 [cited 2023 02/02/2023]; Available from: https://www.globenewswire.com/en/news-release/2022/10/10/2530630/0/en/Digital-Health-Market-Size-to-Reach-Valuation-of-430-52-Billion-by-2028-Telehealth-Generates-38-Market-Revenue-VMR.html.

[5] Research GV. Europe digital health market size, share and trends analysis report by technology (Tele-healthcare, mHealth, healthcare analytics, digital health systems), by component, by region, and segment forecasts, 2022-2030, in Europe digital health market size and share report. 2022. Available from, https://www.grandviewresearch.com/industry-analysis/europe-digital-health-market-report.

[6] Badowski M, Michienzi S, Robles M. Examining the implications of analytical and remote monitoring in pharmacy practice. Clinical Pharmacist 2017;9(6):184—92.

[7] World Health Organization. Classification of digital health interventions v1. 0: a shared language to describe the uses of digital technology for health. World Health Organization; 2018. Available from, https://apps.who.int/iris/bitstream/handle/10665/260480/WHO-RHR-18.06-eng.pdf.

[8] Patient trust must come at the top of researchers' priority list. Nature Medicine 2020;26(3):301. https://dx.doi.org/10.1038/s41591-020-0813-8.

[9] Martin A, et al. The evolving frontier of digital health: opportunities for pharmacists on the horizon. Hospital pharmacy 2018;53(1):7−11. https://doi.org/10.1177/0018578717738221.

[10] International Pharmaceutical Federation (FIP). FIP Digital health in pharmacy education. 2021. Available from, https://www.fip.org/file/4958.

[11] Chakravorti B, Bhalla A, Chaturvedi RS. Which Economies showed the most digital progress in 2020?. 2020. Available from, https://hbr.org/2020/12/which-economies-showed-the-most-digital-progress-in-2020?ab=hero-subleft-3.

[12] Robinson R. Trend: voice assistants. 2018 [cited 2023 02/02/2023]; Available from, https://www.pharmavoice.com/news/2018-11-voice-assistants/612524/.

[13] Alvarez P. This infographic shows the rise of mobile device subscriptions worldwide. 2022 [cited 2022 02/02/2023]; Available from, https://www.weforum.org/agenda/2022/10/mobile-device-subscription-rise-technology/.

[14] StatisticsTimes. World population. 2021. Available from, https://statisticstimes.com/demographics/world-population.php.

[15] Pew Research Center. Mobile fact sheet. 2021 [cited 2023 02/02/2023]; Available from, https://www.pewresearch.org/internet/fact-sheet/mobile/.

[16] Statista. Smartphone user penetration as share of population in the United States from 2018 to 2025 [Graph]. Statitsa; 2020. Available from, https://www.statista.com/statistics/201184/percentage-of-mobile-phone-users-who-use-a-smartphone-in-the-us/.

[17] GSM Association. The mobile economy Europe. 2022 [cited 2023 03/02/2023].

[18] YPulse. 3 Stats on how gen Z is being raised on smartphones. 2022 [cited 2023.

[19] Oyster. The employee expectations-report 2022. 2022. Available from, https://email.oysterhr.com/hubfs/The-Employee-Expectations-Report-2022.pdf.

[20] Pew Research Center [cited 2023 02/02/2023]; Available from, https://www.pewresearch.org/internet/2021/06/03/mobile-technology-and-home-broadband-2021/; 2021.

[21] Bhargava R, Ollis S. How digital transformation is driving action in healthcare. 2022 [cited 2023 02/02/2023]; Available from, https://www.weforum.org/agenda/2022/09/health-information-system-digital-transformation-healthcare/.

[22] Appleby C, et al. Digital transformation: from a buzzword to an imperative for health systems. 2021. Available from, https://www2.deloitte.com/us/en/insights/industry/health-care/digital-transformation-in-healthcare.html.

[23] e-Estonia. We have built a digital society and so can you. 2023. Available from, https://e-estonia.com.

[24] Rehman U, et al. Persuasive technology in games: a brief review and reappraisal. In: HCI in games: experience design and game mechanics: third international conference, HCI-games 2021, held as part of the 23rd HCI international conference, HCII 2021, virtual event, july 24−29, 2021, proceedings, Part I. Springer; 2021.

[25] Guerrero E, Kalmi P. Gamification strategies: a characterization using formal argumentation theory. SN Computer Science 2022;3(4):291.

[26] folio3. Gamification and the healthcare industry. 2022 [cited 2023 02/02/2023]; Available from, https://digitalhealth.folio3.com/blog/what-ways-can-gamification-be-used-in-the-healthcare-industry/.

[27] Bassanelli S, et al. Gamification for behavior change: a scientometric review. Acta Psychologica 2022;228:103657. Available from, https://www.sciencedirect.com/science/article/pii/S000169182200172X.

[28] Ponsoldt J. The circle [film]. 2017.

[29] Adapa K, et al. Augmented reality in patient education and health literacy: a scoping review protocol. BMJ Open 2020;10(9):e038416. https://doi.org/10.1136/bmjopen-2020-038416.

[30] Talboom-Kamp EP, et al. From chronic disease management to person-centered eHealth; a review on the necessity for blended care. Clinical eHealth 2018;1(1):3−7.

[31] Rad D, Rad G. Theory of change in digital behavior change interventions (Dbcis) and community-based change initiatives-A general framework. Technium Social Sciences Journal 2021;21:554.

[32] Sheppard S. FDA approves prescription video game for ADHD. 2020 [cited 2023 02/02/2023]; Available from, https://www.verywellmind.com/a-new-video-game-has-been-approved-by-the-fda-to-treat-adhd-5069615.

[33] Gordon K. Researchers explore an unlikely treatment for cognitive disorders: video games. 2022. Available from, https://www.npr.org/2022/04/15/1092804764/video-games-developed-to-treat-cognitive-disorders.

[34] Bonefeld-Dahl C. Available from, https://www.digitaleurope.org/resources/a-digital-health-decade-driving-innovation-in-europe/; 2022.

[35] Gentili A, et al. The cost-effectiveness of digital health interventions: a systematic review of the literature. Front Public Health 2022;10:787135.

[36] TelehealthHHS.gov. Telehealth and COVID-19. 2023 [cited 2032 02/02/2023]; Available from, https://telehealth.hhs.gov/patients/telehealth-and-covid/.

[37] Joseph S. Digital health's burden of proof: compelling ROI in A new economic reality. 2022 [cited 2023 02/02/2023]; Available from, https://www.forbes.com/sites/sethjoseph/2022/06/22/digital-healths-burden-of-proof-compelling-roi-in-a-new-economic-reality/?sh=1e4973624e17.

[38] Rahimi K. Digital health and the elusive quest for cost savings. The Lancet Digital Health 2019;1(3):e108–9.

CHAPTER 8

Zesting the internet of pharma things*

Timothy Dy Aungst

Department of Pharmacy Practice, MCPHS University, Worcester, MA, United States

It is a capital mistake to theorize, before one has data.

Arthur Conan Doyle

Zesting is performed on the outermost skin layer of citrus-based fruits. These skin parts are different colors, as seen with oranges, lemons, and limes. The colors of these fruits provide aroma and flavor. Note, however, that while we are still touching the outside, we still get a lot of potencies. The Internet of Things (IoT) is a zest to healthcare's potential futures and opportunities. So while we are still on the outside, much can be enjoyed. And as we end up going deeper into the fruit, we will discover other vibrant flavors.

The IoT can be defined as a structure of interrelated mechanical and digital devices, objects, animals, or people, each featuring unique identifiers and the ability to transfer their respective data over a digital network without requiring human-to-human or human-to-computer interaction [1].

A "thing" in the IoT is always assigned an Internet Protocol address and can be, for instance, a pet with a biochip transponder, a light bulb with a Wi-Fi connector, a person with a heart monitor implant, or a smart refrigerator that alerts when food is starting to spoil or needs replacing. Fig. 8.1 shows how the principle of the IoT works.

Identification of every "thing" is closely tied to IoT governance, security, and privacy (see Chapter 17 for more information on compliance). Different forms of identification are key components of multiple layers of the IoT, from those embedded in the user's device to those enabling data routing and discovery (QR Code 8.1).

QR Code 8.1
Internet of Things explained.

---

*In this chapter, you will read about data in the Internet of Health and how to turn them into value, the use of digital biomarkers, the blooming future of integrated personal health records, the need for FAIR data, and the interoperability of healthcare applications, facilitated by HL7-FHIR.

Pharmaceutical Care in Digital Revolution. https://doi.org/10.1016/B978-0-443-13360-2.00001-0

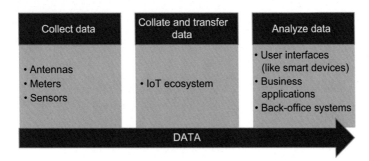

Figure 8.1
How the IoT works.

Rather than using the term IoT, some prefer to talk about the "internet of everyone and everything" (IoEE), as the IoEE connects all separate nodes into one cohesive whole. It's not just about allowing devices to talk to each other; it's also about allowing everything (people and devices) to talk about each other [2]. The expansion of the use of technology for remote services and work during the pandemic highlighted the ability of IoT infrastructure to be used for multiple personal needs.

As such, IoT connectivity has created radically different paradigms of infrastructures in our society; for example, it enabled the development of smart cities, smart metering, disruptive e-commerce, and far-reaching home automation, which has large implications for healthcare.

IoT explosion

Market research by the International Data Corporation (IDC) in 2017 projected that an average person's interaction with connected devices anywhere in the world would increase from about 200 times per capita per day in 2015 to nearly 4800 times per day in 2025—basically one interaction every 18 seconds [3].

The IDC estimates that by 2025 there will be 55.9B connected devices, with over 79.4 ZB of data generated [4]. Much of this technology will encapsulate products integrating IoT services around a user's life. Motor vehicles, appliances, household products, toys, and many more will expand to connect to an online platform that interchains with social media and related profiles. Personalization of a user's preferences and needs will expand and place the user at the center of personalized needs and wants, whether with the aim of commercial targeting or related business opportunities. This will also have a push into the realm of healthcare-related services.

Internet of Health

The healthcare industry has been somewhat slower than other industries to adopt IoT technologies, though in recent years has been accelerating adoption. The Internet of

Health (IoH), or Internet of Medical Things, is expected to help monitor, inform, and notify not only caregivers, but will also give healthcare providers actual data that will enable them to identify health problems before they become critical or to allow for earlier invention. The IoH refers to the connected system of medical devices and applications that collect data that is then provided to healthcare IT systems through online computer networks. In early 2018, there were 3.7 million medical devices in use around the world; these devices are connected to and monitor various parts of the body to inform healthcare decisions [5].

Fig. 8.2 depicts the scope of the device types that are integrated into the IoH. Additional concerns now relate to incorporating IoT health data into other infrastructures, such as genomics, and how to tie all data into a relevant means of exploring patient health journeys [6].

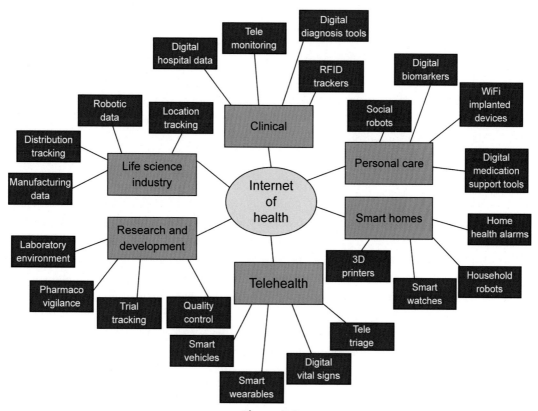

Figure 8.2

The Internet of Health. *Adapted from Romeo S, Corey T, reportInternet of health—Beecham research report 2017. Available from: https://internetofbusiness.com/wp-content/uploads/2017/05/IoHEALTH-Market-Brief-17-Final.pdf.*

The explosive growth in medical monitoring applications is predominantly driven by the following:

- broad adoption of wearable tools and medical products, for example, smart watches, bracelets, and clothing;
- alternative data from novel measurement scores (e.g., Light Detection and Ranging, voice);
- attachable biosensors and measurement tools (e.g., electrocardiogram sensors, continous glucose monitoring);
- new types of measurements for the advancement of medical treatments;
- reduction in size and cost of devices and proliferation of device types; and
- availability of semiconductors and MEMS (micro-electromechanical systems) technologies.

These monitoring devices create a data sea on digital biomarkers, which are defined as consumer-generated physiological and behavioral measures collected through connected digital tools that can be used to explain, influence, and predict health-related outcomes. The Digital Medicine Society has been working extensively to help identify and create a library of sensors that may be used for siteless clinical trials and for remote patient monitoring (RPM) services.

Health-related outcomes can vary from reporting disease states to predicting drug responses to influencing fitness behaviors. In general, patient-reported measures (e.g., survey data), genetic information, and data collected through traditional medical devices and equipment may be stored digitally but are not digitally measured or truly dependent on software and thus are not regarded as digital biomarkers [7].

Ultimately, the digital health monitoring platforms (as described in Chapter 7) may replace a large swath of activities that now take place physically in various healthcare facilities. Connectivity and interoperability will allow for better-connected, more efficient care in a better-informed stakeholder landscape. This push for RPM may subsume an area of pharmaceutical care whereby patients may be monitored for medication benefits and safety. Newly started medications or changes in doses may have their effects monitored through biosensors to measure and track clinical impact. The need to have patients in the clinic or hospital may be pushed toward treatment in the home, which has coined the term the "hospital-at-home" model, focusing on the patient's home as the center of care [8].

Internet of Pharma Things

IoT technology and pharmacy automation will also shift the focus of tomorrow's pharmaceutical care providers. For example, many pharmacies worldwide already use electronic pharmacy record (EPR) databases, often connected with information systems of general practitioners and hospitals, that is, electronic medical records (EMRs).

Several EPR platforms also provide connectivity to supply chain automated solutions to achieve good distribution of medications, for instance, by connecting radio frequency identification data (on medication), production data, and distribution data (e.g., from robotic medication dispensing systems). In addition to generating a lot of interesting data, the latter solutions help reduce counterfeit medication and recall situations. In the coming years, these platforms may be further augmented by digital health data derived from the devices mentioned in subsequent chapters in this book.

Through the connectivity of these different data sources, the Internet of Pharma Things (IoPT) will grow into a powerful medium that enables in-depth data analysis, stratification, and precision medicine.

For instance, it will help optimize and monitor adherence (which we address in Chapter 6), thus resulting in one of the largest areas of improvement in the adequate use of drugs. This can be seen especially in the cardiometabolic space, with the rise of continuous glucose measurement technologies to help modulate the use of insulin for diabetes management.

Fig. 8.3 illustrates how IoPT connectivity can empower pharmaceutical care providers through better data on precise medication adherence.

Successful IoPT platforms, like the concept shown in Fig. 8.3, will incorporate continuous feedback loops that, through monitoring, measurement, and scale, can facilitate dashboards that support circular pharmaceutical care.

IoPT platforms will give the various stakeholders an action perspective, contributing to better and well-informed decision-making. In addition to being medication experts and excellent communicators, tomorrow's pharmaceutical care providers are envisioned to be data analytic translators who, based on dashboards derived from data as shown in Fig. 8.3, can respond in real time to emergencies and provide risk-based analysis of patients' profiles. The rise of at-home real-time assessments of patients response to medications will be key. This includes the utilization of medication for adherence, tracking biological response through sensors, and then communication on what changes may need to be made remotely. The essential competencies required to perform in these changing roles are discussed in Chapter 19.

Data in the Internet of Things

IDC forecasts that by 2025 with the rise in connected devices, the global data sphere will grow to 163 zettabytes (10^{21}). The astounding growth comes from both the number of

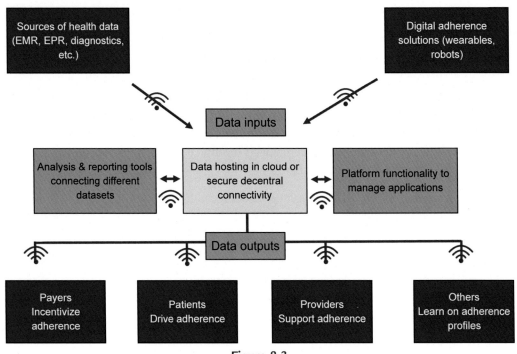

Figure 8.3
Internet of pharma things: An example of adherence.

devices generating data and the number of sensors in each device. As just an example of how much data are generated in normal life, a car like a Ford GT, for instance, carries 50 sensors and 28 microprocessors and can generate up to 100 GB of data per hour [3].

Thus, the amount of data we produce every day is truly mind-boggling. At our current rate, 2.5 exabytes (10^{18}) of data are created each day, and the pace will accelerate with the growth of the IoT. Over the past 2 years alone, 90% of the world's data was generated [9,10].

The enormous amount of data generated are often referred to as big data, which are data sets that are so big and complex that traditional data-processing application software cannot structure them appropriately.

The challenge here is to turn big data into "smart data." Processing and organizing big data has become complex, as countless sources are involved. Many of these sources use different data collection methods, including various sensors, automated reports, and historical trend analysis. The analogy can be made by calling data the next big thing since oil. However, oil cannot be simply dredged from the ground and placed into an airplane, it needs to be refined, and data refinement to a useable stream of clinical utility needs to be addressed.

Big data comprises five dimensions:

- **Volume** refers to the huge amounts of data currently being collected.
- **Velocity** refers to how fast data can be produced and processed (speed of connection, e.g., 4G or 5G technology, as well as the maturity of applications).
- **Variety** refers to the different content of data sets, whether structured, semi-structured, or unstructured.
- **Veracity** refers to the uncertainty of data (related, e.g., to biases, noise, abnormalities, ambiguities, and latency).
- **Value** refers to the ability to convert data into meaningful value.

How the balance between these big data dimensions in a particular business area like pharmaceutical care is defined depends on whether the available and relevant data can be absorbed, processed, and examined within a time frame that meets a particular business's requirement.

For instance, if data on a patient's wearables are considered to be essential to track medication responses, the value of the data is highly dependent on whether ongoing data can be obtained; the speed at which the data is transferred into, for example, an EPR environment; whether the wearables collect fixed data (like heart rates) or spoken information; and whether the data are collected by a regulatory-approved, safe, and secure health device.

Data in the health ecosystem

As previously discussed, the healthcare industry is generating a vast amount of data that is driven by a wide range of medical and healthcare functions, including data from wearable devices, clinical records, health-and-wellness apps, medical images, genomic data, clinical decision support tools, disease surveillance, and public health management.

Again, estimates differ according to definitions and to ongoing insights; according to a Stanford Medicine Stanford white paper in 2017, 153 exabytes (10^{18}) of health data were produced in 2013, and an estimated 2314 exabytes (10^{18}) will be generated in 2020, translating to an overall rate of increase of at least 48% annually [11].

In general, an EMR is meant to contain medical and clinical data gathered in a healthcare provider's office. An EPR contains pharmaceutical data gathered in a pharmaceutical care provider's space.

Electronic health records (EHRs) go beyond the data collected in an individual provider's office. They include more comprehensive patient history, connecting different providers (e.g., EMRs and EPRs) and other data sources (e.g., digital health data or diagnostics). When building an EHR, it is vital to address the mechanics of creating a health record and concepts such as a single logical health record and managing patient demographics and externally generated (including patient-originated) health data. Data may be captured using standardized code sets or nomenclature (which is crucial for using the data in further digital derivates), depending on the nature of the data, or captured as unstructured data, like open fields or even speech.

QR Code 8.2

Example of a personal health application.

With the patient's well-being at the center of decision-making, an EHR is ideally an ecosystem where all data are accessible for relevant care providers and the environment is managed by the patient, with the patient able to authorize care providers to see, use, and review data as required. Chapter 6 refers to this environment as a Personal Health Application (PHA). PHAs can be developed on autonomous platforms but also within existing environments, like the Apple example in QR Code 8.2.

⚠️ A single record for each patient should always be identified and maintained, as this is needed for legal purposes, as well as to organize care unambiguously for all stakeholders. A so-called Single Point of Truth (SPoT) on the patient's health information is created by connecting all different health data from the unique patient with the unique identifier. All stakeholders can then use this SPoT in the health ecosystem as a joint knowledge position to organize a well-aligned and optimized individual health management plan for the patient. There is still an ongoing debate about whether this SPoT should reside in one place (e.g., one server) or can be created by getting access to the constituting data and being generated and maintained at various locations.

By connecting EHRs, PHAs, EPRs, and data such as behavioral, claims, and socioeconomic data, we will be able to create a 360-degree, "digital-twin" overview of patient profiles, compare them with other populations, and make hyperpersonalized care plans that extend beyond the canned information that is linked to current rather siloed systems.

Exogenic data like social determinants of health, psychological profile, exercise patterns, metabolism, literacy level, and so on can further help determine an individual's care needs. Once connected to a genetic profile—which companies like Helix and 23andMe have offered customers since 2016—a personal health dossier can be constructed that provides a complete and holistic overview of a person's life, well-being, health risks, and opportunities.

HL7-FHIR and the interoperability of healthcare applications

Currently, many healthcare applications are not yet standardized and interoperable, so health research and patient data are still redundantly collected and not shared or collected by different methods and formats that are not interchangeable. Thus, the SPoT cannot be created on individual health information. A large part of this is derived from medical data and information not being optimally standardized.

Many standardization initiatives have been introduced in past decades to resolve this problem, such as the Clinical Data Interchange Standards Consortium, the International Statistical Classification of Diseases and Related Health Problems and Health Level Seven (HL7). All coding and classification systems aim to develop and incorporate industry standards that improve the way different healthcare computer systems share data, have uniform interpretations, and allow for consolidated analysis. Also, some health systems use coding systems for reimbursement and resource allocation.

HL7 is an international community of healthcare subject matter experts and information scientists who created a framework (and related standards) for the exchange, integration, sharing, and retrieval of electronic health information to increase the effectiveness and efficiency of healthcare information delivery. HL7 collaborates with other standards development organizations and national and international sanctioning bodies (e.g., ANSI and ISO) in the healthcare and information infrastructure domains to promote the use of supportive and compatible standards [12].

HL7 developed (as a follow-up on HL7-V3 standards) the FHIR structure, which is a standard describing data formats, elements, and an application programming interface (API) for exchanging EHRs. FHIR facilitates the real-time exchange of data using web technology. FHIR can construct and deconstruct Clinical Document Architecture documents from various data sources and systems [13].

With FHIR as the standard format for cloud EHRs, patient-facing mobile applications and wearables, telemedicine platforms, analytics platforms, and care coordination systems, interoperability of healthcare applications has come to a new phase, by solving many problems associated with healthcare domain complexity, data modeling, medical data storage, and custom integrations with legacy systems that resulted in long development cycles and high costs.

One of the latest efforts in 2018 toward interoperability is the Argonaut Project, which is a private sector initiative to advance industry adoption of modern, open interoperability standards. The Argonaut Project aims to develop a first-generation FHIR-based API rapidly and Core Data Services specification to enable expanded information sharing for EHRs and other health information technology based on internet standards and architectural patterns and styles [14].

FAIR data exchange

One of the other grand challenges of data-intensive science is to facilitate knowledge discovery by—in an open structure—assisting humans and machines in their discovery of, access to, integration and analysis of task-appropriate scientific data and their associated algorithms and workflows. The aim of having open health data exchange may be twofold: on the one hand, facilitating transparency of the health sector effectiveness and, on the other hand, providing a valuable resource that can drive science, innovation, and outcome measurement.

To develop valuable and reliable AI applications, organizations often need access to massive training data sets (see also Chapter 11). Making predictive models requires enormous data sets, which is why tech giants like Facebook, Amazon, Microsoft, and Apple and China's Baidu, Alibaba, and Tencent are leaders in the field of AI. But for many other companies, obtaining these large data sets can be challenging. The rise of neural networks and natural language processing AI, such as GPT3, may pave the way toward novel technologies impacting how patients and healthcare providers interact with medical data and manage conditions.

Emerging blockchain companies have dived into this problem by reimagining internet services and access to decentralized data, proposing a way to create data marketplaces that democratize access to AI training data. These marketplaces would coordinate users offering their data with projects in need of it—and because the exchanges are on a blockchain, there are no middlemen handling files, ensuring that the shared data stays secure. More information on blockchains can be found in Chapter 16.

Because not all data being shared are curated, often it is not the lack of appropriate technology that creates the hurdle for developing smart AI tools; the reason more often is that digital objects do not receive the careful attention they deserve.

Therefore, in order to make data reusable and feasible for research, it is recommended to ensure that data comply as much as possible with the FAIR principles [15], which are as follows:

- Findable
- Accessible
- Interoperable
- Reusable

As of 2018, although in many healthcare institutions, the goal for large data integration exists, the key challenges for using and connecting health data sets are to

- ensure that personal data are confidential and protected;
- guarantee high quality and FAIR data;
- maintain control mechanisms for access;
- warrant data are used in an integral way; and
- make data useable for all.

Turning health data into knowledge

Connecting different data sets creates infrastructures that are set up for better dissemination of knowledge by making research data publicly available so that many research groups throughout the world can start working on them.

However, data must be turned into knowledge to use the information to make well-informed decisions. This requires standardization of information models as previously described, but also an approach for modeling of knowledge and knowledge-based processes. In these models, a consistent and systematic way is needed to deal with semantics, files, processes, and information modeling. Only with this structured approach can a SPoT for health data be created.

An interesting example in this respect is Health-RI in the Netherlands, whose goal is to bundle and connect a wide range of resources, including biobanks, IT technologies, facilities, and data collections, into one large-scale research infrastructure [16].

ⓘ The ICT backbone of Health-RI is largely built as a "life science and health workflow and data exchange," which supports seamless access, interoperability, reuse, and trust of data among all the resources contained within the infrastructure. Highly specialized reasoning algorithms help process data as part of migrating research workflows, making it possible to go beyond observation, theory, and simulation into exploration-driven science by mining new insights from vastly diverse data sets.

The Health-RI approach may eventually give pharmaceutical care providers access to data that will help produce more effective treatment evaluations.

Imagine the possibilities if a Health-RI-type initiative is ultimately linked to broader health-wellness-socioeconomic data sets, in which case even more extensive integrated research will be possible, such as calculating the actual societal benefits of drugs, as described in Chapter 3.

Considerations for future IoT uptake

While IoT devices clearly offer new benefits for healthcare provider organizations, adoption is lagging compared to other industries. In addition, healthcare system stakeholders still have several key concerns about the IoT, such as missing standards, inadequate security, difficult interoperability and compatibility, and the high cost of interlinking all devices.

The siloed ecosystem of many healthcare systems worldwide does not make the adoption of IoT devices easy, as most healthcare providers have their own goals and roles to play. Systems are not set up to create a fully uniform approach (e.g., in some countries, systems purposely adopt a free market strategy, which results in different providers competing for the same pot of software development money and thus potentially developing different ecosystems for the same purpose).

Getting them connected is not enough to achieve alignment in all the health optimization initiatives. The connectivity needs to do something more; it needs to add true value to the healthcare chain (the fifth "V" in the five dimensions). Suppose patients see the PHA as the holy grail to getting the best possible care and policymakers are convinced that this is the way to reduce waste and harm in the system. In that case, these factors may drive the pressure required to really achieve interoperability.

Privacy and security

In general, privacy and data protection and information security are complementary requirements for IoT services. In particular, information security is regarded as preserving information's confidentiality, integrity, and availability.

General information security requirements should apply for IoT; however, since IoT is more of a vision than a concrete technology, it is still difficult to properly define all the requirements. More information on the background of privacy and security with a focus on the healthcare industry can be found in Chapter 17 and the Appendix.

To conclude, one has to admit that the largest manmade "zest" is, to say the least, an impressive "thing" and will be followed closely in the coming years. Provided that mankind ensures the proper conditions, then IoT will be a zest for all the digital health technologies described in Chapters 9—16.

This means for blended pharmaceutical care:

- The IoT can be defined as a structure of interrelated mechanical and digital devices, objects, animals, and/or people.
- Data as such are only as valuable as the way they are used; therefore, the challenge is transforming big data into smart data.
- Data has five dimensions, volume, veracity, velocity, variety, and value, and in principle, they must be findable, attributable, interoperable, and reusable.
- Health data are tracked in many scattered databases, such as EHRs, pharmacy and paramedic databases, and decentralized digital tools.
- Connecting all these different health data sets may result in the integrated PHA, which is a 24/7—accessible, secure integrated environment with all personal health data from all providers, managed by the patient.
- A crucial factor for developing PHAs is standardization in data recording and facilitation of interoperability of healthcare applications, for instance, by the adoption of Health Level Seven-Fast Healthcare Interoperability Resource standards.
- Digital biomarker data are defined as consumer-generated physiological and behavioral data collected through connected digital tools.

References

[1] Berte D-R. Defining the IoT. In: Proceedings of the international conference on business excellence, vol 12; 2018. p. 118—28. https://doi.org/10.2478/picbe-2018-0013. Available from.

[2] Iske PL. Combinatoric innovation: Navigating a complex world. KnocoM; 2017. Available from, http://www.chairedelimmateriel.universite-paris-saclay.fr/wp-content/uploads/2012/06/3-IC8_Iske.pdf.

[3] Rydning DR-JG-J, Reinsel J, Gantz J. The digitization of the world from edge to core, vol 16. Framingham: International Data Corporation; 2018. Available from, https://www.seagate.com/files/www-content/our-story/trends/files/idc-seagate-dataage-whitepaper.pdf.

[4] Reinsel D. How you contribute to today's growing DataSphere and its enterprise impact. IDC; 2019. Available from, https://blogs.idc.com/2019/11/04/how-you-contribute-to-todays-growing-datasphere-and-its-enterprise-impact/.

[5] Marr B. How much data do we create every day? The Mind-Blowing Stats everyone should read. 2018 [cited 2023 28/01/2023]; Available from, https://www.forbes.com/sites/bernardmarr/2018/05/21/how-much-data-do-we-create-every-day-the-mind-blowing-stats-everyone-should-read.

[6] Agrawal R, Prabakaran S. Big data in digital healthcare: lessons learnt and recommendations for general practice. Heredity 2020;124(4):525—34. https://doi.org/10.1038/s41437-020-0303-2.

[7] Wang T, Azad T, Rajan R. The emerging influence of digital biomarkers on healthcare. 2016 [cited 2023 28/01/2023]; Available from, https://rockhealth.com/insights/the-emerging-influence-of-digital-biomarkers-on-healthcare/.

[8] Leff B, et al. Hospital at home: feasibility and outcomes of a program to provide hospital-level care at home for acutely ill older patients. Ann Intern Med 2005;143(11):798—808.

[9] Marr B. Why the internet of medical things (IoMT) will start to transform healthcare in 2018. 2018 [cited 2023 28/01/2023]; Available from: https://www.forbes.com/sites/bernardmarr/2018/01/25/why-the-internet-of-medical-things-iomt-will-start-to-transform-healthcare-in-2018.

[10] Madsen LB. Data-driven healthcare: how analytics and BI are transforming the industry. John Wiley & Sons; 2014.

[11] Minor L. Harnessing the power of data in health. Stanford Med Heal Trends Rep 2017. https://med.stanford.edu/content/dam/sm/sm-news/documents/StanfordMedicineHealthTrendsWhitePaper2017.pdf.

[12] HL-7. HL7. 2023 [cited 2023 28/01/2023]; Available from, https://www.hl7.org/.

[13] HL7-FHIR. HL7-FHIR. 2023 [cited 2023 28/01/2023]; Available from, https://www.hl7.org/fhir/.

[14] Argonaut. Argonaut project home. 2023 [cited 2023 28/01/2023]; Available from, https://confluence.hl7.org/display/AP/Argonaut+Project+Home.

[15] Wilkinson MD, et al. The FAIR Guiding Principles for scientific data management and stewardship. Scientific Data 2016;3(1):160018. https://doi.org/10.1038/sdata.2016.18.

[16] Health-RI. Health-RI. 2023 [cited 2023 28/01/2023]; Available from, https://www.health-ri.nl/.

[17] Romeo S, Corey T. Internet of health—Beecham research report. 2017. Available from, https://internetofbusiness.com/wp-content/uploads/2017/05/IoHEALTH-Market-Brief-17-Final.pdf.

CHAPTER 9

The spice rack of health apps*

Ravi Patel

University of Pittsburgh School of Pharmacy, Pittsburgh, PA, United States

> *My powers are extraordinary. Only my application brings me success.*
>
> *Isaac Newton*

Spices alone do not make for a tasty dish. They must complement features of dishes or cultural cuisine to come together on the palate. Finding the right mixture of spices cannot come from experience or practice alone. Patient engagement, clinical value, regulatory guidance, and reimbursement frameworks are all mixing in the dishes of health apps that more and more pharmaceutical care (PC) providers and finding in practice. Finding the right mixture of these "spices" in health apps will help complement the meal that is art and science of the digital revolution.

Technology

There are over 4.8 million apps available across the most popular operating systems. In 2022, Android held a 70% market share, and iOS held a 28% market share globally [1]. In each of the millions of apps between both the Android and iOS ecosystems, more than 350,000 of those apps are related to health and healthcare. While apps that support general wellness comprise most health-related apps, a growing number of apps focus on management or support of specific disease states or health behaviors. With the growing numbers of apps and lengthening time in existence, the evidence, regulations, and clinical utilization of apps have grown [2].

A mobile app is a computer program designed to run on a mobile device such as a smartphone or tablet computer. The term "app" is a short version of the term "software application." Since its inception, an entire industry has emerged to support the

---

*In this chapter, you will read about healthcare apps and their use in the pharmaceutical ecosystem. You will also learn how to decide which ones are relevant, safe, and secure for pharmaceutical care and how to develop a sustainable future for health apps.

Pharmaceutical Care in Digital Revolution. https://doi.org/10.1016/B978-0-443-13360-2.00016-2

use of mobile health technology. The launch of the iPhone in 2007 and the iTunes Appstore in 2008 helped the mobile phone become a channel for health information, communication, and interventions [3]. This Appstore connected developers of technology to the large population of smartphones users. As the adoption of the hardware and devices grew, so did apps' diversity, potential, and clinical relevance to influence health [4,5].

Categories of health apps

The roles of health apps mirror the variety of forms they take. Some categories can reflect the different forms, functions, and goals of health applications, including (adapted from Atluri et al. [6]) the following:

- **Quantified self and wellness** apps that help patients improve their lifestyle via behavioral tools (see Chapter 7)
- **Patient portals that serve** to facilitate services such as accessing disease and treatment information or functions such as scheduling (see Chapter 12).
- **Clinical transparency** related to clinical decisions supports an individualized, holistic health view (see Chapter 6).
- **Disease and/or deterioration prevention** to support both the maintenance and improvement of health
- **Transparency in healthcare** for processes and expenses and makes insurance flows easier.
- **Healthcare information apps** that disseminate research and professional knowledge to clinician population or patient populations in an easy and accessible way.
- **Digital therapeutic apps** that act as a classified healthcare intervention (see Chapter 15).

These multiple functions and goals have to compete with the need to integrate seamlessly with the devices used by patients and healthcare providers. Moreover, this integration must take place while still maintaining the dynamic interoperability standards and developing regulations (see Chapter 8).

Impact on pharmaceutical care activities

Health apps have had both indirect and direct impact on activities of PC (see Chapter 6). The impact of health apps can play a significant role across domains of activity of PC, including communication, data flow, and interventions.

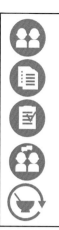

A. **Professional relationship between PCPs and patients:** Increasingly, information and communication flows via digital applications

B. **Adequate collection and recording of health data:** Apps allow for better insight of individual, 24/7 remotely obtained health data

C. **Review health data and provide adequate PC proposal:** This involves a broader health data spectrum for PC planning, one that specifies how to use health app data to optimize outcomes

D. **Patient alignment and facilitate execution of PC plan:** Use shared app data to augment human pharmaceutical support

E. **Circular management of PC plan:** Use optimized remote monitoring, with a focus on prevention and easier adjustment of the PC plan based on individual patient outcomes, retrieved via apps

Medical and pharmaceutical reference apps

The time it takes medical literature to double in quantity is shrinking rapidly [7]. This dynamic scientific landscape adds to the responsibility of PC providers to be "lifelong learners." When working with significant volumes of medical information, the challenge comes in curating and delivering appropriate references at appropriate times. PC providers engage with information such as medication dosing, practice guidelines, scientific literature, and news related to their practice. Apps have allowed medical and drug reference literature to be curated in its form of delivery. Platforms that were historically well established either in print or on the web have found a challenge and balancing their approaches. These references must either duplicate their efforts (in their historical format and in an app) or develop an asymmetric approach. Platforms such as Lexicomp, iPharmacy, and Micromedex have proved to be an advancement in the generation, curation, and delivery of medication information, updates, and continuing education. The span of information may include both education and clinical decision support. These functions differ significantly in the inputs of data and clinician users' needs. The current products, and the growing field of developing clinician decision support systems, must balance the exponential growth of scientific data and the growing variation of user needs. The present and future challenge for existing resources will be delivering timely information in a user-friendly manner. As these libraries struggle to define their role in a world shifting well away from paper and the growing functions of health apps, they will also find compounding challenges in balancing information curation and information delivery.

Medical records apps as gateways to patient information

The history of personal health records has demonstrated distinct challenges when coordinating patients and the health systems that serve them. As early as 2007, there have been various examples of approaches toward personal health record systems by companies such as Microsoft (2007, HealthVault) and Google (2008, Google Health). These products sought to enable patients' contribution, maintenance, or review of data such as activity history, medication lists, lab results, and clinical documents. These approaches by large companies to connect patient health data included attempts to engage with health systems when integrating data across large electronic health records. These attempts resulted in poor user experiences and limited adoption. Ultimately, these products were discontinued by 2011. The rise of the Fast Healthcare Interoperability Resource (FHIR) and planned adoption following 2019 requirements are suggested to drive further adoption of transferable patient records [8]. The growth of patient portals and connected devices raises the question of form factor preferences of web-based portals or apps when accessing records. While growing, the overall use of patient portals is often limited. Despite these low adoption rates, the use of portals may limit patients' use of health record apps and subsequently limit the impact of health record apps in PC settings. With these initial challenges to engaging patients through apps regarding health records, developing data standards will foster further potential opportunities. The Apple iOS 16 operating system includes the Health app. This app features functions that include means to track medications and receive alerts related to interactions [9]. As the apps that bridge consumer technologies and devices continue to grow in variety (see Chapter 7), the greater the importance and adoption of standards will facilitate sharing of records between patients and PC settings.

Apps in pharmacy workflow and prescription management

The roles of health apps include support of PC workflow. This impact extends to the experience of both healthcare professionals and patients. Apps that tie directly to workflow allow for prescription renewals to be set, as well as the potential option for communication with providers and insurance reimbursement. These functions still exist alongside legacy communication methods, including in-person interactions, phone calls, faxes, text messages, messaging platforms (such as WhatsApp), and website interactions (see Chapter 7). In an ideal setting, these various interactions remove administrative burdens from the workflow. In practice, these multiple channels may create variation, often lead to more complex and challenging workflow variations. For example, patient interactions with interactive voice response systems have led to changes in how patients frame their interactions via phone.

Similarly, apps that directly connect patients to their pharmacy records systems (see Chapter 12) or facilitate the renewal of prescriptions can change how patients leverage their mobile devices to interact with them. Health systems are growing sources of apps developed for a variety of functions specific to their workflows or clinical needs in that health system [10]. Some direct impact on workflow includes apps such as Pilleye (from

Medility Inc, based in Korea) which leverages a cellphone or tablet computer to support counting in a dispensing workflow. As pharmacies balance their own workflow optimization, they will continue to face the challenge and opportunity to find, implement, assess, and scale the use of apps as directed by local needs, constraints, and resources.

Disease management apps

The potential benefits of health apps seem particularly compelling for managing chronic conditions such as chronic obstructive pulmonary disease (COPD), heart failure, diabetes, and hypertension, from which, in 2030, about half the global population is expected to suffer. Using a disease management app, patients regularly monitor their vital signs (generally, blood pressure, blood glucose, and weight), other specific symptoms, and their adherence to taking medications on time. Using such apps results in an earlier awareness of health issues and less need for a physician's support.

Also, in complex manageable, multifactor diseases, like oncological and orphan disorders, structured guidance in disease-specific apps may provide relief in both logistics and the knowledge level of patients, caregivers, and providers.

The technology for these chronic disease management apps offers both breadth and depth of impact on disease state management. Many supportive apps for each part of the patient pathway (as described in Chapter 7) have been developed. Often, country-level overviews of the top-rated apps in specific disease areas are available.

An abundance of adherence improvement apps

When the mobile phone was introduced, the pharmaceutical sector sent reminder SMS (Short Message Service) messages to improve adherence to drug treatment profiles. In practice, those reminder services might have been valuable for individual patients or certain disease areas, but research shows mixed outcomes when such services are used as standalone interventions. A review of adherence across apps found some modest positive trends, but the longevity of the adherence behavior and impact on health-related outcomes remains limited [11−15].

With the availability of smart mobile data platforms that allow devices to directly connect to the internet (such as 5G connections), intuitive apps now empower patients to self-manage their medication regimens and appointment schedules from their mobile and tablet devices. When connected to cloud-based platforms, these technologies allow healthcare providers to communicate with patients to clarify their understanding of conditions, complex drug regimens, and potential side effects; likewise, patients can more easily connect with healthcare providers about questions, suggestions, and so on.

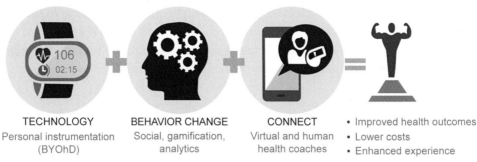

Figure 9.1
Optimal adherence environment [16a].

On the other hand, when setting up a digital adherence improvement program, we know that it is preferable to build a connected adherence ecosystem that is a multifaceted combination of a digital tracking and alerting device, a behavioral modification app, and a connected (human) healthcare environment [16].

Fig. 9.1 shows what an ideal integrated adherence environment looks like.

The development of applications and devices to improve drug adherence has come from both big corporate organizations and startups. These solutions make adherence support easier, and they often link the data directly into electronic pharmacy records to allow for timely and appropriate ordering of refills, checking on contraindications, and making the management of chronic conditions much less complex.

The adherence apps take a variety of different approaches to improve adherence to adequate drug use and address both intentional and unintentional nonadherence (refer to Chapter 6 for classification of adherence problems).

Some examples of action profiles of adherence apps are

QR Code 9.1
Example of medication adherence innovation.

- preferred adherence pattern built into a serious game (refer to Chapter 7 for more info on gamification);
- explanation of set-up and interaction with smart dispenser or adherence device to reduce confusion (see also QR Code 9.1);
- calendar-based alarm notifications via mobile device apps as well as health wearables and virtual personal assistants (see Chapter 12);
- avatars (as well as robots) that support adequate drug intake; and
- remote quality of life measurement after dose intake.

As noted, different applications can be used in parallel in a multifaceted approach and may create synergy in outcomes. While features offer the tailored functions patients prefer in care, the technical difficulties account for negative user experiences that may limit adoption or long-term use [17].

ⓘ Many informal and scientific studies seek to review the hundreds of adherence apps. Some reviews find a high-scoring evaluation of Medisafe, MyTherapy, Dosecast, and SwissMeds. While favorably scored, the limitations of regulations, security, or long-term impact limit recommendations by providers in practice [18].

Considerations

In the spice rack of health applications, it is easy to get lost, as the example box of the dilemma of pharmacists reflects. Nevertheless, PC providers can play an essential role in selecting and offering digital services that really matter to patients. Providers may decide to build their own apps (that meet all the requirements) or choose the best one available (certified and warranted) via one of the many online providers. Following are a couple of important considerations to increase the likelihood a health app's data will have real value in the PC process.

App dilemmas of pharmacists

Suppose a community pharmacy has about 10,000 patients registered. Hypothetically, the number of diseases covered by these patients may be about 130.

Now assume that all these individual patients have different apps to manage their disease. All these apps are requested to be linked to or integrated within the pharmacy information system to allow health data synergy, as described previously.

The dilemma occurs: Is the pharmacist responsible for ensuring the app data are reliable and securely stored? And would they need to check timely updates of the app? Who is responsible for organizing connectivity and compatibility?

And what if the cohort of COPD patients in this pharmacy wants to use 10 different refill-ordering apps or 15 different COPD medication support apps?

What knowledge level does a pharmacist need in regard to all these apps?

Responsibility for connecting and working with health apps

PC providers are confronted with prescription drugs from many different companies, regardless of whether they are active in a hospital or in a retail pharmacy. Often, due to the nonharmonization of apps, a new app connected to an individual product is introduced nearly every time a new drug is dispensed, frequently with different levels of connectivity with the individual patients' devices as well as with prevailing pharmacy software [19].

In addition, patients may be enthusiastic about the health apps they are using and request that their data are linked to the electronic pharmacy records, as described in the example box.

 This brings a number of questions that the PC provider needs to consider:

- Does the app **comply with privacy, quality, and security** regulations, as referred to in Chapter 17, and is the **informed consent** process transparent for both the patient and the provider?
- Does the app gather data that are **FAIR** for researching and augmenting electronic pharmacy records (as indicated in Chapter 8)?
- Is the app **interoperable** with the pharmacy information system; for example, is data transfer HL7-FHIR-standardized?

These considerations must incorporate an awareness of the app's content, the technological conditions a specific app should meet, the health app's validation, and the potential availability of alternatives.

The following sections and subsequent chapters will help provide some of the answers, but in general, a systematic approach to adopting and advising on the merits of health apps will face further development needs and challenges across variations in regulations as they further develop.

Assessing the quality of a health app

QR Code 9.2

Example of an app library that provides resources for patients and clinician.

The number of apps has spawned the creation of assessment frameworks to help patients, caregivers, and healthcare professional users navigate the challenges of interpreting quality. Health app review platforms target user segments to review and assess available health apps and rate their feasibility for use (QR Code 9.2). Formal frameworks for assessment have been developed in scientific settings, by regulatory authorities, and through industry collaborations. While harmonizing approaches to creating standards has been progressing, the still-developing road to success has encountered many barriers.

Notable progression of platforms included the National Health Service of the United Kingdom, which once offered a Library of apps in a central resource. This library was decommissioned at the end of 2021. Now, recommended apps are centralized through the

National Health Service (NHS) website or within the NHS app [20]. The development of standards such as the CEN ISO/TS 82304-2, published in 2021, outlines requirements for quality and defines the quality label to visualize the quality and reliability of health apps [21,22]. Platforms and frameworks may focus on disease areas and may use subjective review input from patients and healthcare providers. Other platforms incorporate a multifaceted, robust examination of quantifiable evidence and data.

Elements that are considered in app review processes are

- the rationale for why an app was developed and whether it aims to improve patient outcomes;
- compliance with global and local standards and regulations on privacy, quality, and security (see Chapter 17 for more information);
- functionality with regard to the purpose;
- evidence base and transparency of their algorithms; and
- level of user-friendliness and ease of integration in a disease management program.

Examples of app review platforms and frameworks

 The global list of review platforms and medical app checklists is too extensive to include in this chapter, but here are some inspirational examples:

- Orcha: www.orcha.co.uk (UK, provider of health and care app reviews and assessments).
- iMedicalApps: www.imedicalapps.com (US, a platform that provides reviews, research, and commentary by health professionals).
- Health Navigator: www.healthnavigator.org.nz/app-library (NZ, peer-reviewed recommendations by medical experts).
- Xcertia: mHealth App Guidelines https://www.himss.org/sites/hde/files/media/file/2020/04/17/xcertia-guidelines-2019-final.pdf (US, developed and disseminate mHealth app guidelines in 2020).
- Digital Health Assessment Framework: https://dhealthframework.org/ (US, open framework for adoption of health technologies)
- mHealthBelgium: https://mhealthbelgium.be/apps (BE, library of apps available via the national platform)
- American Psychiatric Association App Evaluation model: https://www.psychiatry.org/psychiatrists/practice/mental-health-apps/the-app-evaluation-model
- ISO/TS 82304-2:2021 https://www.iso.org/standard/78182.html (Standards to define a health app quality label, free abstract, paid full access)

In addition to evaluating content on the online review platforms, before making recommendations to patients, healthcare providers are advised to perform a thorough, structured approach to determining which health app is most appropriate for a given patient, as follows [23]:

- Review scientific literature, if available.
- Search app clearinghouse websites for potential certification details.
- Search app stores on availability.
- Evaluate app descriptions, user ratings, and review platforms.
- Conduct a social media query within the profession and, if available, patient networks.
- Pilot the app within your own environment.
- Elicit user feedback from patients.

Certification of healthcare apps

There has been a recent growth in the number of health apps, often used in clinical programs or as digital therapeutics (see Chapter 15), that are certified and validated. As global bodies and regulatory frameworks grow to incorporate dynamic criteria of patient needs, the need for evidence of function and safety can be more clearly assessed compared to past app review frameworks. This certification process can include clinical trials and is often considered expensive and time consuming. Most apps do not yet (have to) follow a single constrained regulatory process, depending on their function. Many countries now have regulations that specify how apps must be registered and whether they need to have a CE mark or certification.

In the EU, the Medical Device Regulations of 2020 set forth more stringent regulations than previous criteria addressing health apps. The definition of a medical device requires an assessment of the use of an app as a standalone (compared to use with a device), documentation requirements of clinical evaluation, and technical documentation [24]. The Food and Drug Administration (FDA) revised its guidance on regulating health apps and apps that can function as medical devices in February 2015. The FDA looked to take a tailored, risk-based approach to focus on the small subset of mobile apps that met the regulatory definition of "device" and intended to be used as an accessory to a regulated medical device or that transform a mobile platform into a regulated medical device [25]. In 2017, the FDA announced that it had chosen nine companies out of more than 100 for its Software Precertification (Pre-Cert) program. The primary goal of this program was to support the development of a regulatory model that assesses the safety and effectiveness of software technologies without inhibiting patients' quick access to these technologies [26]. This model took on significant challenges, leading the agency to conclude that it was "not practical to implement" in the current authority in 2022. Future regulation and oversight related to software as a medical device are expected from the Digital Health Center of Excellence within the Center for Devices and Radiological Health (CDRH), formed in 2020, and the Medical Device Innovation Consortium [27]. Further discussion of these definitions of a medical device, when specific regulations are in place, is explained in Chapter 17.

⚠ An additional complexity is how a healthcare provider monitors the maintenance and use of an app after it has been recommended and patients use it. As discussed in Chapter 6, digital PC implies that the provider is responsible for adequate use of drugs and the tools to accomplish this. That begs the question: who is responsible or even liable if errors occur during usage or, for example, if updating of the health app is ignored, which means that the app can no longer be used in a secure and quality-warranted way (with the possibility of pharmaceutical emergencies being missed)? Responsibility probably should rest jointly with the app manufacturer, the healthcare provider, and the end user. Such questions require that new legal frameworks be developed. Initial libraries and platforms have found some adoption in Europe. As these systems come up against the constraints of real-world application, the iterations of these systems will hold new approaches to the dilemmas presented locally and globally.

Much more information on regulating digital health technology can be found in Chapter 17 and the Appendix.

Are apps as effective as they promise?

Although many apps promise to support patients and improve outcomes, a significant number of versions still seem to have basic technological flaws. In 2015, after evaluating more than 400 apps and user-testing 100 of the best-rated ones, researchers noted that nearly 25% of the top-scoring adherence apps could not mitigate a basic nonadherence function (like issuing a medication reminder), could not be installed by a student healthcare professional, or had other barriers to appropriate use (e.g., compatibility issues) [28]. Beyond these initial challenges to user onboarding, the structure of apps to facilitate meaningful change may underutilize behavioral models. One review of 166 apps found that only 12 of 96 potential behavioral techniques were present. This review demonstrated limited use of established behavior change techniques used in medication adherence apps [29]. Even with the addition of more rigorous evaluation, another systematic review and metaanalysis of 172 studies found that there is a weak positive outcome for the use of apps, but the evidence of long-term impact is limited. The notable gap between the evidence to demonstrate the ability to improve health-related outcomes is made even more evident by the variation in intervention and limited consistency applied to define outcomes across disease states [30]. Challenging the progress of efficacy is the complementing challenge of regulatory oversight that may be generalized in the development progress and punitive in identifying potential inaccuracy or risk of harm. The United States Federal Trade Commissions provides best practices regarding advertising, claims, and data security [31]. A number of apps have faced fines and removal based on these criteria [32].

Reimbursement of apps

It is obvious that health apps have not yet lived up to their full potential, which relates not only to efficacy but also to the reimbursement systems in which they exist. Digital health apps are difficult to sell directly to patients; thus, the leading buyers are providers (health systems or primary care practices) or payers (self-insured employers or health insurers). Yet payers worry that patients will not use these apps as regularly as required to manage their disease effectively, so outcomes may be suboptimal.

To succeed under these circumstances, health app developers must first consider who their technologies' primary (that is, paying) customers will be [33]. They may then develop an approach to ensure that a customer's willingness to adopt an app also translates into sustained use of the app and results in relevant clinical outcomes. Moreover, as long as many healthcare systems face a predominant fee-for-service reimbursement system that pays substantially more for seeing a patient in person than for managing care electronically and remotely, adopting remote app technology may also be hindered.

New regulatory and reimbursement models have been introduced in various national settings. Through Germany's Digital Healthcare Act in 2019, the digital health application category (DiGA) was introduced [34]. In 2022, more than 30 applications were included on the registry as a mix of permanent and preliminary listings. In this framework of review, registration, and reimbursement, the value of a simplified pathway is balanced by a need for evidence reporting, return on cost for values, and outcomes beyond controlled settings [35]. Similarly, Belgium adopted a national framework that established an approach for evaluating and reimbursing apps through the mHealthBELGIUM platform. As these national platforms find their initial adoptions, the question of pricing and standardization across multiple countries may guide future reimbursements for health-related apps [36].

In conclusion, we can say that the spice rack of apps is becoming more passable, but there are still sufficient challenges in this dense environment. So for now, there is a vision of a race between the tech giants, in which each tries to come up with the ultimate app, a single program that everyone will find incredibly easy to use and that will do everything we want it to do.

In the next Chapter 10, one can read how data from wearables are converted to useable information in apps.

This means for blended pharmaceutical care:

- Health apps can have different objectives, scopes, and functions, such as supporting the quantifying self, disease self-management, clinical transparency, holistic health overview, disease prevention, disease insight, financial transparency, and provision of professional background knowledge.
- Before recommending a health app to patients, a care provider is advised to use a structured approach and assess the app's privacy, quality, security, and feasibility level.
- Globally, app platforms and developing frameworks are growing as resources that offer insights in validating health apps.
- Authorities are continuing to develop regulations to certify app software as medical devices. Some broad and progressing examples are expected to help define pathways for regulation and reimbursement to align in the upcoming years.
- More research is required to determine the true cost-effectiveness of health apps and define the alignment of value these apps offer clinically and financially

References

[1] StatCounter. Mobile operating systems' market share worldwide from 1st quarter 2009 to 4th quarter 2022. Chart. 2023. Available from: https://www.statista.com/statistics/272698/global-market-share-held-by-mobile-operating-systems-since-2009/.

[2] Aitken M, Nass D. Digital health trends 2021: innovation, evidence, regulation, and adoption. Slideshare; 2021. https://www.slideshare.net/RicardoCaabate/digital-health-trends-2021-iqvia-global. [Accessed 8 June 2022].

[3] Ventola CL. Mobile devices and apps for health care professionals: uses and benefits. Pharm Ther 2014;39(5):356−64.

[4] Fiordelli M, Diviani N, Schulz PJ. Mapping mHealth research: a decade of evolution. J Med Internet Res 2013;15(5):e95. https://doi.org/10.2196/jmir.2430.

[5] Lee G, Raghu TS. Determinants of mobile apps' success: evidence from the app store market. J Manag Inf Syst 2014;31(2):133−70. https://doi.org/10.2753/mis0742-1222310206.

[6] Atluri V, et al. How tech-enabled consumers are reordering the healthcare landscape. McKinsey & Company; 2016.

[7] Bornmann L, Mutz R. Growth rates of modern science: a bibliometric analysis based on the number of publications and cited references. J Assoc Inf Sci Technol 2015;66(11):2215−22. https://doi.org/10.1002/asi.23329.

[8] Dameff C, Clay B, Longhurst CA. Personal health records: more promising in the smartphone era? JAMA 2019;321(4):339−40.

[9] Inc, A.. See more of yourself in health. 2023. Available from: https://www.apple.com/ios/health/. [Accessed 31 January 2023].

[10] Lieser T, Huang Y, Sezgin E. The current state of mobile apps owned by large pediatric hospitals in the United States: systematic search and analysis on Google play and Apple app stores. JMIR Pediatr Parent 2022;5(4):e38940. https://doi.org/10.2196/38940.

[11] Armitage LC, Kassavou A, Sutton S. Do mobile device apps designed to support medication adherence demonstrate efficacy? A systematic review of randomised controlled trials, with meta-analysis. BMJ Open 2020;10(1):e032045. https://doi.org/10.1136/bmjopen-2019-032045.

[12] Kashgary A, et al. The role of mobile devices in doctor-patient communication: a systematic review and meta-analysis. J Telemed Telecare 2017;23(8):693−700.

[13] Kenyon CC, et al. Controller adherence following hospital discharge in high risk children: a pilot randomized trial of text message reminders. J Asthma 2019;56(1):95−103. https://doi.org/10.1080/02770903.2018.1424195.

[14] Pérez-Jover V, et al. Mobile apps for increasing treatment adherence: systematic review. J Med Internet Res 2019;21(6):e12505. https://doi.org/10.2196/12505.

[15] Tao D, et al. A meta-analysis of the use of electronic reminders for patient adherence to medication in chronic disease care. J Telemed Telecare 2015;21(1):3−13.

[16] Choudhry NK, et al. Effect of reminder devices on medication adherence. JAMA Intern Med 2017;177(5):624. https://doi.org/10.1001/jamainternmed.2016.9627.

[16a] Cognizant. 2016. Medication adherence in the real world. Available from: https://www.slideshare.net/cognizant/medication-adherence-in-the-real-world-63632949. [Accessed 3 May 2018].

[17] Park JYE, et al. Mobile phone apps targeting medication adherence: quality assessment and content analysis of user reviews. JMIR mHealth uHealth 2019;7(1):e11919. https://doi.org/10.2196/11919.

[18] Backes C, et al. Digital medication adherence support: could healthcare providers recommend mobile health apps? Front Med Technol 2020;2:616242.

[19] Loiselle CG, Ahmed S. Is connected health contributing to a healthier population? J Med Internet Res 2017;19(11):e386. https://doi.org/10.2196/jmir.8309.

[20] NHS. NHS app library. 2022. Available from: https://digital.nhs.uk/services/nhs-apps-library. [Accessed 5 November 2022].

[21] Essén A, et al. Health app policy: international comparison of nine countries' approaches. Npj Digit Med 2022;5(1). https://doi.org/10.1038/s41746-022-00573-1.

[22] ISO. ISO/TS 82304-2:2021 Health software—part 2: health and wellness apps—quality and reliability. 2023. Available from: https://www.iso.org/standard/78182.html. [Accessed 31 January 2023].

[23] Boudreaux ED, et al. Evaluating and selecting mobile health apps: strategies for healthcare providers and healthcare organizations. Transl Behav Med 2014;4(4):363−71.

[24] Keutzer L, Simonsson US. Medical device apps: an introduction to regulatory affairs for developers. JMIR mHealth uHealth 2020;8(6):e17567. https://doi.org/10.2196/17567.

[25] FDA. General wellness: policy for low risk devices draft guidance for industry and food and drug administration staff. 2019. Available from: https://www.fda.gov/downloads/Training/CDRHLearn/UCM569275.pdf.

[26] FDA. Digital health software precertification pilot program; 2017. Available from: https://www.fda.gov/media/106563/download. [Accessed 3 March 2023].

[27] FDA. The software precertification (Pre-Cert) pilot program: tailored total product lifecycle approaches and key findings. 2022. Available from: https://www.fda.gov/media/161815/download.

[28] Heldenbrand S, et al. Assessment of medication adherence app features, functionality, and health literacy level and the creation of a searchable web-based adherence app resource for health care professionals and patients. J Am Pharm Assoc 2016;56(3):293−302.

[29] Morrissey EC, et al. Behavior change techniques in apps for medication adherence: a content analysis. Am J Prev Med 2016;50(5):e143−6.

[30] Iribarren SJ, et al. Effectiveness of mobile apps to promote health and manage disease: systematic review and meta-analysis of randomized controlled trials. JMIR mHealth uHealth 2021;9(1):e21563. https://doi.org/10.2196/21563.

[31] Commission FT. Mobile health app developers: FTC best practices. 2016.

[32] Dy Aungst T. How to evaluate a mobile app and advise your patient about it? Springer International Publishing; 2023. p. 149−61. https://doi.org/10.1007/978-3-031-10698-9_9.

[33] Huckman R, Stern A. Why apps for managing chronic disease haven't been widely used, and how to fix it. Harv Bus Rev 2018.

[34] Stern AD, et al. Advancing digital health applications: priorities for innovation in real-world evidence generation. Lancet Dig Health 2022;4(3):e200−6.

[35] Lantzsch H, et al. Digital health applications and the fast-track pathway to public health coverage in Germany: challenges and opportunities based on first results. BMC Health Serv Res 2022;22(1). https://doi.org/10.1186/s12913-022-08500-6.

[36] Schudt F, et al. A comparative overview of digital health applications between Belgium and Germany. Curr Dir Biomed Eng 2022;8(2):509−11.

CHAPTER 10

Infusing wearables *

Claudia Rijcken
Pharmi, Maastricht, The Netherlands

I have no doubt that in the future, wearable devices like Fitbit will know my blood pressure, hydration levels and blood sugar levels as well. All of this data has the potential to transform modern medicine and create a whole new era of personalized care.

Michael Dell

The integration of wearable devices with healthcare can revolutionize how medical conditions are diagnosed, monitored, and treated. Infusions in cooking and healthcare wearables can be compared to the process of steeping tea leaves. Just as steeping tea leaves in hot water extracts the flavor and benefits of the tea, healthcare wearables "steep" in a patient's daily life, extracting valuable health data and information.

"Like" different tea leaves can be combined to create unique blends with various flavors and benefits, data from wearable devices can be combined and integrated to create a comprehensive health picture. The end result of both infusion processes is a flavorful and beneficial outcome. In cooking, the infused liquid becomes a tasty beverage, while in healthcare, the extracted health data become a valuable tool for improved patient care and outcomes.

Technology

Wearables are smart electronic devices with microcontrollers that can be worn on the body, in clothing, in accessories, and even in tattoos. Wearable devices provide an alternative pathway to clinical diagnostics by exploiting various physical, chemical, and biological sensors to mine physiological (biophysical and/or biochemical) information in real time (preferably continuously) and in a noninvasive or minimally invasive manner [1].

---

*In this chapter, you will read about how digital biomarker data are mapping the status of the human body with wearables and insideables, you will learn how this broad range of health parameters can augment pharmaceutical care, and what are the vital conditions required to integrate these digital biomarkers successfully in pharmaceutical care.

Pharmaceutical Care in Digital Revolution. https://doi.org/10.1016/B978-0-443-13360-2.00013-7

Global end-user spending on wearable devices is expected to amount to about 81.5 billion US dollars in 2021, with forecasts suggesting that the spending will reach more than 90 billion dollars by 2022. Smartwatches, head-mounted displays, and ear-worn devices are the products that lead the growth of the market. The wearables market also includes wristbands, smart clothing, and smart patches [2].

The first wearables were sports bracelets and fitness trackers, which essentially were a sort of advanced pedometer for counting steps. The bracelets allowed individuals to track data like the number of steps taken, distance traveled, calories burned, and sleep patterns.

Integrating these assessments within a smartwatch opened up opportunities for improved user experience. Many more features have been added, including, for example, GPS linking, detection of abnormal heart rate, blood pressure, and sleeping pattern.

ⓘ Other examples of innovative wearables are orthopedic wearables that determine walking patterns, earbuds that measure temperature, and a smart ovulation tracking bracelet that provides real-time detection of a woman's 5.3-day fertile period and also rehabilitation gloves to reduce joint stiffness due to rheumatoid arthritis, headbands to enhance the effectiveness of meditation, and devices that measure stress levels via the skin pores on our fingertips.

In the future, wearable devices are expected to become much more sophisticated, with the ability to continuously monitor multiple health parameters simultaneously and provide real-time data to healthcare providers. Medical wearables collect body metric−derived so-called digital biomarkers (for definition, see Chapter 8). As such, the devices can help prevent disease and can monitor specific diseases, particularly chronic diseases such as Parkinson's, dementia, chronic obstructive pulmonary disease, cancer, and heart failure; they can, for example, also monitor pain management and improve early intervention. The efficacy of medical-grade devices is being intensively studied, as they must undergo thorough clinical research and meet strict regulatory requirements, which we address in Chapter 17 [3].

Another area of growth for wearable technology in healthcare is telemedicine. Wearables equipped with cameras, microphones, and sensors can allow for remote consultations with healthcare providers, enabling patients to receive medical care from their homes.

Thus, wearables, in the meantime, have advanced far beyond wellness tracking. Fig. 10.1 exemplifies the evolution of the wearable ecosystem up till the assessments that can be measured in today's world.

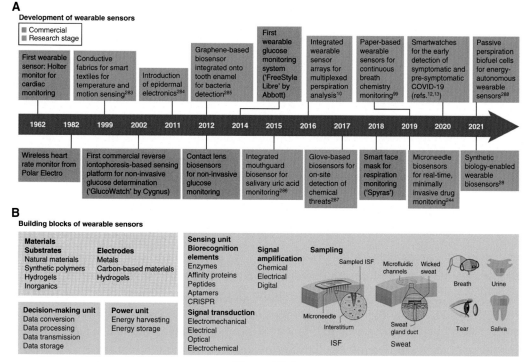

Figure 10.1

The evolution of wearables. A) Development of wearable sensors. B) The building blocks of wearable sensors. *Source: https://www.nature.com/articles/s41578-022-00460-x*

 Here are some of the concrete benefits derived from using health wearables:

- **Continuous and convenient health insights**: Health wearables allow for continuous monitoring of vital signs, physical activity, and other key health parameters, providing real-time data that are accessible and actionable at any time.

- **Personalized disease management**: For individuals with chronic conditions, health wearables can provide customized insights and guidance for managing the condition, leading to better health outcomes and improved quality of life.

- **Promoting healthy habits**: By tracking physical activity and sleep patterns, health wearables can provide feedback and motivation to help individuals develop and maintain healthy habits, leading to improved overall health and wellness.

- **Early health issue detection**: By continuously monitoring health data, health wearables can detect potential health issues early on, enabling earlier intervention and treatment.

- **Empowering self-care**: By providing access to health information and allowing for remote consultations with healthcare providers, health wearables empower individuals to control their health and well-being.

- **Streamlined healthcare delivery**: By providing real-time health data, health wearables can improve the efficiency of healthcare delivery and reduce the burden on healthcare providers and the healthcare system as a whole.

Insideables and implantables

Technological advancements do not end with devices worn on the body. So-called insideables and implantables—i.e., microcomputers that function inside the body—are being developed specifically for medical applications. So far, smart implants have mainly been used to support the function of organs such as the inner ear, heart, or brain. In addition, scientists are developing models that improve the healing process in complex bone fractures, for example, as well as microchips that monitor values such as blood glucose levels directly under the skin.

Also, smart pills, sometimes called "insideables," are already in advanced testing stages. They are swallowed in the form of a hard capsule to send measured values or images, for example, of the intestinal flora, directly from the digestive tract. Researchers are also working on using smart implants to automatically dose active ingredients in the body or monitor the intake of medications in this way. Since implantables and insideables are only just emerging, they will dominate healthcare trends even more in the future.

Insideables: Digital pills

The first drug with an ingestible sensor was "Abilify MyCite," a product developed by Otsuka Pharmaceutical Co. and Proteus Digital Health. It is an ingestible sensor-based medication management system designed to help improve patient compliance with their medication regimen. The system consists of an ingestible sensor that is embedded within a medication tablet, which sends information to a wearable patch worn by the patient. The patch then transmits the information to a mobile application, allowing both the patient and their healthcare provider to track medication ingestion and monitor adherence to the prescribed regimen. Abilify MyCite was approved by the US Food and Drug Administration (FDA) in 2017 and is intended for individuals with schizophrenia, bipolar I disorder, and depression.

Otsuka withdrew the marketing application in Europe after the European Medicines Agency (EMA) informed the company it had some concerns. Its provisional opinion was that Abilify MyCite could not have been authorized in patients with schizophrenia and bipolar I disorder.

The EMA said in a document: "The agency could not assess how well the tablet with the integrated sensor, the patch, and the app work together as only limited aspects of usability and technical performance were investigated.

"There was not sufficient evidence that Abilify MyCite is able to reliably measure the intake of the medicine in the target population."

Insideables: Digital pills—cont'd

It added: "From a safety point of view, there is a risk the patient could take too many doses because the digital medicine system may not work reliably. In addition, the patch can cause skin and subcutaneous tissue reactions" [4].

In the United States, the product is available in 2023 to treat different psychiatric disorders [5]. Yet, despite the landmark FDA approval, digital pills have not exploded in pharma. Privacy and logistical concerns have lingered, especially while studying such applications for vulnerable populations.

Implantables

An implantable device is a medical device designed to be surgically placed inside the body and left in place for an extended period, typically for therapeutic purposes. Implantable devices can range from simple devices such as pacemakers and defibrillators, which regulate heart rhythm, to more complex devices such as artificial joints, cochlear implants, and spinal cord stimulators, which can help to manage various conditions and improve quality of life.

Implantable devices can offer a number of advantages over other types of medical devices, including more precise control of the therapy being delivered, improved convenience and comfort for the patient, and the ability to monitor and adjust therapy in real time. However, implantable devices also have some risks and limitations, including the need for surgery to insert the device, the potential for complications or adverse reactions, and the need for ongoing maintenance and monitoring.

An interesting example of an implantable is AngelMed Guardian, the first and only FDA-approved heart-attack warning system. Guardian is indicated for use in patients who have had prior acute coronary syndrome events, including heart attacks, and who remain at high risk for recurrent events. In addition, Guardian offers continuous monitoring and detection of abnormal changes in heart activity, including silent heart attacks.

It immediately alerts to a heart attack onset and provides an emergency alarm comprising a loud beeping, red flashing light, and a vibration in the chest indicating one should call emergency and be transported to an ER. Speed-to-ER can save a life. In the ALERTS study, Guardian patients arrived at the ER with a median time that was 5.7 h earlier when compared to relying on symptoms alone [6].

As we know that a number of medications may cause potentially harmful ST-segment elevation (as a side effect due, e.g., to hyperkalemia), concomitant use of a cardiac insideable for high-risk profile patients may effectively alert patients and providers before serious adverse cardiac events occur, a concept that fits optimally into a preventative, circular pharmaceutical care model.

Impact on core responsibilities in pharmaceutical care

Using data from wearables and insideables may provide insight into the data of how the body is responding to a medication intervention, thus, on the safety and efficacy of the medication.

It may allow pharmaceutical care providers to assess more real-world data that are representative of patients' responses to medication and general quality of life.

Here is the general impact that wearables and insideables are expected to have on the five domains of pharmaceutical care provision (refer to Chapter 6 for a more detailed discussion).

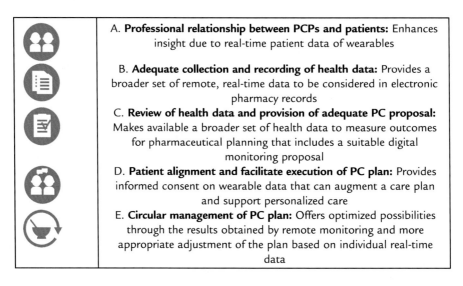

A. **Professional relationship between PCPs and patients:** Enhances insight due to real-time patient data of wearables

B. **Adequate collection and recording of health data:** Provides a broader set of remote, real-time data to be considered in electronic pharmacy records

C. **Review of health data and provision of adequate PC proposal:** Makes available a broader set of health data to measure outcomes for pharmaceutical planning that includes a suitable digital monitoring proposal

D. **Patient alignment and facilitate execution of PC plan:** Provides informed consent on wearable data that can augment a care plan and support personalized care

E. **Circular management of PC plan:** Offers optimized possibilities through the results obtained by remote monitoring and more appropriate adjustment of the plan based on individual real-time data

Implementation in daily practice

As with health apps, wearable and insideable devices are meaningless without the applicable use of the data collected. The use of dynamic APIs and powerful artificial intelligence, health metrics from multiple wearable devices connected in a personal health application with, among others, hospital and pharmacy data could provide valuable insight into patients' health and disease status. Individual data can also be compared against anonymous averages of millions of people with the same characteristics (e.g., age, gender, and genetic predispositions), thus creating the possibility for a clinical benchmark.

Because more people are tracking different data with regard to their health, many healthcare providers and organizations are seeking how to leverage wearable data best to help guide and augment their clinical care practices.

In Chapter 3, we already reflected on the concept of "The Quantified Self," which is characterized by the use of technology to acquire data on various aspects of a person's daily life, including those related to input (food consumption, quality of surrounding air), state (mood, arousal, blood oxygen levels), and health, whether mental, physical, or social. Moreover, these data are often tracked via wearables or home robotics. The Quantified Self movement is still active in 2023. Nevertheless, the principle has somewhat shifted toward the concept of the Digital Twin. See QR Code 10.1 for an explanation of the promise the digital twin concept brings to healthcare.

QR Code 10.1
Applications of digital twin to transform the healthcare industry.

A digital twin is a virtual representation of a physical object, system, or process created using data from sensors and other sources. It is composed of the following three elements:

- a physical entity in real space;
- the digital twin in software form; and
- data that links the first two elements together.

Digital twins can be used to model and simulate real-world scenarios and conditions. For example, digital twins can be used in healthcare to model and simulate the human body, allowing healthcare providers to understand a patient's health better and develop personalized treatment plans.

For example, a digital twin of a patient's heart could be created using data from imaging scans and other diagnostic tests (and data from wearables) and then used to simulate the effects of various treatments or to predict the likelihood of certain conditions, such as heart disease.

In general, digital twins offer a number of benefits, including improved accuracy, reduced costs, increased efficiency, and the ability to make more informed decisions. However, it is important to note that digital twins are not a replacement for real-world testing and validation and that their accuracy and usefulness are highly dependent on the quality and completeness of the data used to create them. Thus, understanding the quality of the health wearable used is an important aspect to be taken into account when striving to use digital biomarker data from wearables.

Pharmaceutical care providers as consultants on the use of health wearables

In a landscape filled with thousands of health wearables, it is difficult to determine which ones meet the requirement to strategically augment a pharmaceutical care plan and provide reliable, specific, and sensitive health data. With patient stratification being central to emerging concepts such as precision medicine and population health management, providers need a better understanding of the wide range of regulated and clinically vetted wearable technologies that can seamlessly capture reliable vital signs and selectively package the wearables most critical for the management of specific diseases.

There are still limited databases or oversights that depict and compare health wearables and provide a structured review, as is increasingly available for health apps (refer to Chapter 9).

Healthcare providers need a platform that compares health wearables, as shown in Fig. 10.2, and that can help them enable care providers and patients to select the most appropriate devices to augment clinical and pharmaceutical care plans.

Specific requirements for the privacy, quality, and security compliance level for wearables are discussed in detail in Chapter 17.

Manufacturers of wearables, academia, and digital health training centers may even consider developing an educational literacy roadmap for healthcare providers who want to work with innovative wearables and insideables, something that in many countries is not available in regular medical training programs or in postacademic medical educational settings.

A future health wearables comparison platform would show most important features and may give relative scores on the following domains:

Features	User experience	Potential disease support
Accuracy	Health benefits	Medical classification
Validity	Trials	Certification status
Quality assurance	Maintenance	Security
Privacy	Price	Reimbursement
Interoperability		

Figure 10.2
Key features of a wearable comparison platform.

Wearables that empower pharmaceutical care providers' work

An upcoming group of wearables does not focus on tracking health data but on easing a healthcare provider's workload. They are in general AI-powered devices that, among other things, help providers handle paperwork by updating a patient's electronic health record, for example, by listening to a provider's conversation with a patient. The device can even come up with an action plan based on the knowledge it collects about the provider's preferences and pharmaceutical practice guidelines. More information on these applications can be found in Chapter 12.

Also, body-worn cameras powered by AI technology (e.g., augmented reality glasses; see Chapter 13) may augment the future role of pharmaceutical healthcare providers, which will enhance triage and communication skills with real-time facial and body recognition and allow predictive alerting of events that deviate from the desired health situation.

Although these supportive tools are definitely in their adolescence phase, they may offer pharmacists already an opportunity to augment the dialogue with patients about their pharmaceutical care and reduce the administrative burden as spoken data can be directly transferred into the electronic patient records (EPRs). In addition, this will increase the time pharmacists can spend with their patients and reduce the amount of time they spend in front of a computer, thereby providing the opportunity to enrich the quality of the human—pharmaceutical support interaction.

Considerations

The threshold to track health data has lowered over time as smart watches, bracelets, and rings have become more affordable. At the same time, as reflected above, the features and possibilities of health wearables are fast expanding, and more people are using the devices, which is increasing the collection of valuable data.

Retention and engagement wearables use: Bring Your Own health Device

Many patients nowadays may have more than a decade of experience with wearable devices connected to their smartphones and other digital applications that add value to their life. However, a younger cohort of adopters, most of whom fall into the 25—44 age range, are most often focused on fitness and wellness wearables. In contrast, adopters between 45 and above are more focused on maintaining and improving their overall health and extending their lives.

Studies found that the attrition rates for fitness devices are rather high; that is, users report increased physical activity after purchasing a sensor, but the longer they own it, the less they use it. Nearly one-third of all users cease tracking activity 6 months after purchasing a device. Qualitative analyses of the reasons for this behavior include forgetting to wear the device, discomfort during exercise, lack of aesthetic appeal, and loss of interest. In some cases, users report they have met their fitness goals and no longer rely on the device [7].

Attrition can occur for a variety of other reasons, including technical issues with the device, a lack of perceived value or benefit, or difficulty integrating the device into the user's daily routine.

In the context of healthcare wearables, attrition can significantly impact patient outcomes, as it may reduce the effectiveness of a treatment plan or prevent patients from accessing critical health data. For example, suppose a patient stops using a wearable device that is designed to track and manage their chronic condition. In that case, they may not receive timely reminders or notifications to take their medications or may miss important changes in their condition that could impact their health.

To mitigate attrition, healthcare providers and wearable device manufacturers need to focus on creating user-friendly and practical devices that offer clear benefits and are easily integrated into patients' daily routines. This may involve designing more comfortable devices, improving battery life, or providing more personalized and relevant feedback to users. Additionally, healthcare providers and manufacturers can work together to develop and implement programs and services that support and encourage patients to continue using their wearable devices over time.

As described in Chapter 7, persuasive technology tactics may also improve users' motivation and engagement to stay connected. Moreover, reemphasizing the value of virtual disease management for the prevention of disease or worsening of the disease is an important factor for retention psychology in medical wearable use.

Once experiences have been positive, and retention is achieved, people are often hesitant to switch to a different wearable platform. Therefore, before proposing wearable data tracking as part of the pharmaceutical care plan, healthcare providers may need to assess which wearable device the patient already uses and whether it can connect to the EPR. This is called a Bring Your Own health Device (BYOhD) strategy.

Provided the used devices meet the clinical needs and comply with regulatory data privacy and security requirements, a BYOhD approach may provide the flexibility needed to capture patient data across different systems and channels. In this case, the patient will not have to deal with additional technology that might not be compatible with other devices or with a double add-on situation. During COVID, this concept was significantly used, for example, at the National Health Service in the United Kingdom, where a specific BYOhD guidance was issued for healthcare workers [8].

As we describe in Chapter 8, the growing tendency of wearables to offer interoperability by using standards and global regulatory frameworks is expected to give a boost to the integration of a broad range of digital health products. In addition, it will allow the pharmaceutical care provider to connect wearable data more easily to, for example, their pharmacy information system.

From this perspective, the industry has meanly learned that it is ineffective to force patients to each individual time use a new or additional wearable device or app as part of a "packaged medical intervention," like a medication plus application/wearable package. These "beyond-the-pill" concepts may be valuable to support better outcomes, like the concept of polypharmacy patients who would get a (potentially free) health tracker for each separate medication they need to use. However, a patient would need extra arms after a certain point in time if this concept were further rolled out. Also, continuously switching patients between different devices and forcing patients to use various platforms does create confusion, is labor-intensive, and thus jeopardizes optimal treatment outcomes and the trust of patients.

Therefore, in a "beyond-the-pill concept," using the device that the patient is already familiar with often has the highest likelihood of adoption and, thus, the most valuable data-tracking to optimize the outcome of the pharmaceutical intervention.

Proofing the value of wearables

A recent systematic review of the limited research yet available did not find a clear role of wearables in improving health care outcomes in chronic disease [9]. However, wearables are becoming increasingly popular within the community. As research and development in wearable technology progress, it is anticipated that these devices will play an increasing role in supporting healthy lifestyle modifications for their users.

More research is required to ascertain a clear causality between wearables and health care outcomes, as defined by the Quadruple Aim (see Chapter 4), for people with chronic disease. As the evidence base for the use of wearables in chronic disease management is strengthened, further challenges will need to be overcome to allow widespread adoption in the healthcare setting, including stringent regulatory approval, data privacy and confidentiality, and software accuracy [9].

Next to providing solid research on the outcome improvement by the use of wearables, there are a number of other factors that constraint the possibility of proving the value of wearables. The research by Deloitte US mentions various companies are developing healthcare wearables to meet growing demand. However, widespread acceptance may be slow due to the relatively new nature of wearables. In addition, there are several challenges to their widespread adoption. One of these challenges is doctor skepticism, as they find the technology helpful but report three main drawbacks. These include data utility, data accuracy, and user error and anxiety. Another challenge is data privacy concerns, with 40% of smartwatch owners being concerned about privacy and 60% of those using them exclusively for health tracking. Cybersecurity threats are also a concern, as all connected devices, including health and wellness wearables, are vulnerable to cyber-attacks. Companies must integrate cybersecurity into their product development and software to mitigate these risks. Finally, increased regulation may be a challenge, as regulators could require companies to adhere to more restrictive rules as these devices become integrated into electronic health records [10].

 Thus, before asking the question of whether using a wearable technology can augment a pharmaceutical care plan, it is advised to make a systematic analysis of the potential added value of the wearable:

- In which phase of the patient journey, as described in Chapter 6, could digital biomarker data help optimize treatment outcomes?
- Can these digital biomarker data be tracked reliably by wearables or insideables?
- Which kinds of digital biomarker data of the patient are already tracked?
- Is it possible to use these existing data from a validity, accuracy, interoperability, safety, quality, security, and privacy point of view?
- How are data going to be analyzed to prove that the wearable augments the pharmaceutical care plan?

This means for blended pharmaceutical care:

- Wearable technology or wearables are smart electronic devices (with micro-controllers) that can be worn on the body, in clothing, accessories, and even tattoos.
- Insideables and implantables are the next phases after external wearables; these devices are implanted in the body, digested and integrated into the body, or attached under the skin.
- Most wearables do not understand the data they track and cannot account for the differing health needs of an individual. Wearables' data must be analyzed in a connected application, which can offer actionable health information.
- Healthcare providers would benefit from a structured platform that gives an overview of the characteristics of wearables and insideables to enable care providers and patients to select well-informed and appropriate compliant devices to augment clinical and pharmaceutical care plans.
- A Bring Your Own health Device strategy may increase the likelihood of patient retention of wearables and may be the most customer-friendly and cost-effective way to collect health data for a pharmaceutical care plan.

This means for blended pharmaceutical care:—cont'd

- Tracked health data cannot yet be considered the gospel truth. Depending on the purpose, medical grade device certification should clarify whether data are reliable, accurate, sensitive, and specific enough to augment clinical decision-making
- A patient has and will have the right to refuse to wear digital technology and share health data.

In the next Chapter 11, we will deep-dive into the flavors of artificial intelligence.

References

[1] Ates HC, et al. End-to-end design of wearable sensors. Nat Rev Mater 2022;7(11):887–907. https://doi.org/10.1038/s41578-022-00460-x.

[2] Gartner. End-user spending on wearable devices worldwide from 2019 to 2022 (in billion U.S. dollars) [graph]. Statista; 2021. Available from: https://www.statista.com/statistics/1065284/wearable-devices-worldwide-spending/.

[3] Christopher E, Atreja A. The best digital biomarkers papers of 2017. Digit Biomark 2018;2(2):64–73. https://doi.org/10.1159/000489224.

[4] European Medicines Agency. Abilify MyCite: withdrawal of the marketing authorisation application. 2020. Available from: https://www.ema.europa.eu/en/medicines/human/withdrawn-applications/abilify-mycite. [Accessed 10 February 2023].

[5] Otsuka America Pharmaceutical, Inc. Abilify MyCite. 2023. Available from: https://www.abilifymycite.com/. [Accessed 10 February 2023].

[6] AngelMed. Who is guardian for?. 2023. Available from: https://angel-med.com/guardian-system. [Accessed 10 February 2023].

[7] Fox G, et al. Why people stick with or abandon wearable devices. NEJM Catal 2017;3(5). https://catalyst.nejm.org/doi/full/10.1056/CAT.17.0396.

[8] NHS. Bring your own device (BYOD) guidance. 2022. Available from: https://transform.england.nhs.uk/information-governance/guidance/bring-your-own-devices-byod-ig-guidance/. [Accessed 10 February 2023].

[9] Mattison G, et al. The influence of wearables on health care outcomes in chronic disease: systematic review. J Med Internet Res 2022;24(7):e36690. https://doi.org/10.2196/36690.

[10] Loucks J, et al. Wearable technology in health care: getting better all the time. TMT Predictions; 2022.

CHAPTER 11

The artificial intelligence pizza*

Ardalan Mirzaei

School of Pharmacy, Faculty of Medicine and Health, The University of Sydney, Australia

AI will not replace you. A person using AI will.

Santiago L. Valdarrama

Everyone's heard of pizza, but not everyone is a chef. How we all imagine the best pizza to be is different. There are so many different options for a pizza, and depending on the user, the taste can be very different. Artificial intelligence (AI) is the same as a pizza. We all have heard of it. We can have it in its simplest form, such as a Margherita pizza, which has one or two ingredients and is simple to make. Alternatively, we can have a complex woodfired burger pizza topped with lobster and sauced with handmade ingredients through a recipe passed down from generation to generation. AI algorithms can be simple and used in various situations, or they can be complex creative models focusing on specialized tasks. Each form serves a particular purpose. In patient care and healthcare systems, the potential for AI is similar to a pizza. Everyone has heard of AI, but not everyone is a chef.

Global tech giants are in a race to become the first to develop the ultimate app. This app is envisioned as a single, fully integrated, AI-driven program that will be incredibly easy for anyone to use and that can do everything it is asked to do—in a way, acting like a personal virtual assistant (similar to the chatbots described in Chapter 12). This vision is not as farfetched as it might sound, as our world is increasingly dependent on AI, which is becoming the backbone of the major providers' big data analytic strategy. For example, a World Economic Forum's Global Agenda Council survey on the future of software and society reported that people expect AI machines to be part of a company's board of directors by 2026 [1]. Therefore, let us have a look at what this technology comprises.

---

*In this chapter, you will read about how artificial intelligence is changing healthcare paradigms and the conditions under which algorithms augment pharmaceutical practice and thus drive apothecary intelligence.

Pharmaceutical Care in Digital Revolution. https://doi.org/10.1016/B978-0-443-13360-2.00021-6

Technology

QR Code 11.1

Can a computer pass for a human?

When mentioning AI, people picture a sentient robot indistinguishable from a human. While humanity is not at that stage yet, AI is the art of replicating human cognitive functions. Therefore, the term "artificial intelligence" has a broad meaning but is defined as when a machine mimics "cognitive" or "rational" functions that are associated with human minds, such as learning, anticipation, or problem-solving [2] (QR Code 11.1).

AI is built to solve questions that include planning, reasoning, knowledge, natural language processing, perception, and the ability to move, manipulate, or omit objects. The methods used to build AI rely on statistical methods, computer science, mathematics, cognitive behavioral techniques, psychology, linguistics, and philosophy.

Algorithms are the basis of AI. They can be defined as a process or set of rules to be followed by computers in calculations or other problem-solving operations to generate answers to a problem. Current-day advances in AI are embedded in machine learning (ML) principles.

Terminology

In this chapter, we will use terminologies such as AI, AI model, model, AI algorithm, or algorithm. The current innovations with AI mean that a 'model' is created and used for a particular purpose. For example, we can have a predictive model designed to make 'predictions' when supplied with new data. In health settings, this could provide the AI model with the patient health data and then predict the probability of an adverse event. Alternatively, there can be an explanatory model which is designed to explain why a particular outcome occurs. In the same adverse event example, we create an AI model that looks at the patient health data and determines which patient health characteristics are the most likely cause of the adverse event. This chapter uses the terms AI, model, and algorithm interchangeably.

The promise of machine learning

Since the 1970s, algorithms have "taught" machines how to read documents and answer questions based on their content. However, the machines' capabilities were limited then by their computational power and the amount of data available to feed the machines.

The last 10 years have seen a 50-fold increase in data produced [3]. With more and more content becoming available, there is increased access to a large pool of data. Combined with computers with superfast process, systems have a deeper and more widespread understanding of many topics (QR Code 11.2).

QR Code 11.2
Innovation Japan: world's latest deep learning.

 ML is defined as a subset of AI (see Fig. 11.1) in the field of computer science that often uses statistical techniques to give computers the ability to "learn" (i.e., progressively improve performance on a specific task) with data, without being explicitly programmed [4].

ML, in general, uses an algorithmic approach that takes both structured and unstructured data through a mathematically driven process to generate a model that recognizes patterns and contextual meaning. The dataset has 'features' that an algorithm will use to find and understand a pattern with a corresponding 'label.' ML can be used in both supervised and unsupervised ways, as exemplified in Fig. 11.2.

A "supervised" approach means that the data come with a label or answer. For example, we have a cancer dataset with lifestyle, genetic, and physiological data for patients. This information would be the features. A corresponding label would be whether they had 'cancer' or 'no cancer.' A supervised ML model finds the patterns based on the features and predicts whether a person is likely to develop cancer. As one can imagine, the dataset has to be 'labeled,' which, if done manually, can be a tedious and error-prone process. Unsupervised or semisupervised approaches reduce the need for large, labeled data sets. The AI system can group unsorted information according to similarities and differences in their features even though no categories are provided.

 Unsupervised learning algorithms can execute more complex processing tasks than supervised learning systems and learn from unlabeled data without

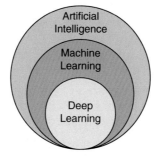

Figure 11.1
Domains of artificial intelligence.

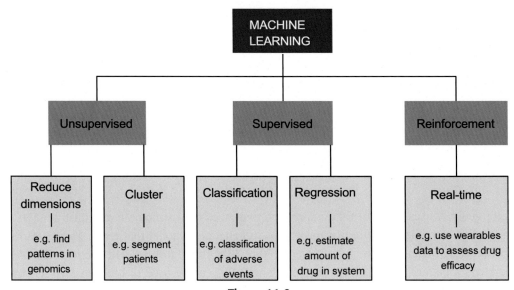

Figure 11.2
Different forms of machine learning.

supervision. However, an unsupervised approach can be more unpredictable than a supervised learning approach. AI algorithms, such as clustering, explore how the database features are related to creating the groups. For example, we can specify the number of groups and let the AI determine which individual case fits each group. While an unsupervised learning AI system might, for example, figure out on its own how to sort black and white cats from Dalmatian dogs, it might also add unforeseen and undesired categories (like stracciatella yogurt pictures), creating chaos instead of order.

Reinforcement learning is an example of an unsupervised technique used to train AlphaGo, the AI system that defeated the world champion of the board game Go. The technique allows algorithms to learn tasks simply through trial and error. For example, good actions get positive rewards and feedback, which the AI model then learns from automatically. In pharmaceutical care, this is a potential technique in which the AI system can learn about the factors that determine patients' adherence profiles and how to deal with them to improve adequate drug use.

While AI capabilities have developed dramatically over time, most instances of AI we encounter today are of the class "Narrow AI" or "Specialized AI." That is, it can handle only a narrow task of capabilities that it has been trained to do. For example, imagine a model used to identify cats and dogs in an image. Suppose we give a dog-identifying AI an image with the word "dog" written on it; most models will not know what to do with that input because the model was trained to pick up 'images' of dogs and not the word 'dog.' Thus, with all the progress in specialized applications of AI, we are still some distance from creating a system on a level with the learning ability of a human baby.

Stream-mining in continuous data stream

A data stream is a flow of information or data sequences that reach a user over time. Working and building models with a continuous and dynamic data stream have challenges that cannot be solved through traditional statistical methods [5]. Stream-mining is the process of working with dynamic data streams to discover the patterns and relationships with the incoming data. Stream-mining is a form of AI that is potentially relevant for pharmaceutical stakeholders. In stream-mining, AI models are programmed over a constant flow of data in a system where individual data does not have to be stored. This capability is valuable in healthcare, for example, in intensive care or home-monitoring situations, where a variety of technologies provide an endless flow of patient health data. Still, only the outliers need to be picked up by care providers and acted on. The potential for this technology is to identify patients with the highest risk for adverse events from medication. Once personal data are shared with pharmaceutical care providers, this can be done continuously. In a home-monitoring situation, there is an example of the Hungry Baby Alarm in QR Code 11.3, where a baby monitoring system was created to monitor the baby for cues of hungry and warn the parents before the infant becomes irritable.

QR Code 11.3
The hungry baby alarm.

AI technology in our current era

The effects of AI implementation on society, in general, have been spectacular. Since its development in 1950, AI has now proven to be capable of matching or surpassing some of the most impressive intellectual feats of humans, including in healthcare, as shown, for example, in QR Code 11.4. Moreover, the big promise of ML is the possibility of exponential learning, as trend analysis and scalability of learning can be done much faster.

QR Code 11.4
The advent of AI in healthcare.

AI has defeated human world champions in chess; the world's most complex game, Go; and poker games. It is already superior to the average person in recognizing faces, videos, or words from speech. And it is also developed as a successful opponent in debating competitions.

AI-enhanced IT systems are used in business to automate increasingly complex tasks that humans used to perform. These include, for example, chatbots that mimic customer service agents and enable new sales channels, loan officers' IT systems that approve and arrange loans, self-driving cars, or security guard systems that automatically check IDs, which are being used extensively at airports. In addition, AI is used increasingly in healthcare to automate structured scientific reasoning, accelerate innovation to find new treatments, and find correlations in previously considered large data sets.

Once all these competencies are combined, a computer is said to have superintelligence, which is an intellect that greatly outperforms the best human minds across many cognitive domains [6].

If computers were to become smarter than the world's entire population, that would prompt what is called a "singularity moment." There are various opinions about the exact time this might happen, ranging from several years to many decades. Mathematician Vernor Vinge predicts it will occur by 2023, and futurist Ray Kurzweil says by 2045 [7]. Recent research suggests there is a 50% chance that AI will outperform humans in all tasks in 45 years and will automate all human jobs in 120 years, with Asian respondents expecting these dates to occur much sooner than North Americans do [8].

The potential is there: different from a human, a machine has (relatively speaking) endless memory, does not forget, does not require sleep, and is backed by ever-increasing technological performance.

Impact on core responsibilities in pharmaceutical care

AI is set to revolutionize pharmaceutical care by connecting different pharmaceutical data sets, analyzing medical and pharmaceutical records platforms, designing holistic treatment plans, or signaling adverse events or nonadherence. Also, AI may help automate repetitive pharmacy tasks, such as checking prescriptions or reviewing poly-pharmaceutical drug profiles (signaling, for example, overconsumption or interactions).

Therefore, it is to be expected that, of all the digital advances mentioned in this book and definitely with the convergence of their data, AI will likely be one that will most significantly disrupt the pharmaceutical care process.

Although AI, in principle, means artificial intelligence, some members of the AI community realized that it was really about enhancing human capabilities and called it augmented intelligence. Taking this concept one step further, we introduce the term "*apothecary intelligence*": augmenting human pharmaceutical expertise.

Here is the general impact that AI is expected to have on the five domains of pharmaceutical care provision (refer to Chapter 6 for a more detailed discussion):

A. **Professional relationship between PCPs and patients:** This will be enhanced due to more integrated health data insights

B. **Adequate collection and recording of health data:** This becomes a stronger prerequisite for feeding pharmaceutical AI in the most optimal way

C. **Review health data and provide adequate PC proposal:** The PC plan will need a roadmap denoting which data and which AI to use

D. **Patient alignment and facilitate execution of PC plan:** Involves discussions on whether data and AI intelligence are accepted and how they augment the human care provider's role

E. **Circular management of PC plan:** The care plan will be adjusted based on outcomes of personalized predictive and prescriptive monitoring models driven by AI

Implementation in daily practice

Creating a good AI model needs a large amount of data. One of the rate-limiting steps of AI in healthcare is the lack of access to large enough training data sets. Another limitation is that health data sets that a patient generates are stored in scattered technological applications, such as separate electronic medical records, pharmacy data, claims data, genetic profiles, and digital health trackers. This type of health data sets are experiencing exponential growth, and imagine what will happen if all these data sets are converged, as described in Chapter 8. With the current pace of advancements in AI, it is, for example, assumed that by 2028 algorithms that analyze these big data sets will outperform humans by 80% regarding classified diagnosis.

AI's impact on healthcare activities

The impact of AI and its use cases occur in three phases [9]. In the first phase, solutions try to address the optimization of tasks by tackling administratively heavy and repetitive work. For example, ML can support analytical tasks like disease detection, diagnosis, automation, advice provision, and process flow.

Some of this first-phase work includes work in imaging. For example, in image recognition, as part of disease detection, AI models have learned to identify images containing certain diseases by analyzing large training image databases manually labeled as "cancer" or "no cancer."

The second phase of AI solutions marks technologies used in home-based care rather than hospital-based care. Innovation is no longer restricted to a clinician's work but is used in conjunction with the patient. For example, in Chapter 12, we discuss using virtual personal assistants and digital pharmacists in Pharmi. Other innovations can include using health apps (Chapter 9) for remote monitoring or in combination with wearable tech (Chapter 10) to create AI-powered alerting systems [10].

In the final phase, AI would be an integrated part of clinical decision support tools. Evidence derived from clinical trials would support AI adoption into clinical practice. A paradigm shift would lead to patients seeing AI technology as essential to how care is delivered and used. Organizations and legislators would have developed frameworks and policies to utilize datasets and integrate datasets better while managing risks and protecting patient data.

Impact areas

A McKinsey report in 2020 highlighted the six areas of impact of AI in healthcare [9]. From Fig. 11.3, the areas are chronic care management, self-care/prevention/wellness, triage and diagnosis, diagnostics, clinical decision support, and care delivery.

There are far too many excellent examples of the use of AI in healthcare to mention in this book. Therefore, the following cases are meant for inspiration only in current tasks undertaken in the first phase and do not reflect their ranking in the level of disruption.

Chronic care management

Launched in 2017, Karantis360 is an 'automated personal monitoring system' which uses sensors that are discreetly linked to a 'mobile device which sends reports and alerts to carers and family members.' The technology was developed with IBM Watson and Internet of

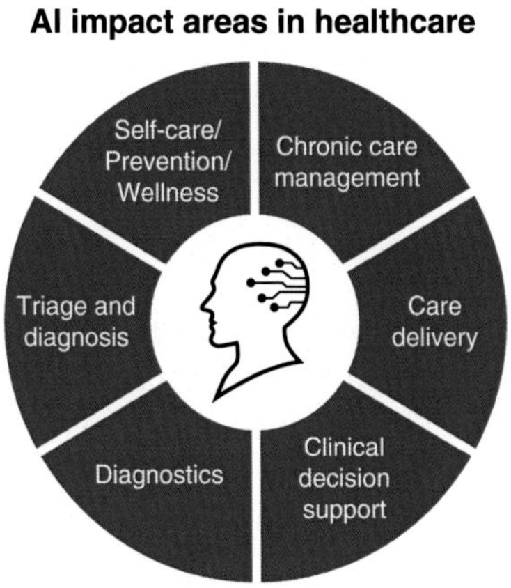

AI impact areas in healthcare

Figure 11.3
Areas of impact for AI in healthcare from the 2020 McKinsey report 'Transforming healthcare with AI.'

Things (IoT) sensors. These sensors track a patient's daily behavior, such as when they go to sleep and leave the house. AI is used to identify when behavior is out of the normal expected outcome and informs the carer or family that something has occurred. For example, the AI system can alert carers if the patient has had a fall, notifying them of the incident. The company aims to help patients who need constant 24/7 care, such as those with cognitive impairment and dementia, and also to remain potentially independent [11].

Self-care, prevention, and wellness

Patients are encouraged to become champions of their health and take ownership of their health and well-being. Companies like AliveCor and Apple have developed technologies to function as personal electrocardiograms in the self-care space. For example, the AliveCor KardiaMobile is either a single or 6-lead device used in combination with an app. The device can monitor heart rhythm and alert when a patient is in atrial fibrillation, bradycardia, or tachycardia. Similarly, the Apple smartwatch is placed on the wrist and a finger on the watch's digital crown. Regulatory bodies have approved both products for the detection of the presence of atrial fibrillation [12].

Diagnostics

In 2018, the first AI-based diagnostic system for the autonomous detection of diabetic retinopathy, a leading cause of blindness, was granted commercialization by the Food and Drug Administration. "The IDx-DR system can be used to provide a fast, immediate, reliable assessment for diabetic retinopathy, including macular edema, during a routine office visit in a primary care setting. It delivers a diagnostic interpretation and associated report, including care instructions that are aligned with the American Academy of Ophthalmology preferred practice pattern for diabetic retinopathy. This enables primary care providers to counsel patients regarding follow-up care while they are still in the office" [13].

Triage and diagnosis

The company Babylon has developed an AI-powered diagnostic triage tool to support patients 24/7 to identify if they suffer from a disease (more extensively discussed in Chapter 12). They published a 2020 paper stating that "their AI was able to identify the condition modeled by a clinical vignette with accuracy comparable to human doctors" [14]. In addition, they found that their AI system recommended triage advice was, on average, "safer than that of human doctors, compared to the ranges of acceptable triage provided by independent expert judges, with only a minimal reduction in appropriateness" [14].

A study in 2016 at Beth Israel Deaconess Medical Center and Harvard Medical School showed that AI is not so much about humans versus machines as it is often thought to be. For example, researchers trained an algorithm to identify metastatic breast cancer by interpreting pathology images. Their algorithm reached an accuracy of 92.5%, whereas the pathologists reached an accuracy of 97%. But used in combination, the detection rate approached 100% (approximately 99.5%). Thus, the synergy between human knowledge and AI capacity is currently considered the most optimal situation [15].

Clinical decision support

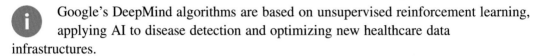 Google's DeepMind algorithms are based on unsupervised reinforcement learning, applying AI to disease detection and optimizing new healthcare data infrastructures.

For example, DeepMind Health entered into an agreement with the UK's National Health Service (NHS) to access patient records to train detection and prevention algorithms. DeepMind Health now works with NHS on mobile tools and AI research to help get patients optimally from test to treatment. Apps use mobile technology to send immediate alerts to clinicians when a patient's condition deteriorates, thus allowing physicians to take faster and more personalized action [16].

Scientists from Verily (formerly called Google Life Sciences) have also discovered "a new way to assess a person's risk of heart disease by analyzing scans of the back of a patient's eye. The AI is able to accurately deduce data, including an individual's age, blood pressure, and whether or not they smoke. Converged data can then be used to predict their risk of suffering a major cardiac event—such as a heart attack—with roughly the same accuracy as current leading methods" [17].

The specific disease areas where Google is studying diagnostics and disease management include, among others, ocular diseases, diabetes, Parkinson's disease, and heart diseases. In addition, there are many initiatives to research aspects of medication, and more developments in the pharmaceutical environment may follow.

Google faced challenges in the United Kingdom for using deidentified health data, which do not ordinarily require an individual's consent [18]. However, this type of research is also expected to go through rigorous medical research approval processes. This partnership had privacy and legal implications discussed further under the privacy, quality, and security section below.

Care delivery

Beta Bionics is a biotechnology company that has built the bionic pancreas called 'iLet.' The technology aims to mimic the human pancreas by monitoring blood sugar levels and controlling the insulin delivery rate. The technology is vital for patients with type 1 diabetes who may have difficulty adhering to strict insulin management regimes. The platform has been described as 'designed to use adaptive, self-learning, control algorithms, together with continuous glucose monitoring and pump technology, to autonomously compute and administer insulin and/or glucagon doses and mimic the body's natural ability to maintain tight glycemic control' [19]. Currently, the trials of the technology show promise by significantly reducing a patient's HbA1c, causing no change in the risk of hypoglycemia, and providing patients with more time in a day to do other activities [20].

AI to fuel "pharmacy-as-a-service" platforms

Introducing AI technology to analyze existing electronic pharmacy records (EPRs), combined with other data sets derived from technologies described in Part 2 of this book, will create huge opportunities to build apothecary intelligence and deliver "pharmaceutical-care-as-a-service" platforms.

Conditional to success will be to identify at first whether unique and anonymized patient identifiers can be established to create a secure (patient) data platform on which AI can be built while respecting the privacy of individuals. For instance, more standardized use of citizen identification numbers may create opportunities to combine all available data into one personal health application (preferably governed by the patient), as described in Chapter 8.

With the use of a unique patient ID, different data sets may be connected to feed the AI, whereas working with open health databases and adopting standardized interconnectivity standards like HL7-FHIR, as noted in Chapter 8, are vital prerequisites to make a convergence of data and technology happen.

Many pharmaceutical care teams are used to working in an EPR environment that connects with general practitioners' data, specialists' data, hospital data, wearables, and other digital health information.

 These connected pharmaceutical data sets can be analyzed by AI technology, augmenting the pharmaceutical professional in various ways:

- **To support getting better patient outcomes:** For example, having access to the genomic profile of a patient and linking it to the data set of various other health data can provide professionals with a detailed prediction on how individuals are going to respond to medication and where to put extra attention to prevent, for example, nonadherence, adverse events, deterioration in illness, or suboptimal dosing.

- **To move from evidence-based to intelligence-based healthcare:** Although AI algorithms in the next decade most probably will not replace the need for clinical trials or postlaunch evidence data generation completely, significant insight on disease and behavioral patterns can be derived from real-world data analyses gathered by consolidating large amounts of connected IoT healthcare devices.
- **To (re)organize patient routes or treatment plans more personalized:** This will be based on historical data, characteristics, and preferences of the individual.
- **To better inform physicians on optimal treatment:** This will involve AI results to augment existing clinical guidelines and balanced treatment decisions.
- **To create voice-controlled pharmaceutical coaching systems for patients:** This will emerge as natural language processing becomes increasingly more sophisticated and smart AI devices like chatbots can be managed via voice control (as described in Chapter 12). In addition, various types of heterogeneous data sets may be added to these virtual coaches (e.g., scientific literature vs. Facebook feeds vs. facial recognition, each of which has very different contextual, semantic, and linguistic characteristics).

How to start tomorrow with AI?

In Chapter 20, the structured Digital-by-Design (DbD) approach is explained to identify whether technology can solve a certain pharmaceutical care issue. In the case of AI, not all business challenges require AI solutions, as statistics and database research often can do the job and may be much easier and less expensive to implement.

Suppose AI is found to be a suitable option after running the DbD model. In that case, it does make sense to collaborate with data science experts at a project's early stage, for example, with consultancy companies, academia, and big corporations, as well as with AI-in-healthcare startups, which are growing in number.

Most AI-in-healthcare startups in recent years were found in the imaging and diagnostic area. Like the example box of Pacmed, the number of these promising startups aboard may supersede the development speed of the big corporate AI vendors, offering simpler and faster options to implement AI technology. Also, they are increasingly able to work with unprepared and incomplete data, as often is the case in healthcare.

AI healthcare startup Pacmed

Currently, evidence on the effectiveness of treatments is often based on average results on a very small number of patients, which is not always representative and does not cover the complexity and variety of the population a doctor sees in practice.

Patients and doctors generate more data daily, allowing doctors to learn directly and objectively from every patient. Pacmed builds decision support software for doctors based on analyzing those observational health data. By combining medical expertise and ML techniques, the software computes and presents expected outcomes of relevant treatment options for the patient a doctor is seeing. Unlike other sources of medical knowledge, Pacmed algorithms learn every time they are applied in practice.

Pacmed identified the treatment of urinary tract infections at the General Practitioner (GP) level in the Netherlands as the most feasible starting point for ML in the consultation room. The software that helps GPs choose the best treatment, based on data from over 250,000 urinary tract infections, is currently being used by over 100 GPs in a scientific implementation study. Pacmed is also developing software for optimal, personal, and outcome-based treatment choices in hospital intensive care units, oncology, cardiology, and psychiatry.

The enormous wealth of smart healthcare AI startups is too broad to mention in this chapter, particularly as some are predominantly locally focused. However, before considering or even starting a new initiative in your pharmaceutical care pathway, it does make sense to run an analysis on available solutions in the market before starting from scratch to build the next own AI.

Kaggle to answer pharmaceutical AI questions

An interesting platform to consider for a pharmaceutical care problem that an AI solution may solve is the Kaggle platform (QR Code 11.5).

Kaggle is a global crowdsourcing platform with public data sets for predictive modeling and analytics competitions. Companies and researchers post data, and statisticians and data scientists compete to produce the best models for predicting and describing the data.

QR Code 11.5
What's Kaggle |
Kaggle.

This crowdsourcing approach relies on the fact that countless strategies can be applied to any predictive modeling task and that it is impossible to know at the outset which technique or analyst will be most effective. Contributors come from a wide variety of backgrounds, including fields such as computer science, computer vision, biology, medicine, and even glaciology.

Competitions have resulted in many successful projects, including furthering state of the art in HIV research, chess ratings, and traffic forecasting.

Challenges to crowdsourcing in 2018 in the healthcare environment are—among others—the complex and heterogeneous data sets and the sensitivity of dealing with patient data [21].

Individual pharmacists of pharmaceutical care groups or chains may consider posting their pharmaceutical care questions (and strict anonymized data sets) on Kaggle or other competing platforms, initiating an environment where experts in big data programming can use their expertise to develop algorithms to solve the problem.

Considerations

Within the optimism about AI's opportunities, there is also more room for realism. AI has existed since the last decade of the 1950s. Although the current speed of computers and our advanced scientific approaches have increased the pace of applicability, there are still a number of hurdles to overcome before AI has a secure, integrated, and trusted place in healthcare.

Bias and responsible data science

AI-based systems are as smart as the data that go into them and the programmers who build them. Thus, two forms are of specific relevance here: the bias caused by the programmer's vision and the bias caused by (poor) decisions in the past. The latter is particularly relevant for healthcare, as inadequate or skewed therapeutic guidelines, unequal gender admission in clinical trials, and many other selection biases may have led to inadequate outcomes in the past, which, if fed into an AI program, will reintroduce the bias. Being conscious of this phenomenon is essential when interpreting the results and further developing AI algorithms.

Additionally, AI systems may be skewed by variations and biases in diverging population data so that models trained in one pharmaceutical pathway may not be applicable in another, especially if they are in a different geographical region or disease population. And good data are hardest to collect in places that need it most, including low and middle-income countries lacking developed healthcare infrastructures. Critical data remain especially scarce in developing countries where electronic health records are not yet widely used.

In this respect, to develop future-proof, responsible data science methods, more foundational research is globally needed, focusing on FACT, which means questions related to Fairness, Accuracy, Confidentiality, and Transparency.

Lack of differentiation in AI providers

The huge increase in startups and established providers—all positioning themselves to offer AI products—is sometimes confusing to end users. For example, in 2018, more than 1000 healthcare providers in the Western world with applications and platforms described themselves as AI vendors or said they used AI in their products. In contrast, differentiation between focus areas is not always transparent.

To build trust with an end-user organization like pharmaceutical care providers, AI providers are recommended to transparently publish research reports and case studies on the methods used and results achieved when implementing AI techniques. This will enable end-users to select an AI provider that best fits their needs and provide a reliable solution for a pharmaceutical problem.

Proven, less complex machine-learning capabilities can address many end-user needs

Advancements in AI, such as deep learning, are getting a lot of buzz but may eclipse the value of more straightforward, already-proven approaches. It is always recommended that programmers and researchers use the simplest approach to accomplishing a job rather than cutting-edge AI techniques.

This means that for pharmaceutical purposes, many questions may already be answered by (relatively) simple, adequate statistical analysis of claims data, connected electronic health databases, or prescription record databases built for pharmacoepidemiological outcomes.

For decades, database analysis has created insight into disease epidemiology and provided the contextual background for designing clinical trials. It can also provide evidence on safety outcomes, effectiveness, drug utilization patterns, the burden of diseases, patient journeys, and adherence relatively easily. Additionally, different types of studies using longitudinal and real-life patient data have already helped us understand the management of health risks. They have provided solutions for decision-makers in the market access, health economics, and health outcomes sectors.

If processes are running well and solving the problems posed, sophisticated, complex AI and ML techniques are not always necessary.

Ethical challenges

To ensure a sustainable balance between artificial and human intelligence, AI applications must remain under meaningful human governance and be used for socially beneficial

QR Code 11.6
AI for good—ethics
in AI

purposes, as has been extensively emphasized by many stakeholders globally (QR Code 11.6) [22].

Data privacy is a twofold challenge when developing AI models. One element of ethics would be to consider using the lowest amount of data to build a model, that is, only using what is required and nothing more. However, most companies are becoming 'big data' companies where they try to collect all available information. The more data points you have, the more accurate model you can build. In some early-stage mode development, you collect all the information you can, as 'you don't know what you don't know' [22]. The second concern is data leakage due to building complex and specific models. That is, the AI model is fed so much specific training information that it no longer observes general population patterns but specific observations of individuals. This leakage can lead to privacy violations [23].

Technology is not value neutral, and in the slight overhyping that has been put on AI in the last years, society asks technologists to take responsibility for their work's ethical and social impact. Understanding what this means in practice requires rigorous scientific inquiry into the most sensitive challenges we humans face and the inclusion of many voices throughout to avoid misconception, misuse, and human rejection of AI implementation [24].

Also, transparency in how unsupervised learning mechanisms work, how algorithms are developed, and what human oversight is warranted are essential to creating societal trust when working with AI. As noted in Chapter 16 regarding the use of robotics, to create trust, our future machines should be able to transparently communicate how their algorithms are programmed, how they are learning, and how suggestions, recommendations, and actions are being posed.

Additionally, as AI will help pharmaceutical stakeholders make better predictions, it is important to realize that we humans make decisions using both prediction and judgment (see Chapter 19). We have never really unbundled those aspects of decision-making. Separating the process in the machine making the prediction makes the distinct role of judgment in decision-making clearer. As the value of human prediction decreases due to AI, the value of human judgment should go up because that is something AI does not do.

The first big initiatives to warrant human governance in AI have already started. One interesting example is the installation of the Partnership on AI initiative launched in 2017, working "to advance responsible governance and best practices in AI" [25]. Another is the Global Partnership on AI launched in 2020 by the Organisation for Economic

Co-operation and Development, which aims to "guide the responsible development and use of AI" [26].

Also, the Future of Life Institute, founded in 2014, has a "strong mission to catalyze and support research and initiatives for safeguarding life and developing optimistic visions of the future, including positive ways for humanity to steer its own course considering new technologies and challenges." They have developed 23 principles to work responsibly with AI [27].

Much more information on how pharmaceutical care professionals deal with ethics in AI can be found in Chapter 18.

AI impact on the workforce

Many have feared that AI will cause one 'to lose their job' and that they will not be able to find their place in the world.

In Box 11.1, there are five considerations noted in exploring the impact of AI on the future of workers in healthcare. One consistent aspect is that a healthcare professional's role and 'job' will change.

For example, imagine asking about a patient's health status and having a computer generate a response. The vast patient medical data are simplified and condensed to a reply that provides the health professional with what they need. In this scenario, the health professional still has a role, whether the doctor, nurse, or pharmacist. However, their function has adapted from exploring medical data and histories to reach a decision, to one, where the information is already consolidated for them. Roles that will likely be replaced require repetitive and autonomous functions. Yet, we know that most of these roles are already reducing, and the professionals that are not learning and adapting are seeing the fear of the impact of AI on healthcare.

Another area of need can be the personalization of healthcare. With readily available information, patients can suffer from information overload or constantly search for the right information [28]. Health professionals can assist a patient's journey by personalizing the information.

The quote from Santiago at the beginning of the chapter notes where the role of AI will be in the future of the workforce. This ability to adapt was mentioned in the foreword of this book as a crucial skill needed for pharmacists. AI systems can help improve work functions without entirely replacing the individual. ChatCPT (https://chat.openai.com/chat) generated the information in Box 11.1 from OpenAI by asking it, "what are the considerations in exploring the impact of AI on the future of workers in healthcare." It may be that the role of an author or writer may have to be adapted and subject to change.

Box 11.1 Five considerations for exploring the impact of AI on future healthcare workers.

There are a number of considerations that should be taken into account when exploring the impact of AI on the future of workers in healthcare, including the following:

- The tasks that are most likely to be automated: Some tasks, such as data entry and analysis, are more easily automated than others, such as patient care and counseling. It is important to understand which tasks are most likely to be automated and how this will affect the demand for labor in different areas of healthcare.
- The potential for job displacement: Automation has the potential to displace some jobs, particularly those that are routine and repetitive. It is important to consider how job displacement will be managed and how affected workers will be supported to transition to new roles or industries.
- The potential for job creation: AI also has the potential to create new job opportunities, particularly in areas such as data analysis and ML. It is important to consider how these new job opportunities can be developed and how workers can be trained to take advantage of them.
- The impact on job quality: The adoption of AI may also affect the quality of jobs in healthcare, including factors such as job security, pay, and working conditions. It is important to consider how these factors will be affected by the adoption of AI and to ensure that workers are protected and treated fairly.
- The ethical implications: The use of AI in healthcare also raises a number of ethical considerations, such as fairness, accountability, confidentiality, and transparency. It is important to consider these ethical implications and to ensure that AI is used in a responsible and transparent manner.

Competencies and skills to evaluate, build, and deploy AI solutions

Many organizations, including healthcare institutions, are currently built on traditional competency frameworks since they are experts in their own professional fields and may have had limited exposure to data science, ML, and platform management. However, data sets, analysis, and adequate use are only as good as their creators; thus, organizations need to adopt skills to ensure the future workforce is familiar with data science and understands algorithms and the different ways of decision-making.

To work adequately with AI data sets, pharmaceutical care providers may need to increasingly combine their pharmaceutical knowledge with technology perception and data science skills. Detailed information on the proposed competency profile of the future for pharmaceutical care stakeholders can be found in Chapter 19.

Privacy, quality, and security

While increased data collection and analysis in pharmaceutical practice may offer numerous benefits to patient care and healthcare business operations, these advantages also can come with a risk. As more sensitive patient data and algorithms are stored online, cyber threats present a growing challenge for the healthcare industry, as the example of the NHS reflects. As another example, a 2017 study by Accenture found that patient data theft is the most likely security risk to occur in pharmacy practice [28A].

In addition to causing financial loss due to legality issues, these breaches also decrease patient trust in pharmaceutical care stakeholders who aim to use digital health technology. Thus, the detailed information on how to warrant security, privacy, and quality conditions by making a compliance blueprint prior to starting off—as discussed in Chapter 17—is noteworthy.

Exposure to patient medical data

Institutions must be careful when housing patient data and how this information is provided to third parties.

The Royal Free NHS Foundation Trust got reprimanded in 2017 for passing personal data on 1.6 million patients to Google's UK-based AI unit, which taught the world that when working with AI platforms, informed consent and data privacy regulation is as valid as the previous manual on epidemiologic research (see also Chapter 17) [28B]. As has been done in other AI big data research, Google used deidentified data, which do not ordinarily require individual consent, but it still needs to go through a rigorous medical research approval process.

The Australian health insurer 'Medibank' had their data systems breached, exposing the details of 10 million patients [29]. The information included patients' personal information and medical records, such as medical conditions and operations. This breach exposes the company to fines, legal suits, and public image damages, let alone the patients suffering identity theft or blackmail [30]. The technical details of how the breach happened are left to security professionals. However, it is essential to consider how patient data are stored and how they are accessed. When working with sensitive patient information, it is necessary to ensure access is restricted to those who need it, and that data are encrypted.

By now, it should be clear why the pizza analogy was used. Although AI is heard and known by most, the intricacies of working with it require proper chefs.

The true beauty of AI in pharmaceutical care lies in the balance between the synergy of its decision support system and human healthcare leadership, making AI a true apothecary intelligence.

AI's biggest influence in the upcoming years is the creation of smart virtual assistants, which is the topic of Chapter 12.

 This means for blended pharmaceutical care

- AI technology can feed pharmacy-as-a-service platforms, providing it can access complete, adequate, and holistic health data sets.
- Apothecary intelligence is the use of AI to augment human pharmaceutical care.
- AI technology is not always required as a solution, as sometimes traditional statistical database research can do the job better and faster.
- Often it is not necessary to use AI technology at the starting point, as big platforms and a wealth of startups have much AI experience to offer.
- When developing AI, algorithm transparency, detection of data bias, competency building, and ethical considerations are crucial conditions for success.
- Ensuring data privacy, quality, and security of both analysis and output is crucial to generate trust in AI algorithms.
- AI may help automate repetitive pharmaceutical care tasks and augment personalized care plans with integrated decision support systems. This will increase providers' value for what they do best: make the human judgment and provide empathic care.

References

[1] World Economic Forum. Deep shift technology tipping points and societal impact—survey report. In: Global agenda council on the future of software & society; 2015. Available from: https://www3.weforum.org/docs/WEF_GAC15_Technological_Tipping_Points_report_2015.pdf.

[2] Mintz Y, Brodie R. Introduction to artificial intelligence in medicine. Minim Invasive Ther Allied Technol 2019;28(2):73—81. https://doi.org/10.1080/13645706.2019.1575882.

[3] IDC and Statista. Volume of data/information created, captured, copied, and consumed worldwide from 2010 to 2020, with forecasts from 2021 to 2025 (in zettabytes). Chart 2021. Available from: https://www.statista.com/statistics/871513/worldwide-data-created/.

[4] Wikipedia Contributors. Machine learning. 2023. Available from: https://en.wikipedia.org/w/index.php?title=Machine_learning&oldid=1131287733. [Accessed 7 January 2023].

[5] Ramírez-Gallego S, et al. A survey on data preprocessing for data stream mining: current status and future directions. Neurocomputing 2017;239:39—57. https://www.sciencedirect.com/science/article/pii/S0925231217302631.

[6] Bostrom N. Superintelligence: paths, dangers, strategies. Oxford: Oxford University Press; 2014.

[7] Ross A. The industries of the future. New York: Simon & Schuster; 2016.

[8] Grace K, et al. When will AI exceed human performance? Evidence from AI experts. arXiv preprint arXiv:1705.08807 2017.

[9] Spatharou A, Hieronimus S, Jenkins J. Transforming healthcare with AI: the impact on the workforce and organizationsvol 10. McKinsey & Company; 2020.

[10] Eippert J. News: apple watch saves the day (and a life). Emerg Med News 2019;41(11):29. https://journals.lww.com/em-news/Fulltext/2019/11000/News__Apple_Watch_Saves_the_Day__and_a_Life_.7.aspx.

[11] Karantis 360 Ltd. About Karantis360. 2023. Available from: https://karantis360.com/about-karantis360/. [Accessed 7 January 2023].

[12] Halcox JPJ, et al. Assessment of remote heart rhythm sampling using the AliveCor heart monitor to screen for atrial fibrillation. Circulation 2017;136(19):1784−94. https://www.ahajournals.org/doi/abs/10.1161/CIRCULATIONAHA.117.030583.

[13] U.S. Food and Drug Administration. FDA permits marketing of artificial intelligence-based device to detect certain diabetes-related eye problems. News Release; April 2018.

[14] Baker A, et al. A comparison of artificial intelligence and human doctors for the purpose of triage and diagnosis. Front Artif Intell 2020;3. https://www.frontiersin.org/articles/10.3389/frai.2020.543405.

[15] Kritz J. Artificial intelligence achieves near-human performance in diagnosing breast cancer. 2016. Available from: https://www.bidmc.org/about-bidmc/news/artificial-intelligence-achieves-near-human-performance-in-diagnosing-breast-cancer.

[16] Suleyman M. Working with the NHS to build lifesaving technology. DeepMind; 2016. Available from: https://www.deepmind.com/blog/working-with-the-nhs-to-build-lifesaving-technology.

[17] Poplin R, et al. Prediction of cardiovascular risk factors from retinal fundus photographs via deep learning. Nat Biomed Eng 2018;2(3):158−64.

[18] Shead S. Google and DeepMind face lawsuit over deal with Britain's National Health Service. 2021. Available from: https://www.cnbc.com/2021/10/01/google-deepmind-face-lawsuit-over-data-deal-with-britains-nhs.html.

[19] Beta Bionics. The insulin-only bionic pancreas pivotal trial showed consistent mean HbA1c reductions across a variety of subgroups at ADA's 82nd scientific sessions. 2022. Available from: https://www.betabionics.com/the-insulin-only-bionic-pancreas-pivotal-trial-showed-consistent-mean-hba1c-reductions-across-a-variety-of-subgroups-at-adas-82nd-scientific-sessions/.

[20] Beta Bionics. The iLet® bionic pancreas significantly reduced HbA1c and improved time in range vs standard of care for a diverse range of people with type 1 diabetes. 2022. Available from: https://www.betabionics.com/the-ilet-bionic-pancreas-significantly-reduced-hba1c-and-improved-time-in-range-vs-standard-of-care-for-a-diverse-range-of-people-with-type-1-diabetes/.

[21] Derrington D. Artificial intelligence for health and health care. 2017. Available from: https://www.healthit.gov/sites/default/files/jsr-17-task-002_aiforhealthandhealthcare12122017.pdf.

[22] van Est R, Gerritsen J, Kool L. Human rights in the robot age: challenges arising from the use of robotics, artificial intelligence, and virtual and augmented reality. Rathenau Instituut; 2017. Available from: https://research.tue.nl/nl/publications/64867060-a711-4e79-a161-507094c5678a.

[23] Strobel M, Shokri R. Data privacy and trustworthy machine learning. IEEE Secur Priv 2022;20(5):44−9. https://doi.org/10.1109/msec.2022.3178187.

[24] Tegmark M. Life 3.0: being human in the age of artificial intelligence. Vintage; 2018.

[25] Partnership on AI. How we work. 2023. Available from: https://partnershiponai.org/how-we-work/. [Accessed 7 January 2023].

[26] OCED. The global partnership on AI (GPAI). 2023. Available from: https://oecd.ai/en/gpai.

[27] Future of Life Institute. AI principles. 2017. Available from: https://futureoflife.org/open-letter/ai-principles/. [Accessed 7 January 2023].

[28] Mirzaei A, et al. Predictors of health information seeking behavior: a systematic review and network analysis. J Med Internet Res 2020;23(7):e21680. https://doi.org/10.2196/21680 (preprint).

[28A] News-Medical. Accenture survey highlights healthcare data breaches among english consumers. 2017. Available at, https://www.news-medical.net/news/20170426/Accenture-survey-highlights-healthcare-data-breaches-among-English-consumers.aspx.

[28B] Deepmind. Deepmind. 2023. Available at: https://deepmind.com.

[29] Hyland A. 'This is a business for them': why Medibank should have paid the hackers. In: The Sydney Morning Herald; 2022. Available from: https://www.smh.com.au/business/consumer-affairs/this-is-a-business-for-them-why-medibank-should-have-paid-the-hackers-20221121-p5bzzn.html.

[30] Office of the Australian Information Commissioner. OAIC opens investigation into Medibank over data breach. 2022. Available from: https://www.oaic.gov.au/updates/news-and-media/oaic-opens-investigation-into-medibank-over-data-breach.

CHAPTER 12

Your chef: the virtual pharmaceutical care assistant*

Guido Jongen[1], Claudia Rijcken[2]
[1]*Virtually Human, Pijnacker, The Netherlands;* [2]*Pharmi, Maastricht, The Netherlands*

> *In the music world, "bot" is often a dirty word, conjuring up the tools used by high-tech ticket scalpers. Yet 50 Cent, Aerosmith, Snoop Dogg and Kiss have all deputized chatbots as their automatic, ever-alert greeters on Facebook Messenger, handling the flood of inquiries that would overwhelm any human.*
>
> **Ben Sisario**

The fast incline in computing capabilities and data storage has led to new and ingenious artificial intelligence (AI) techniques that enable machines to execute and learn with minimal human supervision.

In the last decade, more innovations than ever have been introduced in the virtual assistant space are innovations that can automate and engage in human-like conversations with a user. The experience offers that users can fulfill needs from homecare situations without having to always move to physical, human interaction. The concept has already been successfully applied to a number of industries, including banking, retail, marketing, and others.

As people generally do not like to go to a doctor, health care is an industry that may also be ready for so many use cases of the virtual assistance space. As mentioned in Chapter 1, doctors are increasingly becoming home-oriented care providers. In addition, with the rise of virtual assistant innovations, a growing amount of patient care can be offered via virtual personal assistants (VPAs) like chatbots or digital humans, allowing more time to be freed up for human interaction.

---

*In this chapter, you will read about how conversational AI is disrupting health care, how it can enhance patients' care experiences and knowledge of healthcare providers and which challenges hinder the fast maturation of this technology.

Pharmaceutical Care in Digital Revolution. https://doi.org/10.1016/B978-0-443-13360-2.00003-4

Concepts all aim to support health in the virtual space and act as your healthcare menu's chef. And if the doctor is in the virtual space, why not have the pharmacist there, too?

Technology

The shift from traditional bots to advanced conversational platforms is a much-needed natural evolution for organizations dealing with consumers and patients. In years to come, speech recognition via conversational AI technology is foreseen to feature rich standardized output object, like for example ChatGPT [1], to be accessible to a large population, to be scalable, and to support rich multilingual requests. Humans and machines are expected to collaborate seamlessly, allowing machines to learn new words and speech styles organically. Conversational AI technology will add value like fast scalability from a technology and content point of view. It can always be available for the user, as long as the device the user uses has its battery charged and internet access.

The global voice recognition market size has an enormous impact on the healthcare business of the future, as it is forecasted to grow from 10.7 billion U.S. dollars in 2020 to 27.16 billion U.S. dollars by 2026 [2].

The technology behind conversational AI has evolved in the last decades, as summarized in the paragraphs below.

Chatbots

A chatbot is an application designed to simulate a digital conversation with human users through AI that may act via textual or auditory methods. Initially, chatbots were text-based, requiring a certain level of literacy to use them.

Chatbots have been around for decades, but only in recent years have they become more popular. Joseph Weizenbaum created the first chatbot in 1966 to stimulate the patient-psychiatrist conversation [3]. As the bot was called, Eliza responded to basic commands by giving responses based on pretrained list keywords.

In this same period, Alan Turing developed the Turing test. The Turing test is a test of a machine's ability to exhibit intelligent behavior that is indistinguishable from a human. The Turing test is based on the idea that a machine can be considered intelligent if it can fool a human into thinking that they are interacting with another human rather than a machine. To conduct the test, a human evaluator is placed in a room with a machine and another human. The evaluator is then asked to engage in conversation with the machine and the human without knowing which is which. If the evaluator cannot tell the difference between the machine and the human, then the machine is considered to have passed the Turing test.

Being rule-based, keyword-based and text-only without an "own" brain was the main limitation for the first wave of chatbots (or faq-bots or menu-bots). User input was only recognized if it exactly matched the training data (keyword matching), and responses were limited to questions and answer pairs only. These early chatbots were not particularly intelligent and could not understand the nuances of human conversation.

This limitation in technology also held back the use cases for these types of bots, as only the most straightforward questions could be answered. For example, think of asking for opening hours without the capability to distinguish between different branches, Holidays or other variables.

Conversational AI

The basis of conversational AI is rooted in natural language processing (NLP). NLP combines linguistics and computer science to analyze and automatically represent the human language [4]. That is, textual data can be analyzed through AI techniques, as discussed in Chapter 11, and the relationships between words, sentences, and grammar can be related for a computer to understand. NLP has also formed the basis for other advances such as language translations and text-to-speech programs [5] and, more recently, been used to tell stories from a series of supplied images [6].

Chatbots require data inputs, which through NLP and AI, are translated into knowledge relevant to users. AI algorithms must understand the grammar in the language, and they also have to grasp the context in which they interpret the language, as in many languages, semantics are well known for their ambiguity and may be easily misinterpreted, which in health care has the potential to lead to disastrous, deadly results. Thus, accuracy in health care is of utmost importance and, therefore, subject to strict regulation.

Conversational AI can be best described as the part of a machine's "brain" that allows it to learn, understand, analyze and reply to human language. Intelligent virtual assistants filled with new talents have digitized human–machine interactions enabling them to do anything from answering factual questions to playing games and supporting routes.

Unlike conventional bots that depend upon sensitive keyword data from a predefined database, conversational AI chatbots use NLP and AI algorithms to process the dialogue in a conversation. Then, it uses this information to form better and more natural responses to customers' concerns and queries. In simple words, conversational AI is bringing conversations to life. In combination with an avatar that provides the corresponding empathic experience, conversational AIs will come closer to forming humanistic interactions.

Typically, conversational AI will communicate with humans. However, applications are also being developed where two bots can communicate with each other. This might be relevant for recreational, educational or chatbot training in the future days.

The first conversation-based chatbots had a questionable reputation, as they might lack full and broad understanding. Moreover, users considered their support unhelpful and irritating, even more so once the bot had again not been able to understand the question, e.g., was of poor quality and lacked empathy.

Some additional reasons why the initial user experience of conversational AI was not meeting the expectations in the early days:

1. The back end of the conversational AI should ultimately be kept up to date to gain and maintain a user's trust. If users feel the information the AI is providing is not correct and outdated, this leads to frustration and abandonment of the application.
2. The machine learning models (see Chapter 11) did not function correctly, as AI is meant to learn over time. The bot needs to be enabled to learn from past interactions and improve itself. Early chatbots were simply not as advanced as they are today.
3. Initially, chatbots were not fulfilling the expectations of users, as users' expectations of automation were higher than the chatbots' capacity for automation. As expected, users felt irritated and stopped using chatbots. However, we have now grown in understanding and are digitally integrated well enough such that chatbots serve a specific purpose. And when chatbots are unsure or feel that a human follow-up is required, they can transfer to human support seamlessly.
4. The balance between conversational and human interaction has to be discovered, and it is still evolving. Not every human is suited to work with conversational AI, and not every topic can be handled by chatbots yet. Finding the balance per ecosystem is a journey that requires structurally analyzing experiences and optimizing the approach.

Conversational AI has many use cases, including customer service, e-commerce, and personal assistants. In customer service, conversational AI can be used to answer frequently asked questions and assist customers with their inquiries. In e-commerce, conversational AI can be used to recommend products and assist with the purchasing process. And in personal assistants, conversational AI can be used to manage schedules, set reminders, and provide information. Use cases in healthcare will be described later in this chapter.

Speech as an additional feature

While the conversational AI got smarter, adding speech to the interface made more sense.

The development of speech recognition technology has come a long way in the past few decades. In the early days, speech recognition systems were based on traditional acoustic models that required large amounts of training data to recognize speech accurately. As a result, these systems were often limited in their ability to understand different accents and dialects and were not very robust in noisy environments.

However, as technology has advanced, speech recognition systems have become much more sophisticated. One key development has been using large sets of training data to improve speech recognition accuracy. By using large datasets, speech recognition systems can learn the characteristics of different accents and dialects, as well as the variations in individual voices, to improve their accuracy.

Another important development has been using deep learning algorithms to improve speech recognition. Deep learning algorithms are a form of machine learning models that can learn complex patterns and relationships in data, allowing speech recognition systems to become more accurate and efficient.

The current state of speech recognition technology is highly advanced. For example, modern speech recognition systems can accurately transcribe speech into text in a wide range of environments and with various accents and dialects. As a result, these systems are used in multiple applications, including voice-activated assistants, transcription services, and accessibility tools for individuals with disabilities.

Voice user interfaces

Voicebots and VUI (voice-user-interfaces) are two related technologies transforming how people interact with machines. A voicebot is a type of AI designed to understand and respond to spoken words, allowing people to interact with machines using their voice. A VUI, on the other hand, is the interface that allows people to interact with voicebots and other AI systems using their voice.

One of the key advantages of voicebots and VUI is their convenience. By allowing people to interact with machines using their voice, these technologies make accessing information and performing tasks easier and faster. For example, a voicebot can be used to answer questions, provide directions, or play music, all without the need for the user to type or click on anything.

Another advantage of voicebots and VUI is their accessibility becoming a valuable tool for individuals with disabilities who may not be able to use a traditional keyboard or mouse.

Smart speakers with voice assistants like Google Home or Amazon Alexa are increasingly popular and essential in daily lives due to their convenience of issuing voice commands.Nearly gone are the days of typing in a search query. Approximately seven out of 10 consumers prefer to use voice searches to conduct a query over the traditional method of typing [7].

Despite more advanced features, voice search capability's most popular usages remain restricted to more basic features, like queries and information requests. This is because users like to use voice searches to do basic tasks like checking on the weather, playing music, and setting a reminder. Given the potential and benefits of voice search, it's no wonder it's growing in popularity, also in healthcare.

An increasing number of companies are integrating voice-user-interfaces into their e-commerce strategies, individual (care) robot systems and other communication platforms. VUIs can be programmed at the literacy level of the user, meaning that personalized advice on specific content and literacy level can be provided. This is a very powerful tool in health care as well, as a correct understanding of the complex content of healthcare management programs is a serious challenge, as described in Chapter 2 on Single Point of Truth creation.

Developing a VUI in healthcare can be challenging, as several steps need to be followed:

- Defining the data sets to be used for filling the back-end "brain" of the VUI
- Describing the compliancy level to be achieved and the regulation to be followed
- Preparing dependencies in programming languages like Python or C+
- Importing the data
- Training models on large, diverse big datasets
- Designing conversational flows
- Integrating the conversational flows into a (human-feeling, empathic) avatar interface
- Deploying the models in a scalable and regulatory consistent, and compliant way
- Updating and maintaining the VUI based on a standard of care and user experiences

There are a number of possible approaches to training a chatbot or, in this case, VUI algorithm (from public health and medication data). The early chatbots learned through the use of preprogrammed rules and scripts. These rules and scripts are written by developers and provide the chatbot with a set of predetermined responses (direct answers and decision trees) to specific inputs. While this learning method can be effective in some cases, it can also result in rigid chatbots that lack the ability to adapt to new situations.

As chatbots and VUIs have evolved, so has the way they learn. An important development in the field of VUI learning is the use of deep learning algorithms. These algorithms are based on neural networks designed to mimic the structure and function of the human brain. Deep learning allows chatbots to analyze complex data and make more accurate predictions and decisions.

Another significant development is reinforcement learning (see Chapter 11), which allows chatbots to learn from their user interactions. In this approach, the VUI receives feedback on its performance and adjusts its behavior accordingly. This can help the VUI to understand better and respond to user inputs over time.

Natural Language Generation (NLG) algorithms allow VUIs to generate human-like responses to user inputs, making their interactions with users more natural and conversational. One of the most powerful NLG algorithms is GPT-3, which stands for Generative Pretrained Transformer 3. This algorithm is trained on vast amounts of data and can generate high-quality text that is difficult to distinguish from human-generated content. By using GPT-3, VUIs can produce responses that are more sophisticated and engaging than ever before.

Looking into the future, knowledge graphs and NLG will play a huge role in the automation of conversations. A knowledge graph is a structured dataset representing real-world entities and their relationships. This data is typically organized in the form of a graph, with nodes representing entities and edges representing the relationships between them.

One of the main advantages of knowledge graphs compared to traditional models is their ability to capture the complex and often ambiguous relationships between entities. Traditional models, such as relational databases, are limited by their structure and not well-suited to represent real-world data's nuances. For example, if a user asks a VUI about the capital of France, the VUI can use a knowledge graph to determine that the capital of France is Paris. The knowledge graph may also provide additional information, such as the population of Paris and its location within France. This additional information can help the VUI to provide a more detailed and accurate response to the user.

Use case of patient leaflet transformation in a VUI

With the supervised route, in which the available data are manually encoded into domain-specific information categories, an algorithm subsequently analyses this information and creates knowledge maps. Often referred to as an "inventory of knowledge," these maps are organized using various interconnected nodes to make it easy to know where to look for information. However, the coding can be labor-intensive and requires solid, standardized information classification and knowledge mapping.

This approach is relevant in pharmaceutical care, for example, in the case of converting data from a patient information leaflet into a VUI application. Currently, the patient information leaflet derived from Europe regulatory-approved "Summary of Product Characteristics (SPC)" text is restrictedly coded and classified. Thus, to use this information in a VUI, it still has to be manually coded, so it can understand the context uniformly and convert the ingoing data into something called "a Single Point of Truth (SPoT) of patient information."

An increasingly structured and coded, and thus, manual classification is less required.

Once structured, it facilitates machine learning, which is the more statistical approach in which the computer is given a magnitude of structured and coded SPC samples and, thus, is able to identify patterns across this information, that convert into question-and-answering models. Thus, intelligent VUI context can be developed more or less automatically. However, this method requires an enormous amount of training data and computer power and also definitely in the initiating process even more human checks for accuracy than the supervised learning does.

Because a VUI in health care is considered a safety-critical application, tolerance for algorithm and technology mistakes should ideally be reduced to zero. Thus, the AI's conversion of data-to-knowledge process and output needs to be fully transparent and thoroughly regulated by humans—before the release of every new version—as the example in Box 12.1 reflects.

Box 12.1 The complexity of learning AI

The more data varieties a VUI gets, the more it has to learn. That means that if—for example, in healthcare—patients have a specific verbal accent not yet known by the bot, at the first interaction, a VUI chatbot will have to verify whether the patient asked that specific question known by the algorithm, however, with a variable accent. Once the patient agrees that the question was correctly interpreted, the computer will store this information ("learn"), and the next time, will understand the question in that specific accent at once and will not repeat the verification process.

In this respect, one can imagine the complexity of making healthcare VUIs work reliably for - for example - verbally impaired people (e.g., aphasia in dementia, speech problems after stroke, etc.) using semantics and accents that are not generally understood. Therefore, this type of VUI learning requires programming-and-learning restrictions and thorough human oversight.

Specific regulations for VUI algorithms have recently intensified like in Europe in the Medical Device Regulation and the United States in the FDA Software-as-a-Medical Device Regulation (see Chapter 17). These regulations are instrumental in ensuring patient safety and exposing the technology's current limitations.

Digital humans

Digital humans present the further evolution of the VUIs, because they have a "physical", "nearly human" representation on screens, bringing empathic, more meaningful connections to the digital world.

Digital humans are interactive representations with some of a human's characteristics, personality, knowledge and mindset, typically rendered as digital twins, digital avatars, humanoid robots or conversational user interfaces. They can interpret speech, gestures and images and generate their own speech, tone-of-voice and body language.

Multiple organizations use these digital humans already to act as identified digital agents for customer service, support, sales and other interactions with current and potential customers. In addition, digital humans are integrated into a website or applications that run on telephones or tablets.

Digital humans in healthcare can be viewed as VPAs who can interact with the user on topics regarding, for instance, well-being, experienced health, questions on diseases, and information about healthcare interventions.

When VPAs are developed to support pharmaceutical care processes, they can be called Digital Pharmacists.

We define a Digital Pharmacist as a computer application designed to simulate pharmaceutical care with human users through AI. It may interact via auditory or textual methods. In other words, Digital Pharmacists are VPAs in pharmaceutical care.

Digital Pharmacists may help, for example, in logistical matters with medication supply or optimize treatment outcomes by supporting adherence by guiding the patient through their treatment pathway. They may also support adequate drug use by instructing a patient what to expect during the first weeks a medicine is taken. Another functionality is using the Digital Pharmacist to support rational drug use, for example, by supporting tapering programs like opioid withdrawal by having a blended care approach and motivationally coaching the patient to cope with the withdrawal challenges.

Digital Pharmacists may be present with pharmaceutical services in the Metaverse as well.

Both the prescription supply service as well as the consultation support is envisioned to take place in future days as well in Metaverse-like ecosystems (Box 12.2).

In the Metaverse, people use avatars to represent themselves, communicate with each other and virtually build out the community. In the Metaverse, digital currency is used to buy products as well as services, making both the e-commerce environments as well as healthcare interesting domains to explore. Users can of course also virtually travel through the Metaverse for fun with no goal in mind using a virtual reality headset and controllers.

Box 12.2 Pharmi: a digital human pharmacist

QR Code 12.1
Demo movie Digital
Pharmacist Pharmi.

Pharmi is a conversational AI trained to provide care to rheumatoid arthritis patients. It can answer the most common questions for a range of rheumatic medications, replying with easily accessible content to questions like "can I use alcohol with my drug" "show me an instructional video" or "what kind of disease do I use it for" Pharmi is a Digital Pharmacist in its adolescent years, currently in academic research in the Netherlands [8]. For information, see QR Code 12.1.

Metaverse

Digital humans are expected to play a role in the Metaverse. Gartner predicts that by 2027, a majority of business-to-consumer enterprises will have a dedicated budget for digital humans in metaverse experiences [9].

The Metaverse is an idea that many in the computer industry see as the next step for the internet. It's a single, shared, and immersive virtual space that is persistent and in 3D, where people can experience life in ways not possible in reality. Some of the technology required for accessing this virtual world, such as VR and AR devices, is rapidly advancing, while others, like adequate bandwidth and interoperability standards, are yet to be developed and may never be realized. Nevertheless, the concept of a virtual reality-based internet is not new and dates back to decades, with the term "metaverse" first used in 1992 in the science fiction novel "Snow Crash" by Neal Stephenson [10].

QR Code 12.2
How real and virtual people
connect in the Metaverse.

The Metaverse is not competing with our internet; it builds on it. The internet is something that people "browse" whereas, to a degree, people can "live" in the Metaverse as well (QR Code 12.2).

Considering that avatars are already able to run facial recognition models that can understand customers' moods and at the same time draw a number of conclusions based on people's facial expressions, the technology presents the possibility of always having an understanding virtual pharmacist accompanying you by way of your mobile phone (QR Code 12.3).

Additional use cases in healthcare
More accessible information dissemination to patients

The need to educate people about the facts behind a particular health-related issue, and to undo the damage caused by misinformation, does place an additional burden on medical professionals. VPAs can support this by proactively informing patients how to manage their disease or use their medication appropriately.

QR Code 12.3
Explanation of Metaverse in healthcare by Bertalan Mesko.

Amazon's Alexa added medical advice to its repertoire for developers already years ago. Increasingly, more health skills have been programmed on the Alexa device, for example, a virtual nurse to ask questions, breast-feeding advice, symptoms checkers, and hospital interactions with patients in their homes, reminding them to take their medication and facilitate prescription refills. These types of services are most often available 24/7 for nonemergency needs—like allergies or colds.

Partnerships with telemedicine companies allow users to ask Alexa: "I want to call to a doctor" They will be connected to a call center, and a health provider will call back through the device. In addition, Amazon announced in 2022 that it would allow brands to ask their customers queries, facilitating companies to understand their users better and optimize their products.

There is too limited space in this book to address the current developments in this domain. Nevertheless, as another interesting AI medical assistant example, one may think of Sensely, which combines AI-based triage and support for specific groups of patients under the avatar name Molly. Molly supports patients with, for example, heart failure in their disease management, using direct patient inputs (e.g., quality of life surveys) and inputs from digital health devices and medical records.

VPAs may also support answering frequently asked questions (FAQs) because they may overcome some of the typical challenges of FAQ sections on healthcare providers' websites. For example, patients might struggle to find the most relevant answer to their question because they are not using the exact same terminology as the FAQ list of the healthcare provider. The VPA can help to identify fitting answers faster: they use NLP to understand the intent of the question and to provide understandable answers, even if the way it is asked does not correlate with the exact terminology on-site and varies significantly between users.

Efficient triage and treatment support

The current increasing physician-as-well-as-pharmacist shortage in many countries is expected to double in the next decade. Thus, while conversational AI platforms cannot and should not replace care providers, they have a strong promise to offer relief amid the rising labor shortage in the industry [11].

VPAs focusing on patient-care provider interactions are consultation applications that connect the two groups, for example, to offer diagnosis support with medical triaging applications. Conversational AI can be applied for symptom checking and medical/ pharmaceutical triaging, assigning care priority as needed. In addition, they can be used as step-by-step diagnosis tools, leading the customer through a series of conversational questions and allowing them to input their symptoms in a logical sequence. Some symptoms may point to something serious that requires immediate escalation. However, in most cases, it will be a matter of following the VPA advice or scheduling an appointment with a human doctor for further review.

For instance, Gyant, ADA and Babylon applications are examples of VPAs providing virtual doctor applications. Those types of applications aim to put accessible and affordable health services into the hands of every person around the globe, assuming that a large quantity of physical general practice consultations may be avoidable. By combining the ever-growing computing power of machines with the best human medical expertise, they have created comprehensive, immediate, and personalized health services that handle triage effectively and are available 24/7 for patients.

With this evolution, the efficiency of offering health care providers' knowledge is maximized by reducing the time providers have to spend on questioning the patient, and all administrative triage duties, as the apps store all survey results and patient information directly in their medical records.

As an example of these concepts' clinical effectiveness, Babylon Health researched their Babylon Triage and Diagnostic System, as discussed in Chapter 11. In short, the AI system was able to safely triage patients without reverting to overly pessimistic fallback decisions, and its decision-making was, on average, safer than human doctors [12].

An additional advantage of these VPAs is that they allow easy consulting and triage in remote areas where access to healthcare facilities is difficult. The software may prevent people from having to travel (unnecessarily) for days to reach facilities, and the effectiveness of the applications is increasingly augmented with logistic solutions like drones, which can provide medication remotely efficiently and quickly.

Patient health maintenance support

Patient-oriented healthcare VPAs are applications that help a patient track and make sense of their health data. They can be regarded as the chefs that determine their health menu. Patients can use VPAs to track their progress toward their personal health goals, such as body weight, mood, or fertility in addition to requesting specific information, like what specific actions they should be taking to meet their goals or, for example, when they need to take their medication.

Periodic health updates and reminders help people stay motivated to achieve their health goals.

Secretary and logistic support

Today, care professionals are stretched thin, often having hundreds of tasks to complete before they even have their morning coffee. Unfortunately, rather than helping as it was intended, technology solutions for all these tasks can sometimes stand in the way of getting tasks done, leading to delays and costly errors.

VPAs can be great secretaries, for example, in supporting pharmacists in documenting prescription dialogs, appointment scheduling, or customer-service representation (for example, helping patients with their route through a treatment plan). In addition, staff can easily access a wide range of patient information by voice, such as lab reports, prescribed medications and upcoming appointments, with just a few keystrokes.

For example, the voice recognition software built by companies like Autoscriber is meant to solve the problem of doctors struggling to capture conversations with their patients in a structured way [13]. Companies like this built a speech recognition system and NLP technologies to extract structured data from conversations between physicians and patients with automation at its center and collaboration with doctors at the core.

Ideally, the output of the voice recognition software is automatically connected to the electronic patient dossier and can be integrated in a structured way with all other patient data available.

VPAs can also provide communication solutions, with conversational AI prioritizing and smart-routing requests to the right resource. Efficient resource allocation can save significant time and free pharmaceutical workers to focus on other, more critical tasks.

Impact on core responsibilities in pharmaceutical care

Due to the growing quality of interaction and the 24/7 availability of VPAs, these tools may significantly augment the day-to-day interaction of pharmacists with patients. In addition, they will change the professional task profile from a human-only to a blended care model, providing care digitally where possible. Thus, more time is freed up for the ultimate necessary human care.

Many of the frequent questions a pharmaceutical care stakeholder gets are repetitive, information-based, and have significant commonalities. Thus, these questions may be standardized and offered as digital standardized care to patients as a VPA.

Here is the general impact that VPAs are expected to have on the five domains of pharmaceutical care provision (refer to Chapter 6 for a more detailed discussion):

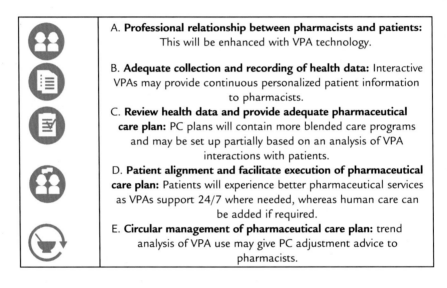

A. **Professional relationship between pharmacists and patients:** This will be enhanced with VPA technology.

B. **Adequate collection and recording of health data:** Interactive VPAs may provide continuous personalized patient information to pharmacists.

C. **Review health data and provide adequate pharmaceutical care plan:** PC plans will contain more blended care programs and may be set up partially based on an analysis of VPA interactions with patients.

D. **Patient alignment and facilitate execution of pharmaceutical care plan:** Patients will experience better pharmaceutical services as VPAs support 24/7 where needed, whereas human care can be added if required.

E. **Circular management of pharmaceutical care plan:** trend analysis of VPA use may give PC adjustment advice to pharmacists.

As indicated previously in this chapter, there are many reasons why pharmaceutical care stakeholders may decide to deploy VPA functionality. Examples are to augment patient service experiences, offer information on drugs, or provide a virtual pharmacist that a patient can consult on a 24/7 basis. In addition, empathic VPAs can solve the more repetitive and easy questions, which allow the pharmacist to handle the most complex problems and may assist in signaling which patients are in the most need of human intervention.

Moreover, VPA updating can be done with the click of a button. Thus, a VPA can scale up quickly and remains always up to date, as long as all relevant new information is integrated in a timely way. This in contrary where in many pharmacies still outdated books or reference documents are used (Box 12.3).

Box 12.3 An example: advantages of a Digital Pharmacist for a patient

Take an elderly person, just having received a new knee, still on an anticoagulant, but happy to be released from the hospital to go home. However, after 5 days in the homecare situation, the patient notices a number of blue spots on his arms and wonders what is causing them. While still immobile, the patient can ask the voice assistant what to expect 5 days after having surgery. The VPA can do a simple triage and reassure the patient that blue spots are known to occur with anticoagulant therapy and that there is no reason to worry.

The blended approach of providing digital pharmaceutical care support where possible, thus more time for caregivers is freed up to provide human care where needed, does offer a patient convenience, while also directing patients to the right level of care in a timely way (e.g., escalation to human care by VPAs is done timely in case of disturbing health signals).

Additionally, providing these forms of virtual care may lower the number of avoidable calls to pharmacies on topics where self-management is possible, resulting in less distraction and more focused time for pharmacists on human care. This is crucial in a healthcare system where age increases and patients use more complex medications for longer.

As it would give patients access to 24/7 self-care, the Digital Pharmacist may also be able to support healthcare commissioners and payers to cut down on any unnecessary patient visits to hospitals and pharmacies and reduce out-of-hour staff costs.

Considerations

 When evaluating the quality of a Digital Pharmacist, a few factors are of particular importance:

- Does it avoid redundant text, as patients may not take a verbose VPAs seriously?
- Does it still work when a patient uses incorrect grammar or typos?
- Does it recognize synonyms, and does it have a sufficient understanding of the context?
- Can or has the VPA dealt with accents, dialects, or diseases that impact the lingual centers in the brain?
- Does it encourage humans to learn or just tell them what they don't know?
- Is the advice given to patients understood by all, and is this sufficiently tested?
- Are the ways the algorithms work transparent, and can they be made public?

- Are retention and engagement rates available to indicate why patients may or may not be satisfied with the service provided?
- Is it possible for patients to refuse a Digital Pharmacist, if they prefer to speak with a human?
- Is optimal privacy and security of patient data ensured?

Security, privacy, and ethics

Data privacy and security challenges are increasing nowadays, leading to strict legal requirements on security and privacy for all digital health devices in the coming years. Also, it is assumed that most patients will want to know transparently how algorithms work and how data are analyzed unbiasedly. Thus, healthcare providers must develop teams that observe regulations, create transparency, and follow data privacy requirements, as explained in Chapter 17.

If VPA technology aims to disrupt healthcare, it has to gain the end user's trust. That trust is primarily built on providing transparency of algorithms and adequate use of data (both storing and analyzing). As noted in Chapter 11, future VPAs may also explain in a transparent way to users how they are structured toward giving recommendations, which data they have used, how the algorithm is programmed, and what data will be shared with whom.

More fundamental ethical questions should also be considered when implementing VPAs. For example, can patients refuse to be triaged by a Digital Pharmacist? Can patients insist on being treated by a human care provider in the future? Can we trust VPAs to make the correct diagnosis and use unbiased data? Can patients ignore the device, and what if the device gives a recommendation they prefer not to obey? Who is liable? A growing set of ethical and moral dilemmas ask for solid guidance. Chapter 18 provides more information on global developments toward developing ethical and moral guidance.

Liability

As mentioned before, triage tools and digital pharmaceutical care coaches are regarded as critical safety systems, falling in many cases under local Medical Device Regulations (see Chapter 17). Therefore, a manufacturer must understand the legal framework before deploying to formulate how to handle once an algorithm is not functioning adequately or how to handle the consequences once a patient is not following VPA advice adequately.

After all, unlike a face-to-face conversation, a VPA cannot yet adopt the full concept of emotional intelligence as humans do and may be less persuasive in convincing patients to follow advice. In the upcoming years, it will also be possible to apply facial recognition to add this feature. However, in the beginning, this feature may still lack the capacity to observe patients and interpret their answers, comfort level, and intuitive feelings based on decades of human experience.

Legislation is required to determine the liability when the advice of a VPA is not well understood, and the patient's well-being becomes at risk due to misinterpretations or other reasons. Additionally, current regulatory systems are yet limited positioned to oversee and review the content of complex healthcare VPAs adequately. As an example, regulators cannot yet determine whether pharmaceutical-focused voice-controlled algorithmic content should be considered an advertisement. In contrast, direct-to-patient advertising is not allowed in many countries. Thus, a regulatory framework in this respect is required as well.

Creating a single point of content truth to improve digital pharmacists

Using VPAs as true pharmaceutical treatment companions—as envisioned in the earlier paragraphs—is still limited. An important reason for this is the earlier mentioned fact that the patient leaflet and additional information resources are currently not yet available as uniform Single Point of Truth (SPoT) medication information in a format that allows integrated conversion to bot-knowledge. In the ideal future situation, all data on medication information as approved by, for example, EMA or FDA would be centrally accessible and maintained as structured data. Structured data would create a pharmaceutical SPoT, which is uniform and always kept up to date on all digital derivatives used by all pharmaceutical care stakeholders, such as pharmacists, physicians, and adherence providers. In order to let these central data sources act as a SPoT, more up-front standardization of coding and classification is required. An increasing number of medicinal product information data fields have already been standardized based on global standards like ICD-10, ATC codes, MedDRA codes, or Snomed.

Manufacturers of medication should be mandated to submit or update product information directly in a SPoT environment via authorized access levels and in a structured approach. That would greatly improve the current submission format, which is often driven by transferring PDF and Word files. Thus, the VPA can be updated simultaneously with new developments and is always a reliable information tool for patients without worrying about outdated information.

Regulatory bodies can use such a SPoT to run all required information content assessments and release information for use by third parties. Notified bodies can easily use the SPoT to assess the content quality and technical tools. Pharmaceutical care providers can use a SPoT as a uniform data feed for digital patient support tools.

This future vision has another advantage as well: the SPoT would not only be the Single Point of Truth but would also create a *single point of trust*, as it would be guaranteed that digital derivatives like VPAs are always up to date and based on the same, validated and approved product information.

In conclusion, there are huge benefits the evolution of VPAs can bring. However, there are still several challenges in development and ethics to overcome before VPA integrations in pharmaceutical care can be scaled broadly.

In the next Chapter 13, we will dive deep into the Personal Health Application and the Electronic Patient Dossier.

 This means for blended pharmaceutical care:

- Conversational AI has undergone huge evolution in the last decade
- VPAs are quickly finding their way into healthcare to support systems and triage, diagnostic, and disease management applications.
- VPAs in pharmaceutical care can be called digital pharmacists.
- Digital pharmacists can support blended pharmaceutical care as an augmentation of human care, for example, by providing drug information, adherence support, or consulting.
- Logistic or administrative VPAs can also help reduce internal administrative burdens, offering pharmacists more time for situations that require human intervention.
- In future, blended pharmaceutical care may also be offered in the Metaverse.
- To ensure sound updating and consistency in the pharmaceutical content of Digital Pharmacists, full coding of medication information is preferred.
- The conditions required for the successful implementation of Digital Pharmacists, like security, privacy and ethical soundness, require an innovative, proactive, and entrepreneurial approach by regulating authorities.

References

[1] OpenAI. [cited 2023 03/02/2023]. Available from: https://openai.com/blog/chatgpt/.
[2] Intelligence M. Voice recognition market size worldwide in 2020 and 2026 (in billion U.S. dollars) [Graph]. 2023, Statista. Available from: https://www.statista.com/statistics/1133875/global-voice-recognition-market-size/.
[3] Weizenbaum J. ELIZA—a computer program for the study of natural language communication between man and machine. Commun ACM 1966;9(1):36—45.
[4] Chowdhary KR. Natural language processing. Springer India; 2020. p. 603—49. https://doi.org/10.1007/978-81-322-3972-7_19.
[5] Hirschberg J, Manning CD. Advances in natural language processing. Science 2015;349(6245):261—6.

[6] Wang E, Han C, Poon J. RoViST: learning robust metrics for visual storytelling. 2022. Preprint arXiv:2205.03774.

[7] PwC. Consumer intelligence series: prepare for the voice revolution. In: Consumer intelligence series; 2018. Available from: https://www.pwc.com/us/en/advisory-services/publications/consumer-intelligence-series/voice-assistants.pdf.

[8] Pharmi. Pharmi products. 2022 [cited 2023 14/01/2023]. Available from: https://www.pharmi.info/en/solutions/pharmi-products.

[9] Moore S. Gartner outlines six trends driving near-term adoption of metaverse technologies. Gold Coast; 2022. Available from: https://www.gartner.com/en/newsroom/press-releases/2022-09-13-gartner-outlines-six-trends-driving-near-term-adoptio.

[10] Tucci L, Needle D. What is the metaverse? An explanation and in-depth guide. 2023 [cited 2023 03/02/2023]. Available from: https://www.techtarget.com/whatis/feature/The-metaverse-explained-Everything-you-need-to-know.

[11] Accenture. Artificial intelligence: healthcare's new nervous system. 2017. Available from: https://www.accenture.com/content/dam/accenture/final/a-com-migration/manual/r3/pdf/pdf-49/Accenture-health-artificial-intelligence-j.pdf.

[12] Baker A, et al. A comparison of artificial intelligence and human doctors for the purpose of triage and diagnosis. Front Artif Intell 2020;3. Available from: https://www.frontiersin.org/articles/10.3389/frai.2020.543405.

[13] Ai.nl. With AI and NLP, Autoscriber is helping healthcare professionals better care for the patient. 2023 [cited 2023 14/01/2023]. Available from: https://www.ai.nl/artificial-intelligence/with-ai-and-nlp-autoscriber-is-helping-healthcare-professionals-better-care-for-the-patient/.

CHAPTER 13

The taste of virtual, augmented, and mixed reality*

Vincent Suarez Takizadeh

Technologies Division, Cloudstone Group, Sydney, NSW, Australia

> *The power of imagination created the illusion that my vision went much farther than the naked eye could actually see.*
>
> **Nelson Mandela**

Taste is often accentuated by herbs and spices, the mix of which creates a harmony of flavor that captures the imagination. Taste buds react to the foods we consume, sending signals to our brains that activate chemical reactions that make us feel joy and satisfaction. The brain can be tricked into believing that something is spicy if we simply suggest it before a meal is consumed. It may be fooled into believing that something is real by simply stimulating the mind. Similarly, technology can be used to trick the brain into thinking that the space that surrounds it is real, and thereby provide the support needed for healthcare practitioners to maintain the health of a patient.

Augmented reality (AR) as well as virtual and mixed reality (MR) are technologies that are quickly changing the perspectives we have on healthcare.

Technology

Virtual reality (VR) is a computer-generated simulation of a three-dimensional environment that can be interacted with using specialized equipment such as a headset and handheld controllers. It enables users to explore, play, and interact with virtual objects and surroundings. The use of haptic clothing, alongside the use of an omnidirectional treadmill, further enhances this experience and allows for an elevated sense of immersion of virtual settings (QR Code 13.1).

QR Code 13.1
VR to educate on the human body.

---

*In this chapter, you will read about the fast-growing potential of virtual, augmented, and mixed reality for performing treatments, augmenting literacy in pharmaceutical care, improving patient experiences, and enhancing educational techniques for pharmaceutical care providers.

Pharmaceutical Care in Digital Revolution. https://doi.org/10.1016/B978-0-443-13360-2.00005-8

QR Code 13.2
What is augmented
reality?

Augmented reality (AR) enhances or blends the real world with virtual elements, such as 3D objects, sounds, or other sensory information. This can be viewed and interacted with through a device such as a smartphone, tablet, AR headset, or smart glasses to either supplement or replace physical reality. AR is related to computer-mediated reality, where a view of reality is modified (possibly even diminished rather than augmented) by a computer (QR Code 13.2). The difference between VR and AR is nicely explained in QR Code 13.3.

Mixed reality (MR) encompasses both AR and VR technologies, as well as variations between them. Both technologies combine to create a hybrid experience where virtual and augmented elements blend seamlessly.

Analysts predict that AR and VR in the healthcare industry are expected to hit $18.5 billion by 2032 [1]. The differences between the three forms of reality are shown in Fig. 13.1.

In general, the concepts of serious gaming (refer to Chapter 7) are frequently integrated in virtual, augmented, and mixed reality (VR-AR-MR) applications.

QR Code 13.3
Difference between AR
and VR.

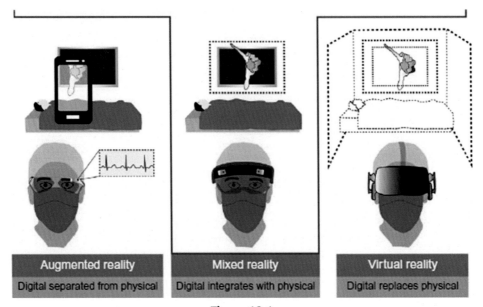

Figure 13.1
VR-AR-MR explained. *Adapted from Silva, JNA, et al. Emerging applications of virtual reality in cardiovascular medicine. JACC (J Am Coll Cardiol): Basic Transl Sci 2018;3(3):420–430. https://dx.doi.org/10.1016/j.jacbts.2017.11.009.*

Impact on core responsibilities in pharmaceutical care

Augmented and VR experiences can help us determine how a drug works, visualize the expected prognosis of a disease or drug effect, translate the most probable experience of a pharmaceutical intervention, and depict a patient's status after adherent (or nonadherent) drug use.

Here is the general impact that VR-AR-MR is expected to have on the five domains of pharmaceutical care provision (refer to Chapter 6 for a more detailed discussion).

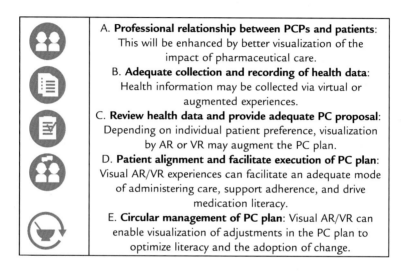

A. **Professional relationship between PCPs and patients**: This will be enhanced by better visualization of the impact of pharmaceutical care.

B. **Adequate collection and recording of health data**: Health information may be collected via virtual or augmented experiences.

C. **Review health data and provide adequate PC proposal**: Depending on individual patient preference, visualization by AR or VR may augment the PC plan.

D. **Patient alignment and facilitate execution of PC plan**: Visual AR/VR experiences can facilitate an adequate mode of administering care, support adherence, and drive medication literacy.

E. **Circular management of PC plan**: Visual AR/VR can enable visualization of adjustments in the PC plan to optimize literacy and the adoption of change.

Implementation in daily practice

Grasping the complex concepts of diseases and drugs can be a challenge for many people. Printed materials, pictographics, and videos can lack the immersive engagement needed for patients to truly understand their health concerns and how best to treat them. Questions like "how a disease represents itself in different organs"; "what does the drug do in the body"; or "what will I experience after having taken the drug" are often explained verbally, provided through written documentation, or sometimes expressed through videos.

Evidence suggests that health literacy plays a significant role in determining how well patients interpret medication labels and whether patients take nonprescription and prescription drugs safely and appropriately [2].

Research also suggests that patient information leaflets (PILs) need to be shorter, better structured, and augmented with visual and textual explanations to improve understanding and empower patients [3,4].

As these technologies allow for the complete integration of sensory information, it can be seen how VR-AR -MR can be used to enhance communication. Moreover, using VR-AR-MR interactivity on the benefits of medications and the risks may ameliorate patients' trust so that they start using the medication and make an effort to go through the PIL information.

VR-AR-MR as a treatment option

VR-based therapy exploits a psychological phenomenon known as "presence"—the illusion that you are really *in* an environment and not just looking at a picture or video of it. They work by tracking the position and orientation of the user's head and display images on screens that adjust in real-time to match the user's movements, creating the illusion of being inside a virtual world. As this is exactly the way in which a brain interprets images through the retina, the brain interprets the virtual environment more realistically [5].

This phenomenon has shown particular benefits in treating psychological orders, such as post traumatic stress disorders (PTSD), anxieties, or stress-related diseases. For example, in 2010, a small study using fMRI brain scans found this kind of VR exposure therapy to be at least as effective as imaginal therapy at damping down the hyperactivity typically seen in a PTSD patient's amygdala and hippocampus—the first being the seat of the fight or flight response, and the second being a key site in memory formation and presumably the source of haunting flashbacks. Both therapies also seemed to restore normal activity in frontal lobe areas that are inhibited in PTSD and may account for the disorder's characteristic emotional numbing and social withdrawal. A much larger comparison with about 200 patients is now underway [5].

The Medical School of Stanford University used Google Glass AR technology to help treat children with autism. It was used to assist them in interpreting the emotions of others. The project is still underway, and it is hoped that this will allow for social relations to develop through the use of memory [6].

QR Code 13.4
Example of VR as treatment.

Anxieties, like the fear of flying and the fear of vaccinations, can be reduced by gradually exposing a patient to a "safe" frightening environment with the use of VR smart glasses. This approach offers vivid forms of distraction and helps the patient to slowly get used to the concept of reducing anxiety to a lower level of dread. Step by step, this treatment reduces the paralyzing effects that anxieties can have and can diminish the need for high doses of anxiolytics, which are known for their serious adverse effects (QR Code 13.4).

The same sort of application is used in the care of severe wounds, where VR headsets offer gaming or relaxation environments that distract patients from the agony of their pain. VR is also used to reduce labor pain and perform drug-free deliveries.

Interactive learning and pharmaceutical care support

People can be overwhelmed when trying to understand and choose the correct over-the-counter medication in a supermarket or pharmacy. In addition, incorrect selections may occur without understanding dietary restrictions, drug interactions, or contraindication information at a glance, leading to further medical issues (QR Code 13.5).

QR Code 13.5
Example of AR smart packaging.

In the future, it is anticipated that people will be able to interact increasingly with products by simply looking at them through AR smart glasses or other smart devices. When hovering over a product with their smart device, people will be able to see information relevant to them, which may be data on allergies, potential food–drug interactions, or possible side effects, to name a few. By providing patients with engaging and immersive experiences and offering new ways to support adequate drug use optimally, manufacturers and care providers can better communicate with patients and distinguish themselves from competitors.

App stores now have numerous medical and pharmaceutical AR/VR applications available to support a patient's educational program. These applications can be used in specific care consultancy, and VR experiences can be offered in general waiting rooms. Medical concepts may provide useful insights, such as why blood clotting is dangerous (e.g., with the Invivo Bloodstream Explorer VR app), how the anatomy of the ear works (e.g., with the Stanford Health Care Anatomy app), or how the human body works (e.g., with the Human Anatomy 4D MR Zone app). Or people can experience how it feels to have a certain disease (e.g., via the Virtual Dementia Tour) or how it feels to have a condition cured (e.g., getting over flight anxiety).

Free AR apps allow students to observe how drugs and proteins interact with each other using smart devices. 3D models of complex drug complexes are shown in real time, allowing students to grasp the interactions better [7].

Furthermore, as noted earlier, when patients start taking a medication, a lot of information is "pushed" through, which means that once they get home, they may find it difficult to recall how to use an asthma inhaler, how to apply ointments, what to expect when beginning a new medication, or when to alert a doctor in case of a serious adverse event. Through VR, a patient can participate in spaces with other patients worldwide, and learn together as a group on adequate drug use, and thus be more engaged as stakeholders in the disease management plan. Those suffering from limited mobility could easily benefit from this, as well as those suffering from social anxiety.

This approach could go as far as explaining, in a home kitchen environment, which foods may interact with individual drugs; for example, if a patient's medication should not be taken with certain foods, the image recognition software in AR technologies could be used to analyze whatever may be presented to it, and inform the patient why the food could cause adverse reactions.

With MR, the technology could be used to inform polypharmacy patients which pill to take next. If they reach for the wrong bottle, they get a warning. When they have the correct medication in hand, they get a green light, along with directions for its use and other relevant information, such as interactions with alcohol, drowsiness risks, and so on.

Virtual pharmacists

The future blue sky scenario for AR will most likely introduce virtual pharmacy coaches in smart glasses that will guide patients through the situations that trouble them, ask them questions, and give them feedback and advice and that will personalize treatment experiences.

How to make this kind of support possible is basically a convergence of AR/VR with technology, which is described in other chapters of this book.

In principle, this support involves programming each condition independently, knowing its various manifestations, tailoring the treatment conditions within an AI algorithm, and then connecting this algorithm with a patient's individual characteristics based on data in the Personal Health Application (PHA), but also potentially on broader societal factors.

Alternatively, Home Medical Reviews can be done through MR, where the patient can interact with their pharmacist directly and even show the medications they are using in real time. The pharmacist can observe how medications are taken or used and suggest ways to improve management and control.

As social isolation continues to be a significant issue for older populations, VR spaces can act to mitigate the feeling of loneliness and improve psychological well-being by providing access to an environment populated with other users suffering from the same condition. These spaces could also see group consultancy being provided by pharmacists who wish to participate and allow for direct consultation to take place in separate virtual rooms if required (and on-demand) [8].

The coaching output may be projected in AR smart glasses but may also fit in a digital pharmacist or in the Metaverse, as explained in Chapter 12. However, the converged package of different technologies is a digital therapeutic on its own (see Chapter 15) and would require regulatory approval, given the sensitivity of risks if inaccurate advice is given.

Dynamic education for pharmaceutical care providers

As part of the medical ecosystem, VR technology is frequently used to assist in complex surgeries. Surgeons are able to perform procedures without having to be present at all. It can be done from any distance, allowing the patient to access specialist surgeons worldwide. According to the Lancet Commission on Global Surgery, the surgical workforce will need to double by 2030 to meet the needs of basic surgical care for low and middle-income countries. Companies that offer VR solutions anticipate that they will be asked to train thousands of surgeons simultaneously in VR. There are already platforms that enable doctors to remotely log into a shared virtual office to discuss patient cases and learn about specific surgical procedures.

Simulation-based education (SBE) is quickly becoming the key tool for medical education, proving to be an effective resource that is both cost-effective and repeatable. This allure is driving innovation in VR education and enables remote, collaborative learning without necessarily affecting the costs associated with running an educational clinic [9]. Clinical pharmacy also benefits from SBE but remains to be an underutilized resource [10]. Core competency developed through practical experience can be completely simulated and possess real-case scenarios that could further enhance skills and understanding. Graduates would then be better prepared when faced with complex decisions that may come their way during their course of work.

Similarly, cardiology teams are taking advantage of VR-AR-MR for education, preprocedural planning, intraprocedural visualization, and patient rehabilitation.

As these technologies are continually improving and assimilating, a doctor in the United Kingdom, with the support of a nurse in India, can assist a doctor in Australia in performing complex procedures in an MR environment. They can guide the doctor every step of the way and lend their expertise without leaving their home.

Extrapolating the VR-AR-MR advantages to the pharmaceutical environment can allow pharmaceutical students to explore the body in VR, visualize in AR how receptors are acting, or even how the mechanisms of drug molecules work (QR Code 13.6).

QR Code 13.6
Example of VR/AR in healthcare education.

An example of how to improve communication in the pharmaceutical profession is through the use of "pharmaceutical mannequins," which are virtual coaches in a training environment that can generate unlimited training scenarios and patient concepts, offering real-life practice on conflict-handling, counseling, and empathy to pharmaceutical stakeholders.

Another future use for VR is one in which pharmaceutical companies will train pharmacists in a global virtual VR community on how new, innovative drugs work, how to administer them appropriately, how to recognize specific side effects, and how to inform patients best.

Pharmaceutical industry representatives may use AR in brochures for tablet-equipped pharmaceutical care providers (PCPs), providing easy access to up-to-date, in-depth drug and disease information. AR can also be used in all future packaging, allowing the patient to view any additional information by simply observing the medication through a smart device or smart glasses.

Supporting the work-around in the community and hospital pharmacy

As pharmacists work with thousands of different prescriptions and bottles daily, there is a real risk of errors to be made. With AR technology, a pharmacist can receive real-time input when a bottle is not filled according to a prescription or if the patient is using the wrong medication. Currently, in most pharmacies, this is done by barcode scanning (an extra step) or visual inspection by peers (resources); however, AR could provide further accuracy and efficiency in the distribution process, thereby increasing productivity.

For products that cannot be distributed via automation, such as preparing injectables or ointments, AR can assist in streamlining the process behind preparation and application. In addition, it can act as a *guiding hand* that informs and directs the user.

Using readily available technology to improve safety when dispensing and compounding medication in everyday practice can create high levels of efficiency.

AR smart glasses can also act as a constant recording device. Besides acting as direct assistants to pharmacists, they can also record the activities that are carried out during the day, making them available for auditing purposes.

Using AR smart glasses in pharmaceutical care consultancy will enable PCPs to view patient information while speaking with the patient and have information at hand about any allergies, previous illnesses, or side effects experienced through a heads-up display (HUD). Additionally, when the AR is connected to the PHA, the PCP immediately goes into an informed care dialogue, focusing on the human aspects of care.

Considerations

Although the promises of VR-AR-MR are huge, a number of factors still limit the full adoption of the tools.

Adoption challenges

These factors are largely related to the global feasibility, affordability, and accessibility of VR-AR-MR technologies and applications:

- For AR smart glasses, people will have to wear such glasses. Not everyone will consider doing so, and for patients who already wear correcting glasses, adding AR will require the need for a separate set of glasses. It may not be finically feasible to buy AR glasses, as the costs associated with procurement are quite substantial.
- AR for smart devices is more sustainable as smartphones have a large adoption rate. Apps are still being developed to exploit this technology better; however, they have yet to break into mainstream use.
- VR headsets are just as costly as AR smart glasses; however, the adoption rate is far greater. A sizable population is already using VR, but wide-scale adoption is still underway.
- MR glasses or smart devices are yet to be fully developed, as AR and VR make up its framework.
- VR-AR-MR applications are not yet available for all diseases and all use cases.
- Patients have limited knowledge about these tools' advantages and may not be open to using their full potential.
- Prolonged use of VR headsets often requires sedentary behavior and a lack of physical activity. This can eventually lead to social isolation and disconnection from the real world. The lockdown periods during the pandemic have exhaustingly been characterized by these behaviors, which may be a turn for those who desire physical connections in the real world.
- The costs of producing these devices, such as the Microsoft HoloLens, the Oculus Quest, and even high-end smart phones, are still relatively high. There are solutions that offer low-cost entry into VR and MR technology such as the Samsung Gear VR and Oculus Go. They are cardboard frames that house smart phones as a means to create a similar experience to a dedicated headset.

Potential adverse health effects of VR-AR-MR

Notwithstanding the excellent opportunities VR-AR-MR can offer for healthcare, there are reasons for health-related caution as well.

One issue known with VR is a phenomenon called vergence-accommodation conflict, which can cause eyestrain. This occurs when the eyes have to focus on an object at a different distance than what they are actually converging on. This can cause visual discomfort and fatigue. The effects of this are usually temporary, though long-lasting effects are worth monitoring, as limited clinical research on extensive VR use has been only done. VR has also been known to cause musculoskeletal pain. Using VR headsets for prolonged periods can cause neck, back, and shoulder pain due to the device's weight. Prolonged use can also disrupt an individual's sense of balance and spatial orientation, leading to eventual disorientation and instability.

VR is also known to potentially affect a person's psychological state, ranging from temporary dizziness and light-headedness to more severe detachment from reality that may last for longer periods. Again, this is probably relevant only when using 3D extensively, but it is important to keep in mind personalized situations when starting to work with VR.

AR has also been correlated with the misjudgment of real-life situations (such as the use of the game "Pokemon Go" where people have ended up in very peculiar environments or situations), underestimation of reaction times, and unintentional ignorance of the hazards of navigating in the real world. Shifting the view to the side of your vision (like when wearing glasses) for too long can distract focus in real-life situations. Even if the temptation to glance at a notification appearing at the edge of the lens is avoided—waiting perhaps until crossing a street—these intrusions still may present a danger, as they tend to distract the user.

AR wearables may also affect how a typical person perceives the world, reducing focus. There are already various natural impairments to vision that affect focusing. For example, presbyopia, farsightedness, and nearsightedness all affect the ability to focus. Diseases like glaucoma, retinitis pigmentosa, and diabetes can create tunnel vision, which may mask objects in the peripheral visual field. Age-related macular degeneration causes the reverse, leaving only clearly defined items in peripheral vision.

A poorly designed AR interface could interfere with vision to the same degree as these ocular diseases. Thus, providing AR for this group of patients and considering the quality of the AR innovation are essential things to keep in mind when working with AR.

Therefore, as more applications become available and are used by a larger population, the boundaries for where to use or not to use particular types of medical and pharmaceutical ARs need to be further investigated. Safety measures are technicalities to consider, for example, the development of AR tools that stop notifications for a user who is moving or may suffer from one of the conditions outlined above. In addition, there should be consideration made toward limiting the use of the technology for children.

Other challenges to solve

Just as malware can attack mobile software and the technologies covered in other chapters of this book, the same may happen with VR-AR-MR platforms. AR HUDs can offer criminals a huge advantage in developing scams that potentially victimize innocent users, especially since healthcare-related data are extremely sensitive. This is why it will be essential for regulatory authorities to be involved and work with users and vendors to minimize any potential harms that could be unleashed on large populations or individuals. There is also the matter of how this information is collected when interacting with these technologies, and where this information is held. Some counties require that information related to privacy is kept within the nation as laws that define security may include storing the information locally.

Like the digital health compliance blueprint for other digital technologies (see Chapter 17), additional regulation may be needed to prevent the disadvantages of medical and pharmaceutical VR-AR-MR applications. Regulatory scrutiny can also limit the technology's evolution, causing a delay in the rollout of potentially life-saving solutions. As certain laws and requirements develop, applications may simply choose to avoid providing solutions that would attract unnecessary censorship that may prevent them from bringing their solutions to the market altogether.

In terms of hardware limitations for communication technologies, the resolution and clarity of the image/audio being produced is strictly dependent upon internet infrastructure and the technology used in said infrastructure. Regardless of how advanced the headset or smart device is, the sensory information will either lag or become pixelated if the internet speeds are slow.

Lastly, as other chapters address, reimbursement for medical and pharmaceutical VR-AR-MR applications is variable among countries. VR-AR-MR is limited in its recognition as a valid therapy or care activity. In order to support the development of more patient-centric tools with a concrete healthcare intervention focus, reimbursement options must be further researched based on the feasibility, reliability, and cost-effectiveness of VR-AR-MR tools.

In summary, these tantalizing insights into the taste of VR-AR-MR show impressive opportunities for the future of healthcare; however, significant developmental work still needs to be done to fully integrate the principles these tools offer in pharmaceutical care pathways.

In Chapter 14, the opportunities regarding pharmacy information systems will be explained.

This means for blended pharmaceutical care:

- VR-AR-MR applications are proven tools that can be used as autonomous patient treatments and are crucial in the future training of physicians as well as other health-care stakeholders.
- VR-AR-MR can support PCPs by visualizing medical and pharmaceutical care concepts, which can lead to a better understanding and improved literacy among medication users, thus reducing mistakes and optimizing outcomes.
- VR-AR-MR technologies may not only support customer services but also augment educational pharmacy programs or the efficacy of daily operations.
- Feasibility, affordability, and accessibility of VR-AR-MR applications are aspects that influence broad global adoption.
- Health risks associated with VR-AR-MR applications should be well considered before integrating the technology into a patient care solution.

References

[1] Global Market Insights Inc. Augmented and virtual reality in healthcare market to hit USD 18.5 billion by 2032. says Global Market Insights Inc; 2023 [cited 2023 05/02/2023]; Available from, https://finance.yahoo.com/news/augmented-virtual-reality-healthcare-market-072100409.html.

[2] Prevention, C.f.D.C.a. Medications. 2022. cited 2023 05/02/2023].

[3] Sciences, A.o.M. Enhancing the use of scientific evidence to judge the potential benefits and harms of medicines. London: Academy of Medical Sciences; 2017.

[4] Van Beusekom MM, et al. Low literacy and written drug information: information-seeking, leaflet evaluation and preferences, and roles for images. Int J Clin Pharm 2016;38(6):1372—9. https://doi.org/10.1007/s11096-016-0376-4.

[5] Waldrop MM. Virtual reality therapy set for a real renaissance. Proc Natl Acad Sci USA 2017;114(39):10295—9. https://doi.org/10.1073/pnas.1715133114.

[6] Hsieh M-C, Lee J-J. Preliminary study of VR and AR applications in medical and healthcare education. J Nurs Health Stud 2018;3(1):1.

[7] Wayne State University. 3D augmented reality app helps pharmacy students study protein, drug reactions. 2018 [cited 2023 05/02/2023]; Available from, https://tech.wayne.edu/news/3d-augmented-reality-app-helps-pharmacy-students-study-protein-drug-reactions-39836.

[8] Lee LN, Kim MJ, Hwang WJ. Potential of augmented reality and virtual reality technologies to promote wellbeing in older adults. Appl Sci 2019;9(17):3556. https://doi.org/10.3390/app9173556.

[9] Pottle J. Virtual reality and the transformation of medical education. Future Healthc J 2019;6(3):181—5. https://doi.org/10.7861/fhj.2019-0036.

[10] Andrews LB, Barta L. Simulation as a tool to illustrate clinical pharmacology concepts to healthcare program learners. Curr Pharmacol Rep 2020;6(4):182—91. https://doi.org/10.1007/s40495-020-00221-w.

[11] Silva JNA, et al. Emerging applications of virtual reality in cardiovascular medicine. JACC (J Am Coll Cardiol): Basic Transl Sci 2018;3(3):420—30. https://doi.org/10.1016/j.jacbts.2017.11.009.

CHAPTER 14

Fusion cooking with pharmacy information systems[*]

Mina Wanis[1], Whitley Yi[2,3]

[1]*Corum Group Pty Ltd, Sydney, NSW, Australia;* [2]*Skaggs School of Pharmacy and Pharmaceutical Sciences, University of Colorado, Anschutz Medical Campus, Aurora, CO, United States;* [3]*Well Dot, Inc, Chapel Hill, NC, United States*

Bringing flavors together

Fusion cooking is a style of cuisine that combines various forms and techniques of culinary traditions originating from different countries or cultures. It is a style that allows the chef to take control of the dish and not stick to a single style of cookery, creating endless opportunities for flavor and ultimately leading to an enhanced customer experience and greater satisfaction with their meal. By extension, this metaphor can also apply to the pharmaceutical dispensary.

The pharmaceutical practitioners, using their knowledge of pharmaceutical culinary techniques, can provide the patient with the best pharmaceutical care according to their needs, utilizing a variety of skills and tools available to them. A fundamental tool in the arsenal of a pharmaceutical culinary master is their Pharmacy Information System (PIS).

It is hard to think of a pharmacy nowadays without a computer. Maybe a small community pharmacy can get away with an old school "cha-ching" style cash register, but there will always be at least one computer for dispensing medication. Consider dispensing a 100 prescriptions per day without software to help manage health records, dispensing histories, drug interactions, stock management and logistics, identifying potential patient needs, running utilization reports, managing payer claiming or rebate transactions, and, most

---

[*]In this chapter, you will read about pharmacy information systems (PIS); what they are, how they came about, and where they are headed. It is important to understand their place in the pharmaceutical kitchen and acknowledge how these platforms are currently and will be, positioned to enable the pharmaceutical chef to provide the best care for their patients. This chapter will cover best practices and considerations to keep in mind when implementing or optimizing the use of PISs.

Pharmaceutical Care in Digital Revolution. https://doi.org/10.1016/B978-0-443-13360-2.00007-1

importantly, accurately, and efficiently dispensing medications. Of course, if that were the case, it would all need to be handwritten work on paper stored in folders and managed in leather-bound ledgers.

Technology

The use and adoption of information technology in pharmacy have exponentially increased over the past 30 to 40 years. Pharmaceutical care professionals have always been regarded as early adopters in the product adoption cycle. And now, with a greater emphasis on patient-centeredness, cost-effectiveness, collaboration and integration, and care pathways, healthcare is becoming more patient-centric, made possible by improved digital information availability. Community pharmacies serve as the community's go-to resource for medication knowledge, but they always run the risk of disruption [1]. Health silos will eventually be eradicated by digital health interoperability, which will also make health partnership-based ventures that span primary care, allied health, community care, and elderly care possible thanks to technology. Well-informed consumers will want health care when and where they need it and will anticipate clinician collaboration and communication [1].

Before the computer

 Prior to the pharmaceutical industry's proliferation in standardizing medication manufacturing, pharmaceutical care professionals were heavily involved in

QR Code 14.1
Before the computer.

medicine compounding at their local pharmacies. The compounding of medicines was time-consuming, given the manual preparation process; the accuracy required to prepare it and the number of records required to be kept were imperative for the day-to-day practice [2]. This took much of the pharmacist's time that could have been spent with the patient. QR Code 14.1 links to a short video developed by the Medical University of South Carolina College of Pharmacy and provides a great summary of the history of pharmacy from ancient times until today.

What is a pharmacy information system

 Before we talk about PIS, let's first talk about what it means to be an information system. An information system can be defined as the integration of interrelated software and hardware components that are used to collect, store, process, and provide access to data, information, and/or knowledge [3]. Information systems are used by organizations to accomplish a wide range of functions. These include supporting operations, interacting with external partners and customers, and driving strategic decision-making. Broadly speaking, there are six types of information systems [4].

- Transaction Processing Systems (TPS)
- Office Systems (OSs)
- Knowledge Work Systems (KWS)
- Management Information Systems (MIS)
- Decision Support Systems (DSS)
- Executive Support Systems (ESS)

Many information systems are also combinations of any or all of the above. However, when it comes to operations, a PIS allows the pharmacy to dispense, label, and organize patient records and medication histories at its most basic functions. The driving factor for their adoption originated from a financial and operational need. As medication became more expensive and various payers and funding bodies became involved in the patient journey, financial management modules were developed to accommodate this industry change. Over time, as the complexity and number of different medicines available increased, pharmaceutical care professionals needed a way to manage the logistics administration of their stock, maintain accurate patient records, and reduce the risk of patient misadventure during the dispensing process due to human error.

When computerized pharmacy systems became available, the uptake by the profession was almost instantaneous. A welcome by-product of this evolution of pharmaceutical care was that the day-to-day became the dispensing of pharmaceuticals as opposed to the compounding of formulations in the dispensary. Therefore, more time was spent with the patient, providing care [5]. However, with the increase in social welfare and the increasing availability of publicly and privately funded medication costs, the rudimentary dispensing and logistics application became the source of all pricing, claiming, and pharmacy financial data.

Complex patient-specific pricing rules necessitated the need to compute the correct pricing to ensure the pharmacy's viability. In countries with publicly or privately subsidized medicines, these rules can become quite difficult to calculate manually, and the PIS is crucial to run a profitable health business. Traditionally, pharmacy systems had simple user interfaces with very little functionality [5]. Of course, computer hardware was a limitation, and the proliferation of technology did not really occur until the late 1980s and early 1990s, when household personal computers became ubiquitous.

How does it relate to other healthcare information systems

The term Health Information System refers to any information system used within the healthcare sector for the provision of care, to support public health initiatives, or to provide any adjacent service. Examples of health information systems include electronic medical records (EMR) or electronic health records (EHR), which capture a patient's medical history and information; practice management systems, which help health clinics or offices manage operations such as scheduling and billing; and patient portals, which allow patients access to data and in some cases, serve as a communication platform between patients and healthcare providers. Health information systems can also include public health registries for disease surveillance and monitoring of outcomes and resource allocation.

As part of the spectrum of healthcare information applications, the focus of the PIS is on prescription management. Traditionally, a patient's medical record will include data points such as vitals, signs and symptoms, and clinical measurements as well as prescribed medication. The PIS, however, helps the pharmacist manage their patient records, but with a focus on pharmaceutics. The PIS has some common features like prescribing systems such as clinical decision support to aid prescribing/dispensing. However, prescribing applications provide no insights into supply, adherence, or postadministration adverse events. This knowledge is contained in the PIS patient record, which provides the pharmaceutical professional with a way to keep track of and report on the patient's dispensed prescriptions and any follow-up notes on adherence, compliance, and adverse events.

However, EMR systems and PISs allow their respective clinicians to access various digital health tools and shared government-sponsored clinical record repositories. In addition, they provide the ability to integrate with the same tools, such as multi-disciplinary team communication tools, and ultimately provide two pieces of the much larger patient health journey.

The one main distinction between the PIS and other clinical systems is regulatory requirements concerning medication supply and government cocontribution entitlements. With the PIS sitting on the side of medicine administration, providing the patient with the correct medicine costs is vital, given their social security status or insurance policy.

What all of these systems have in common is the collection, storage, and utilization of data. Therefore, having timely access to information is vital for health system governance and strategy development. This is further emphasized by the fact that the World Health Organization (WHO) has declared the use of health information systems as critical for achieving Universal Health Coverage [6], due to the role health information systems can play in providing relevant and timely information to key decision-makers at every level, for improving access and quality of care.

How it supports care

The PIS is vital in the workflow and management of dispensing pharmaceuticals in a healthcare setting. These systems are also critical for several reasons. One of PIS's primary functions is to support medication administration logistics. This includes managing the medication inventory, tracking the medication movement from the manufacturer to the pharmacy, and tracking the dispensing of medications to patients. This insight can further provide insights into operational efficiencies, clinically and logistically. For example, the system can track inventory levels and alert pharmacy staff when it is time to restock certain medications. This notification and tracking can help reduce the risk of shortages, ensure that patients have timely access to their medications when needed, and help prevent shortages or errors in the medication supply chain. Improved efficiencies ultimately help reduce serious consequences for patients requiring medicines in need of timely care.

In addition to logistics management, a key requirement of a PIS is to support the clinician in recording normalized patient-specific data. This support is important as it enables the software engineers to provide clinicians with tools to generate reports on their patient's adherence and other relevant insights. This can be especially important for patients with chronic conditions who need to take multiple medications regularly. By tracking how often patients are taking their medications and how well they adhere to their prescribed regimens, clinicians can identify potential problems and provide support to help patients stay on track with their treatment. By extension of this functionality, a PIS can then employ clinical decision support modules to provide algorithmic clinical insights, alerts, or warnings (see Chapter 11).

When a patient is prescribed multiple medications, it is important to ensure that there are no interactions between the medications that could cause harm. Implementing drug interaction modules in a PIS can alert the clinician to potential interactions or contraindications, helping to ensure that patients are taking their prescribed medications as directed.

The PIS can also be used to connect to other sources of patient data, such as reported outcomes or other acute care health information, to help clinicians understand how a patient responds to their treatment or if their clinical conditions dictate a modification to their treatment dosage. This can be especially useful for tracking the effectiveness of medications or identifying potential side effects. As remote patient monitoring tools become more prevalent, integration of their data feed will become standard and eventually part of the dispensing workflow.

Benefits and impact

The benefits of a PIS include reducing medication errors, improving workflow efficiency in drug distribution [7] and facilitating the provision of more pharmaceutical care services [7]. For example, integrating Computerized Provider Order Entry with PISs has been shown to reduce medication error rates by up to 55%−80% [8,9]. PIS also makes possible the ability to leverage machine-readable drug codes on labels and packaging, such as barcodes [10], to help improve accuracy and efficiency in dispensing and administration.

Implementing a PIS allows for the introduction of standardization and safeguards into pharmacy documentation and operations that previously were not possible through a manual record-keeping system. However, even when standards are adopted and utilized for manual systems, they cannot be enforced or monitored without a significant administrative burden. For example, suppose a specific unit of measurement should be used when preparing a medication (e.g., mg/dL vs. mg/mL). However, there is no way to ensure it is documented correctly every time unless each relevant prescription is reviewed manually. However, by implementing a PIS, validation steps can be created in order to enforce inputted data to adhere to a specific structure. This creates guardrails while ensuring data are stored in a useable and interpretable format by all parts of the system, including reporting, inventory management, and clinical applications.

Using structured data elements, medication orders or prescriptions transcribed into a PIS can be mapped to discrete drug codes representing meaningful medication concepts. These drug codes can be linked to other metadata and information about the medication through a drug information database or compendium. When a PIS is integrated with a drug information knowledge base, a prescription record suddenly contains rich, contextual information about that medication that may be useful to the end-user. The system can link that prescription record to the drug's active ingredient(s), pharmaceutical classification, drug–drug interactions, pregnancy/lactation information, adverse reactions, and any other information encoded in the drug information database. Rules and algorithms can be developed to automatically check for drug-drug interactions, patient allergies, or other potential medication errors or red flags. Rules can also be created to provide alerts if a dose is beyond the recommended range or requires routine monitoring. These types of algorithms and alerts are called clinical decision support tools, which are discussed later in this chapter. The ability to have integrated software with clinical decision support tools has demonstrated positive outcomes. Research has shown a 39.8% reduction in medication errors when providing medication therapy management services that are integrated with the PIS [11].

Overall, PISs play a vital role in the care of patients by helping to manage the logistics of medication administration, tracking patient adherence, and providing tools and reports to help clinicians understand how patients are responding to their treatment. By using PIS to support patient care, streamline pharmacy operations, and provide valuable insights into patient adherence, and other key factors, the PIS can improve the quality and effectiveness of the medications dispensed, ultimately leading to improved patient outcomes.

Adoption and perception

One of the concerns with implementing any electronic information management system is the potential for e-iatrogenesis or unintended consequences caused by health information technology. While technology has amazing potential to improve health system capabilities, efficiency, and patient safety, it also has the potential to introduce new variables into a health system that can create different types of errors and safety concerns, such as over-reliance on technology [12] and alert fatigue from clinical decision support tools [13]. Health information technology (HIT)-related errors have been defined as anytime "HIT is unavailable for use, malfunctions during use is used incorrectly by someone, or when HIT interacts with another system component incorrectly, resulting in data being lost or incorrectly entered, displayed, or transmitted." [14] One of those unintended consequences is increased cognitive load and stress when working with health information systems that are not user-friendly. Health information technologies, specifically EHRs, have been associated with clinician burnout [15] due to increasing workload, higher documentation burden, and poor usability.

Do these concerns apply to PISs as well? When looking at acceptability and adoption, the perceived benefit of PISs tends toward being positive overall, but concerns with usability and workflow impacts still exist. A study of pharmacists in Saudi Arabia examined pharmacists' perceptions of the PIS. While respondents reported that the PIS made distributing medications easier, improved the pharmaceutical services they were able to provide and enhanced their workflow, around half the respondents also reported that it increased their workload and responsibilities and made work inflexible [7]. In Sweden, a majority of pharmacists perceived the PIS as improving safety in medication dispensing [13].

Impact on core responsibilities in pharmaceutical care

The PIS is pivotal to improved pharmaceutical care. It provides the clinician with the necessary information to safely and efficiently dispense the pharmaceutical. To align with our fusion cooking metaphor, the clinical data recorded or aggregated in the PIS forms the basis of the dish.

The system will eventually present care providers with the opportunity to visualize their patient's data in context with other external data sources, such as remote patient monitoring, external public health data, eHealth record repositories, and patient input from connected health apps.

This wealth of health data will require a system to transform the collected data into actionable insights for pharmaceutical care provider to make informed care decisions for their patients.

Highlighted below are some of the ways PISs are expected to impact the five domains of the pharmaceutical care provision (refer to Chapter 6 for a detailed discussion).

	A. Establish and maintain professional relationships with patients: The PIS is fundamental to establishing a relationship with the patient. It allows the recording of visits, interactions, and dispensing as it will always inform the PCP's conversation. **B. Adequate collection and recording of health data:** The PIS allows the PCP to collect the required data points to allow them to make a well-informed decision. Maintaining data quality and accuracy is vital to keeping the system relevant and reliable for the PCP. **C. Review health data and provide an adequate Pharmaceutical Care proposal**: Through improved data quality and accuracy, the utility of the information system is improved, and by extension, the system's ability to utilize data to optimize outcomes and suggest opportunities for care. **D. Patient alignment and facilitation of execution of the PC plan:** The PIS will allow the pharmaceutical professional to identify the needs of the patient based on their medicines and help inform any care plans. **E. Circular management of the PCP plan:** The PIS, using all data available, provides the PCP with the ability to record patient feedback or ingest external data feeds with respect to adherence, tolerability, allergies, and preferences to always make the most informed clinical decisions and ultimately improve patient outcomes.

Implementation in daily practice

At its core, the PIS is governed by two main principles that are vital for pharmaceutical care professionals to be aware of: the Data, Information, Knowledge, Wisdom pyramid, and Information System Components comprising Input, Processing, Output, and Feedback.

A primer: DIKW pyramid and information systems

Data are being generated in unfathomable amounts each day. For clinicians, this is as simple as a blood pressure reading or the name of a medication. Once we add different descriptors to the data, a clearer picture emerges, i.e., the medication's context, dose, quantity, dosage form, and directions. Combining all these different data elements starts to give the pharmaceutical care professional a better idea and begins to be transformed into actionable data, i.e., information. When we apply this information in the context of the patient profile as we see it in our PIS, we can make an informed decision about supply, i.e., knowledge. As our PIS becomes more advanced with improved integration of third-party patient tools, primary care records, and other sources to close the medication-management loop, it will become quite difficult to achieve the ultimate state of wisdom (Fig. 14.1).

In light of the above DIKW pyramid, at its core, and name, a PIS is an information system that is governed by a fundamental concept of information systems (Fig. 14.2).

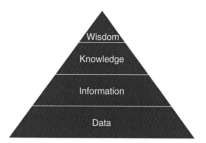

Figure 14.1
DIKW pyramid [16].

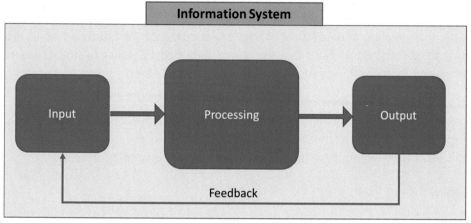

Figure 14.2
Information system components [17].

The Information System Components Diagram is a visual representation of the main components of an information system. The main components of this diagram are

- Input: This component is responsible for collecting and digitizing data from various sources. These sources can be internal, such as data entered by employees, or external, such as data received from other systems.
- Processing: This component is responsible for converting the raw data collected by the input component into meaningful information. The processing component performs various operations such as data validation, data transformation, data analysis, and data storage.
- Output: This component is responsible for presenting the processed information to the end-users in a meaningful format. Depending on what the end-user wants, the output component can make different kinds of output, such as reports, alerts, and visualizations.

- Feedback: This component is responsible for providing feedback to the system about the results of the output component. Feedback can be used to measure the system's performance by improving the Input component.

All these components are interconnected and interdependent to provide useful feedback to the end-users of the system. The diagram represents the flow of data through the system, highlighting the importance of each component in making the information system functional. Input and output are the boundaries of the system, while processing and feedback are at their core, enabling constant improvement and adaptability. In the case of a PIS, this would mean improved patient care, more accurate logistical administration, and improved financial reporting for the organization.

By extension of this logic, third-party integrations for a PIS can add additional data for processing, thus creating a more valuable output. According to the DIKW pyramid theory, integrating third-party applications into the information system allows for the improved transformation of data or information into actionable knowledge.

Pharmacy is a fundamental component of the larger health system and third-party integrations are inevitable. There are many start-ups and scale-ups looking to enter the health technology market through pharmacy. However, the trick is to develop seamless integrations in the PIS without having to leave the clinical workflow and disrupting patient care.

Integrations

A major pain point for healthcare professionals is the need to disrupt their clinical workflow to access third-party applications required in the care of their patients. In the pharmaceutical care realm, the pharmaceutical care professional can be overlooked, despite how crucial third-party native integrations within a PIS are for improving patient care and safety and efficient pharmacy practice. An example of a PIS that has integrated clinical features is FrameworkLTC [18]. This PIS has the ability to integrate with electronic health records (EHRs) like Cerner, Epic, and Allscripts to provide a comprehensive view of the patient's medications and streamline orders. This facilitates the development of effective treatment plans, reduces the risk of adverse drug events, and improves patient outcomes.

Financial integration is also an important aspect of PIS. An example of this is the integration of billing and insurance modules into the PIS, which can help streamline the claims process and reduce errors in claim submission. In Australia, payment platforms, such as Lantern Pay (https://www.lanternpay.com/) and Zephyr Claims (https://zephyrclaims.com.au), have developed claims integrations within the PIS that allow the pharmacy to submit medication claims for various insurance and government rebate schemes to avoid patient out-of-pocket costs. This is a great step for patients, as they are not out of pocket, and the pharmacy is reimbursed instantly. On the other hand, PIS-specific accounting module integrations such as Xero (https://www.xero.com/au/small-businesses/healthcare/) can provide the pharmacy with the ability to reduce the amount of time the accounting function takes from organizations improving flexibility and helping streamline operations.

Marketing integration is another feature that can help pharmacies better understand their customers, which is an essential aspect of customer relationship management. Health platforms such as Carebook have the ability to provide pharmacies with the ability to expand their reach and engagement with patients. They integrate with a PIS and utilize the data feed to enhance the patient-pharmacy relationship and communication. On the other hand, solutions such as Digital Pharmacist (https://www.digitalpharmacist.com) enhance a pharmacy's digital enablement through a cloud-based platform. They combine communications, adherence, digital marketing, and relationship management modules in an integrated cloud platform, allowing the pharmacy to manage its digital footprint, drive operational efficiencies, target new customers, and keep track of current customers.

Integration of medication management systems, such as order entry, administration, and history systems, can also extend the functionality and effectiveness of a PIS. These systems can help reduce medication errors and improve medication safety. An example of a complete medication management solution is the introduction of the Spencer Health medication dispensing aid [19]. This solution provides an end-to-end platform for pharmacies to help manage patient dispensing, usage analytics, and telehealth functionality for long-term care and patients most in need of dosage administration support. The data are fed back to the pharmacy to provide pharmacy teams access to real-time actionable and critical healthcare data, improving adherence rates and reducing misadventures and adverse events. Further information on this solution can be found by scanning QR Code 14.2.

QR Code 14.2
Integration.

Lastly, the ability to integrate interoperability tools into the clinical network enables access to various clinical results that can immediately impact patient care. For example, in Canada, the Fraser Health Authority in British Columbia utilized Altera Digital Health's dbMotion interoperability solution to provide immediate access to lab test results for patients on the Clozapine program as part of the Psychosis Treatment Optimisation Program [20,21]. Before dosing, the pharmacy reviews the patient's lab results and performs a clinical assessment before Clozapine administration. The use of such an integration resulted in overall reduced hospitalization and emergency room visits for the organization but also increased cost savings and improved patient lives.

As the healthcare industry adopts more and more third-party applications, it is becoming necessary to have a standard way of integrating them with PIS; this is where interoperability comes into play. Interoperability is the ability of different systems to work together seamlessly and share data. Improving interoperability makes it easier to integrate new applications with the PIS, which can help improve care and reduce costs.

Striving for interoperability

Ever since the dawn of the healthcare information technology age, there has always existed the utopian dream of seamless interoperability between digital health solutions across the patient care spectrum. Unfortunately, given the proprietary nature of software, interoperability was seen as counterintuitive to commercial success.

Interoperability refers to a PIS's ability to communicate with other services and systems. It depends on having the appropriate telecommunication infrastructure and data standards, as mentioned above. PISs can be connected to electronic health records, prescription databases, and drug information databases. They can also be connected to third-party vendors that provide services such as facilitating communication with prescribers when prescriptions need prior authorization. PISs also allow integration with other dispensing technologies, such as automated medication dispensing systems. These usually involve robotic systems that can count, package, and label medications but may also include more advanced robots that can prepare sterile IV compounds.

The Healthcare Information and Management Systems Society (HIMSS), defines interoperability as the

Ability of different information system, devices and applications (systems) to access, exchange, integrate and cooperatively use data in a coordinated manner, within and across organizational, regional and national boundaries, to provide timely and seamless portability of information and optimize the health of individuals and populations globally. [22].

As discussed earlier in Chapter 8, international for-purpose organizations such as HL7 have developed content standards to help support the interoperability initiatives of various organizations. The development and implementation of clinical terminologies, such as SNOMED CT and ICD-10, have also given clinical information systems the ability to codify clinical data for easier database storage and algorithmic manipulation.

More recently, and to align with the proliferation of API-based communication between systems, HL7-FHIR-based transport standards are becoming more prominent in the health tech space (see Chapter 8). Given the ease of implementing an API-based technical architecture, FHIR terminology standards have allowed the larger health record systems to reach a more advanced level of interoperability. FHIR is structured in a set of "resources," which also cover pharmaceutics, and with the help of local HL7 chapters, the basic set of FHIR resources has been adapted for different countries to align with their needs. For clinical systems not built with interoperability baked in, integrating an FHIR-based API layer into their system architecture presents a significant step forward for overall system interoperability.

FHIR is primarily a data exchange communications standard; it necessitates a structure for messages sent to and from various systems. This is where content standards can be applied to the outgoing messages, of which the most commonly used are the HL7 V2 and the HL7 V3 Clinical Document Architecture (CDA). CDA is a commonly used international structured message; however, it is more data intensive compared to FHIR API request-response transactions.

As pharmaceutical care professionals, we must be aware of the transport and content standards used in our clinical information systems and third-party applications in order to ensure that they are not proprietary and can interact with other environments should the need arise. Unfortunately, the decision for implementation lies with the software vendor and is a fundamental piece of the system used.

What is in our control as care professionals are the ability to ensure the data we capture in our PIS is interoperable and based on standardized data. Essentially, we must ensure we are always using codified data in our PIS instead of free-text additions to our patient notes. To enable automation and improve the accuracy of a PIS, standardizing data based on clinical terminologies is vital. This method captures patient and medication data in accordance with standard formats and conventions. This is where interoperability and integrations provide the most value. In addition, terminology standards such as SNOMED CT and other localized medicines terminologies will enable the standardization of communication.

As discussed in Chapter 8, FHIR standards will become more prominent in clinical systems with a heavy focus on facilitating out-of-the-box interoperability. QR Code 14.3 links to the HIMMS Interoperability page that provides a list of popular internationally recognized standards to be aware of as pharmaceutical care professionals:

QR Code 14.3
Striving for
Interoperability.

It is important to understand what standards drive your systems and how they align with your national or regional digital health strategy. Research is required to understand the standards implemented in your applications so you can make an informed decision about which information system is best for your clinical practice's interoperability needs.

Data standards and vocabularies

One of the key considerations when implementing a PIS is choosing the specific drug terminology and code standards that will be used to encode drug and prescription information. In some instances, the drug code that must be used will be dictated by national standards or billing requirements. For instance, in the United States, the National Council for Prescription Drug Programs (NCPDP) developed and maintains the standards for billing insurance and how drug information should be transmitted as an electronic prescription. The NCPDP standards are based on RxNorm standards and National Drug Code for drug identifiers. Each drug terminology has pros and cons, which must be carefully considered. Equally important is the ability to map between drug terminologies when interfacing with systems that use a different drug vocabulary.

Clinical decision support in pharmacy: today and tomorrow

Clinical decision support systems (CDSS) are algorithmic-based integrations that assist healthcare providers in making clinical decisions by providing relevant patient information and recommendations at the point of care. There are several types of clinical decision support functionality that may be available in the PIS and can impact pharmacy practice.

- **Medication management**: The CDSS can provide pharmacists with information on appropriate medication dosing regimens, drug interactions, and contraindications, helping to reduce the risk of medication errors and improve patient safety.
- **Drug formulary management**: CDSS can provide pharmacists with access to drug formularies and assist in selecting the most cost-effective medications for patients. Clinical guidelines: CDSS can provide access to clinical guidelines and protocols for various medical conditions, which can help pharmacists stay up to date on the latest best practices for medication use and ensure that patients receive appropriate treatment.
- **Clinical alerts**: CDSS can provide pharmacists with real-time alerts for important events, such as abnormal lab values, drug dosages, or interactions, helping to identify and address potential issues quickly and preventing patient misadventures.
- **EHR integration**: Many CDSS are integrated with electronic health records (EHRs), allowing pharmacists to access patient information and decision support tools within the same system. This can improve communication and coordination of care between pharmacists and other healthcare providers.

However, as these tools become more sophisticated, the lines will blur between clinicians' decisions and trusting "the algorithm." Machine learning (ML) and artificial intelligence (AI) are expected to impact the future of PISs significantly (see Chapter 11). It has been shown that when doctors incorporate such technology, such as machine learning and the integration of AI tools, into their practice, they achieve better diagnosis rates and improve patient outcomes [23].

One potential use of ML and AI in pharmacy is to improve medication prescribing and dispensing accuracy and efficiency. For example, ML algorithms could be used to analyze patient data and identify potential drug interactions or contraindications, helping pharmacists avoid errors and ensure patients receive the most appropriate medications [24].

Another potential use of ML and AI in pharmacy is to improve the management of medication stockpiles and inventory. For example, ML algorithms could be used to predict demand for certain medications and help pharmacists optimize inventory levels and prevent shortages [25]. Even though the research may focus on problems that affect the whole industry, the technology will eventually be used in pharmacies.

Additionally, ML and AI could be used to improve the accuracy and timeliness of patient medication lists and records. By analyzing data from EMRs and other sources, ML algorithms could help pharmacists identify and update discrepancies in patient medication lists, reducing the risk of errors and improving patient safety [26].

Other examples include.

- **Population health management**: CDSS can help pharmacists identify and manage patients at high risk for certain conditions, such as diabetes or heart disease, and provide recommendations for interventions to prevent or mitigate these conditions.
- **Natural language processing (NLP) systems**: These systems use AI to analyze and interpret unstructured text data, such as EMRs and clinical notes. NLP systems can help pharmacists identify relevant patient information, such as medication lists and allergies, and can also be used to extract data for use in CDS algorithms.
- **Predictive analytics systems**: These systems use machine learning algorithms to analyze patient data and predict future outcomes, such as the likelihood of a patient developing a certain condition or experiencing a negative drug reaction. Predictive analytics systems can help pharmacists identify patients at risk and intervene to prevent negative outcomes.

As these tools become more ubiquitous, it will be in the PIS that they provide the most value. And so, as clinicians, we should consider if we want to incorporate these tools into our practice to make more informed decisions as opposed to relying on an algorithm for a clinical decision.

Data quality, data sharing and data governance

The increasing use of information systems in healthcare requires that we consider data quality, sharing, and governance as part of our everyday workflow. Information systems help us collect, record, and share patient health data. For these systems to work together seamlessly, the data needs to be formatted in a machine-readable, interoperable standard. However, issues around data accuracy and patient consent arise.

QR Code 14.4
Data quality, data sharing and data governance.

To address these issues, pharmacies and clinics must have data governance policies and procedures in place to ensure data is well-managed and secure, with clear accountability. These principles are essential in a pharmacist's day-to-day workflow, and you can find more information about data governance and quality in the HIMSS resource linked by QR Code 14.4.

Data quality in patient records

Data quality is critical in PISs to provide high-quality care to patients. Accurate and current data are necessary for pharmacists to identify and resolve medication-related concerns, customize treatment recommendations, and address public health challenges. As pharmacists expand their services, accurate data will become even more crucial to monitor patient health and identifying problems. In addition, access to relevant and accurate information is essential to use emerging technologies such as CDS risk stratification algorithms. Therefore, pharmaceutical care professionals must establish a culture of high-quality data collection in their day-to-day practice to improve patient outcomes and save healthcare costs.

Examples of how improved data quality can support pharmacy practice and patient care include.

- Improved data quality can benefit patient care through the identification and resolution of medication-related problems. For example, Porterfield, Engelbert [27] found that using an electronic prescribing system improved the accuracy of medication orders and reduced the rate of medication errors in a primary care setting. Similarly, Agrawal [28] found that electronic systems are vital components of strategies to prevent medication errors, and a growing body of evidence calls for their widespread implementation.
- Improved data quality can also support pharmacists in providing more personalized and targeted care to patients. For example, Hippman and Nislow [29] identified that using pharmacogenomic data (i.e., data about a person's genetic makeup) in conjunction with

EMRs can improve the accuracy of medication dosing and reduce the risk of adverse drug events.

- Improved data quality can also support pharmacists in addressing public health issues. For example, prescription drug monitoring programs (PDMP), such as the CDC's PDMP [30] or The Australian Department of Health and Aged Care Real-Time Prescription Monitoring (RTPM) program [31], are utilizing prescribing and dispensing systems to track patterns of medication use in a population, which can help identify potential issues such as overuse or misuse of opioid medicines.

 Conversely, poor data quality can have severe implications for patient treatment and cause inefficiencies in care delivery. In pharmacy, accuracy, completeness, and timeliness of patient records are crucial factors for providing high-quality treatment and avoiding harm to patients. To improve data quality, healthcare professionals must take the time to evaluate and verify the data carefully and implement best practice data entry and quality control procedures. Improving patient record data quality is essential for pharmacists to deliver high-quality treatment and effectively support their role as healthcare professionals.

Data sharing and patient consent

Data sharing is crucial for improving patient care, informing research efforts, and advancing public health initiatives. However, patient privacy must be protected, and data exchange must be carried out in compliance with relevant laws and regulations. Patients have the right to be informed and give their consent before their data is shared with third parties. Utilizing data in a privacy-preserving way can improve patient care and enable pharmacies to gain insights into medication use patterns and identify trends in patient health outcomes, leading to the development of targeted interventions that enhance medication safety and efficacy. By providing a more complete picture of a patient's health history, for instance, sharing data among healthcare providers can improve patient care [32].

One example of how data sharing can improve patient care is through the use of PDMPs. PDMPs are state-managed databases that collect information on prescriptions for controlled substances, such as opioids. These programs can aid in the identification of patients who may be at risk for opioid abuse and provide information that can guide treatment decisions. For instance, a pharmacist could use PDMP data to identify a patient who has received opioid prescriptions from multiple providers, which may indicate the patient is "doctor shopping" and is at risk for overdose. The pharmacist could intervene and provide appropriate care for the patient using this information in coordination with their primary physician.

Data sharing in health care can have negative consequences if patient privacy is not protected. Data breaches can result in identity theft or discrimination against patients, and unethical behavior can lead to legal action. Additionally, data sharing can raise concerns about ownership and control of the data. Therefore, it is essential to establish clear data-sharing agreements and policies that protect patient confidentiality and adhere to data governance protocols. Healthcare organizations must have a comprehensive data governance strategy in place that prioritizes patient consent and privacy to build trust with patients and ensure the benefits of data sharing are realized.

Data governance

Data governance is a critical process in the healthcare industry to manage and safeguard the sensitive personal and medical information that organizations collect and use. This process involves creating policies and procedures for data collection, storage, usage, and sharing. It also involves assigning roles and responsibilities for data management, as well as implementing systems and controls to ensure data is used correctly and in compliance with applicable laws and regulations.

 Different types of policies and procedures can include.

- **Data quality**: This policy outlines the standards that data must meet in terms of accuracy, completeness, and timeliness, as well as the necessary steps to ensure data quality.
- **Data sharing and patient consent**: This policy outlines the conditions under which data may be shared with external parties, such as other healthcare organizations or researchers. It may also specify the steps that must be taken to ensure the confidentiality and security of shared data.
- **Access control**: who is permitted access to various types of data and under what conditions. For instance, only authorized personnel with valid reasons should be permitted to access patient records.
- **Classification of data**: This policy defines different categories of data based on sensitivity, significance, and other factors and specifies how each category should be handled. For example, sensitive personal or medical information may be deemed "confidential" and require additional safeguards.
- **Data storage and retention**: This policy specifies where and how data is to be stored, as well as for how long. For a certain number of years, patient records may need to be stored in a secure, centralized location.
- **Data breach response**: This policy outlines the actions to be taken in the event of a data breach, including notifying affected individuals and regulatory authorities, conducting an investigation, and implementing corrective measures.

As seen in the examples above, strong data governance policies and procedures are essential in ensuring the quality and integrity of health records, as well as protecting patient privacy and confidentiality. It is also vital for supporting clinical decision-making and research, as well as optimizing healthcare operations and ultimately improving patient outcomes.

Data governance is important for ensuring that data is trustworthy and not misused, especially in the healthcare industry, where sensitive personal and medical information must be kept secure and confidential. Practitioners should have a framework in place to uphold patient data security and confidentiality, and understanding data governance can help with implications such as data requests or hiring temporary staff. Various laws, regulations, and standards outline requirements for data governance in healthcare, such as the Health Insurance Portability and Accountability Act (HIPAA) in the United States, and professional organizations like the HIMSS and the International Association of Privacy Professionals (IAPP) provide guidance and resources for healthcare organizations to reference (see Chapter 17). These organizations often publish best practices, case studies, and other resources that healthcare organizations can use as references for their data governance programs. Practitioners need to research what is most appropriate for their practice environment.

Considerations

The PIS is fundamentally an information system and, in its essence, is only as effective as the data that is captured in it and processed by it to generate actionable outcomes for the pharmacist in the context of operational efficiencies and improved patient care. Just like in fusion cooking, a change to an ingredient can possibly change a dish from a delicious meal to a distasteful mess.

And so, it is vital to make sure we are using the right ingredients, i.e., data and information, in our PIS. When considering the DIKW pyramid, the requirements of pharmaceutical care professionals' PIS will evolve into a knowledge- and, eventually, a wisdom-generating system as their scope of practice expands. Because the PIS will also serve as the primary point of integration for third-party providers, the data we choose to enter into our system will either help or hinder our efforts as pharmacists. We will explore the topics below that have the propensity to affect the PIS.

Electronic workflows and consequences to patient care

As the delivery of care becomes more digitized and the number of third-party integrations increases, paper-based operations in pharmaceutical care will diminish. The integration of various third-party sources of patient data, such as digital health apps, government-sponsored eHealth solutions, direct insurance claiming and payment services, patient communication and outreach tools, virtual care, and interoperable clinician-to-clinician secure messaging, will mean that the workflow of the pharmaceutical care professional will transform to an electronic workflow. Handwritten notes will eventually become obsolete on the dispensary bench, and prescriptions no longer walk in on paper but will be sent by online third-party applications integrated into your dispensing Script-In queue.

The PIS has become the "digital" cornerstone of a pharmacy's electronic workflow. And now, with the rise in electronic prescription adoption globally, the PIS is becoming more important than ever [33]. In light of this, a realistic patient experience with their local pharmacy can take the following shape:

1. Via a telehealth consultation, the patient receives an electronic prescription from their physician as they are not able to have a face-to-face consultation.
2. The patient then sends their prescription to their pharmacy. The pharmacy received the request in their electronic intake queue.
3. Pharmacists confirm the prescription with the patient via telehealth or phone consultation.
4. The pharmacist dispenses the medication, during which the PIS applies CDS tools to the patient profile to make sure it is safe.
5. Once dispensed, the order is sent to a robotic dispenser, and medication is delivered to the pharmacist at their workstation.
6. Upon completion, the order is checked and prepared for delivery through a parcel fulfillment service.
7. The patient receives their medicine delivery at their home.

In contrast to this improved efficiency and access, as we can see above, a digitized workflow has the potential to reduce face-to-face patient interaction. And so, it is important to consider the potential consequences for patient care when face-to-face consultations are avoided, or even eliminated, in favor of alternative methods such as telehealth and online consultations [34].

One potential issue is the lack of personal interaction between the patient and the clinician. For in-person consultations, clinicians have the opportunity to ask questions, react to body language and engage in a dialogue with their patient, which is an important component of the treatment process. Gordon, Solanki [35] found that patients who participated in telehealth consultations with their healthcare providers reported feeling less connected to their providers and less likely to follow through with treatment recommendations compared to those who had in-person consultations.

Another consequence may be the difficulty in fully assessing certain aspects of the patient's health remotely. For example, a healthcare provider may not be able to completely understand the patient's overall health and well-being without physically examining the patient [35]. This could potentially lead to misdiagnoses or inadequate treatment.

Additionally, some patients may not have access to the technology or internet connectivity necessary to participate in telehealth consultations. This can create barriers to care for these individuals and may result in them not receiving the necessary healthcare [36]. Even in 2022, there are still limitations to internet access and technology capabilities of the average person, particularly in rural and remote locations worldwide.

There are also potential consequences for the healthcare provider in a scenario where face-to-face consultations are reduced or eliminated. For example, without the opportunity to see and interact with patients in person, healthcare providers may be less able to build relationships with their patients and may be less able to provide personalized care [35]. This could lead to a decrease in patient satisfaction and an overall decline in the quality of care.

Overall, while alternative consultation methods such as telehealth can be beneficial in certain situations, it is important to carefully consider the potential consequences to patient care when face-to-face consultations are reduced or eliminated. To ensure the best possible care for patients, a balance should be struck between the use of technology and in-person interactions.

Data protection regulations

The pharmacy's PIS and IT technical infrastructure must be secure and dependable. As pharmacies routinely handle sensitive patient information, it is crucial that their systems comply with applicable data protection regulations. We will examine the General Data Protection Regulation (GDPR) in the European Union and the Health Insurance Portability and Accountability Act (HIPAA) in the United States as examples of data protection regulations and measures for pharmacies. Both of these regulations establish guidelines for safeguarding sensitive patient information and provide pharmacies with examples of appropriate security measures to implement.

In Chapter 17, the topic of data protection regulations is expanded upon in further detail including the topics of data privacy, quality compliance, and information security.

For further information on the HIPAA act and its implications on the healthcare system in the United States of America, refer to QR Code 14.5.

QR Code 14.5
Data protection regulations. Health information privacy.

QR Code 14.6
Data protection
regulations.
General data protection
regulation (GDPR).

For further information on the GDPR, refer to QR Code 14.6. In addition, reviewing Act 1 in the GDPR will provide further context on the regulation and its overarching objectives.

By adhering to these guidelines and taking the necessary precautions, pharmacies can ensure that they handle sensitive patient information in a responsible and compliant manner while also safeguarding patients' privacy and confidentiality and reducing the risk of a cyber incident for the organization.

Cybersecurity risks of a digital workflow

As we now know, the PIS contains patient records, prescription orders, pharmacy financial and operations data, patient medical history, and personal identification information. Also, we have identified that the PIS is becoming a more integrated information system, increasingly being exposed to and communicating with external API web services and internet-based resources. With this increased exposure and connectivity, the risk of malicious actors recognizing pharmacy as a potential data honeypot increases.

One of the main risks of PIS security is the possibility of data breaches [37]. These breaches can occur when unauthorized individuals gain access to the system and steal or misuse the stored data. For example, in 2022, a pharmacy group in the United States was the target of a data breach [38]. The attack's perpetrators accessed the system, stole sensitive information, and posted it to the dark web.

QR Code 14.7
Cybersecurity risks of
a digital workflow.

Another risk to PIS security is the possibility of ransomware attacks. Ransomware is a type of malware that encrypts a victim's data and demands a ransom from the victim to restore access [39]. If a pharmacy's PIS is targeted by ransomware, it could disrupt the pharmacy's operations and potentially lead to delays or errors in patient care. In 2018, a pharmacy chain in the United Kingdom was the victim of a ransomware attack that resulted in the temporary shutdown of some of its systems [40]. QR Code 14.7 links to an article detailing a cybersecurity attack on a pharmacy department and how they adapted and adjusted to ensure patients still received the care they needed.

In addition to these risks, pharmacies and PIS systems are also vulnerable to other types of cyberattacks, such as phishing scams, where attackers attempt to trick users into disclosing their login credentials or distributed denial of service (DDoS) attacks, where the attacker floods the system with traffic to disrupt its operations [41]. This can shut down an entire business's infrastructure [42].

To mitigate these risks, it is important for pharmacies to implement strong security measures for their PIS systems. This can include using secure passwords, regularly updating software and security protocols, and providing training to employees on how to identify and prevent cyberattacks. It is also important for pharmacies to have a plan in place to respond to a security breach or other cyber incident, such as having a backup system in place or partnering with a cybersecurity firm to help restore the system.

Overall, the risks of PIS security are significant and can have serious consequences for both pharmacies and their patients. It is important for pharmacies to be proactive in addressing these risks and taking steps to protect their systems and the sensitive data they store.

Data valuation

In the larger information technology space, a larger focus is now placed on putting a dollar figure on the value of the data an organization holds prior to acquisition compared to the past.

Although still considered theory, Short, Todd [43] have recognized three practical steps to help organizations prioritize data value as part of their day-to-day practices. These steps include.

1. Make valuation policies explicit and shareable across the organization
   a. This can be as simple as cataloging the different data sources available in the organization and tracking the usage of the specific data sets.
2. Create internal data valuation expertise
   a. From an organizational perspective, this could mean data being licensed for third-party applications or licensing. In the pharmaceutical care environment, the reverse could also apply, where a value can be placed on the integration of a third-party application to potentially calculate the revenue and value generated from the implementation of the third-party application.
3. Decide which type of valuation processes are the most effective for the organization
   a. There are two types of valuation processes:
      i. Top-down: organizations identify the critical apps and apply a value to the data utilized in those apps by understanding the different linked systems, and third-party applications, that feed into the overarching information system, i.e., the PIS, and measuring the activity that exists between systems.
      ii. Bottom-up: define the value of data heuristically by first drawing a map of where data is utilized across the organization and the directions of data flow and linkages across the organization, producing a detailed pattern of use.

This theory will only become more prevalent as we continue to capture data in and generate from our systems. We will begin to recognize that the data contained within the PIS are an organization asset. And so, as organizations conduct their commercial valuations, either as part of their fiduciary responsibility or for acquisition purposes, pharmaceutical care organizations will eventually need to consider the value of the data captured in their PIS as part of that equation. In the near future, a pharmacy organization's valuation will take the value of the PIS's data into consideration as it becomes even more central to the valuation of the organization.

When the application fails

As professionals in the pharmaceutical care industry, we have a responsibility to keep in mind that our ability to provide care to our patients is directly correlated to the education and experience we have gained in the clinical setting. Technology and information systems are tools that help facilitate this relationship for the patient's benefit, allowing our professional care responsibilities to be enabled and enhanced. However, pharmaceutical care professionals should never put their complete trust in these systems to the point where they feel helpless or unable to provide treatment in the absence of those systems.

Even if the information system is damaged or becomes inoperable, business operations should continue as usual, even if it requires the care professional to record the information and the instructions for the medication dispensing by hand. After the systems have been brought back online, the information will be able to be re-entered into the system. Unfortunately, working with technology and software in general inevitably presents one with this unfortunate reality.

In addition, as cloud computing and communications based on web services become more widespread, software developers will need to incorporate considerations for internet connectivity, connection speed, and, most importantly, offline workflows into the overall architectural design of the system.

Conclusion

To conclude, fusion cooking represents the evolution and creative melding of existing culinary styles to create something new. The PIS forms the basis of a new era of pharmaceutical care. By serving as the technological foundation, a dynamic mix of services, functionalities, and integrations can be built around it, generating new flavors of care.

In next Chapter 15, the inspiring and fast emerging field of Digital Therapeutics will be explained.

 This means for blended pharmaceutical care:

- PISs play a vital role in the care of patients by helping to manage the logistics of medication administration, tracking patient adherence, and providing tools and reports to help clinicians understand how patients are responding to their treatment.
- PIS systems can be used to transform the wealth of health data continuously being generated into actionable insights for the pharmaceutical care provider to make informed care decisions for their patients
- Promoting data quality and adherence to data standards must be a priority, as it is a primary driver for system value and utility
- Key considerations for PIS implementation should include data governance, cybersecurity, and interoperability

References

[1] Guild P. Community pharmacy 2025 framework for change. 2018. Available from, https://www.guild.org. au/__data/assets/pdf_file/0029/69437/15023_PGA_CP2025_framework-change_FA6_web.pdf.

[2] Krantz J, Hartley F. Pharmacy-Encyclopaedia Britannica. 2017. 2017 14/01/2023]; Available from, https://www.britannica.com/science/pharmacy.

[3] Zwass V. Information system. In: Encyclopaedia Britannica; 2022. Available from, https://www.britannica.com/topic/information-system.

[4] Pardal M. Computer science research for the Internet of Things. Lisboa: Instituto Superior Técnico; 2008.

[5] PSA Australia. Pharmacy History-Pharmacy champions of information technology. 2009. 2009/11/1 14/09/2022]; Available from, https://www.psa.org.au/wp-content/uploads/flipbook/13/files/basic-html/page17.html.

[6] World Health Organization. UHC Technical Brief: strengthening health information systems. 2017.

[7] Alanazi A, et al. Factors influencing pharmacists' intentions to use Pharmacy Information Systems. Inform Med Unlocked 2018;11:1–8.

[8] ASHP guidelines on pharmacy planning for implementation of computerized provider-order-entry systems in hospitals and health systems. Am J Health Syst Pharm 2011;68(6):e9–31. https://doi.org/10.2146/sp100011e.

[9] Bates DW. Using information technology to reduce rates of medication errors in hospitals. Bmj 2000;320(7237):788–91.

[10] National Coordinating Council for Medication Error Reporting and Prevention. Recommendations for bar code labels on pharmaceutical (drug) products to reduce medication errors. 2007 [cited 2023 17/02/2023]; Available from, https://www.nccmerp.org/recommendations-bar-code-labels-pharmaceutical-drug-products-reduce-medication-errors.

[11] Alshehri AM, et al. Pharmacist intention to provide medication therapy management services in Saudi Arabia: a study using the theory of planned behaviour. Int J Environ Res Publ Health 2022;19(9):5279. https://doi.org/10.3390/ijerph19095279.

[12] Campbell EM, et al. Types of unintended consequences related to computerized provider order entry. J Am Med Inf Assoc 2006;13(5):547–56.

[13] Hammar T, et al. Swedish pharmacists value ePrescribing: a survey of a nationwide implementation. J Pharmaceut Health Serv Res 2010;1(1):23–32.

[14] Sittig DF. Defining health information technology–related errors. Arch Intern Med 2011;171(14):1281. https://doi.org/10.1001/archinternmed.2011.327.

[15] Poon EG, Trent Rosenbloom S, Zheng K. Health information technology and clinician burnout: current understanding, emerging solutions, and future directions. J Am Med Inf Assoc 2021;28(5):895–8.

[16] Frické MH. Data-information-knowledge-wisdom (DIKW) pyramid, framework, continuum. In: Schintler LA, McNeely CL, editors. Encyclopedia of Big data. Cham: Springer International Publishing; 2018. p. 1–4. https://doi.org/10.1007/978-3-319-32001-4_331-1. Available from.

[17] Bourgeois D, Bourgeois DT. What is an information system? – information systems for business and beyond. 2020. Available from, https://pressbooks.pub/bus206/chapter/chapter-1/.

[18] Warehime N. How pharmacy integration to facility EHR/EMARs benefit pharmacies, facilities, and patients. 2021. Available from, http://blog.frameworkltc.com/how-pharmacy-integration-to-facility-ehr/emars-benefit-pharmacies-facilities-and-patients.

[19] Spencer Health. Spencer health solutions-improving healthcare...from the home. 2020. 2020/12/1 12/11/ 2022]; Available from, https://spencerhealthsolutions.com/.

[20] Allscripts. AllScripts. 2021. 12/11/2022]; Available from: https://www.cvisionintl.com/media/hwibhxjk/hospital-and-health-system-portfolio-brochure-smarter-more-intuitive-and-open-for-everyone.pdf.

[21] Galassini M. Case study: fraser health authority uses dbMotion to improve patient care. 2015. Available from, https://www.linkedin.com/pulse/case-study-fraser-health-authority-uses-dbmotion-care-matt-galassini.

[22] HIMSS International. Interoperability in healthcare. 2020. 2020/8/4 15/12/2022]; Available from, https://www.himss.org/resources/interoperability-healthcare.

[23] Shen J, et al. Artificial intelligence versus clinicians in disease diagnosis: systematic review. JMIR Med Inform 2019;7(3):e10010.

[24] Corny J, et al. A machine learning-based clinical decision support system to identify prescriptions with a high risk of medication error. J Am Med Inf Assoc 2020;27(11):1688–94.

[25] Nguyen A, et al. Data analytics in pharmaceutical supply chains: state of the art, opportunities, and challenges. Int J Prod Res 2021;60.

[26] Choudhury A, Asan O. Role of artificial intelligence in patient safety outcomes: systematic literature review. JMIR Med Inform 2020;8(7):e18599.

[27] Porterfield A, Engelbert K, Coustasse A. Electronic prescribing: improving the efficiency and accuracy of prescribing in the ambulatory care setting. Perspect Health Inf Manag 2014;11(Spring):1g.

[28] Agrawal A. Medication errors: prevention using information technology systems. Br J Clin Pharmacol 2009;67(6):681–6.

[29] Hippman C, Nislow C. Pharmacogenomic testing: clinical evidence and implementation challenges. J Personalized Med 2019;9(3).

[30] Centers for Disease Control and Prevention. Prescription drug monitoring programs (PDMPs). 2022 [cited 2023 17/02/2023]; Available from, https://www.cdc.gov/opioids/healthcare-professionals/pdmps.html.

[31] Department of Health and Aged Care. National real time prescription monitoring (RTPM). 2022 [cited 2023 17/02/2023]; Available from, https://www.health.gov.au/our-work/national-real-time-prescription-monitoring-rtpm.

[32] Lee H, et al. Utility-preserving anonymization for health data publishing. BMC Med Inf Decis Making 2017;17(1):104. https://doi.org/10.1186/s12911-017-0499-0.

[33] Halde R. Global e-Prescribing Market is set to witness an exponential growth of 22% to reach $4 billion in the next 5 years. 2022. Available from, https://www.globenewswire.com/en/news-release/2022/05/16/2444096/0/en/Global-e-Prescribing-Market-is-set-to-witness-an-exponential-growth-of-22-to-reach-4-billion-in-the-next-5-years.html.

[34] Ilardo ML, Speciale A. The community pharmacist: perceived barriers and patient-centered care communication. Int J Environ Res Publ Health 2020;17(2).

[35] Gordon HS, et al. "I'm not feeling like I'm part of the conversation" patients' perspectives on communicating in clinical video telehealth visits. J Gen Intern Med 2020;35(6):1751−8.

[36] Almathami HKY, Win KT, Vlahu-Gjorgievska E. Barriers and facilitators that influence telemedicine-based, real-time, online consultation at patients' homes: systematic literature review. J Med Internet Res 2020;22(2):e16407.

[37] Dowell MA. Pharmacies must take steps to protect against data breaches. 2022. Available from, https://www.uspharmacist.com/article/pharmacies-must-take-steps-to-protect-against-data-breaches.

[38] Diaz N. CVS-owned pharmacy company becomes target of ransomware attack. 2022. 2022/7/7; Available from, https://www.beckershospitalreview.com/cybersecurity/cvs-owned-pharmacy-company-becomes-target-of-ransomware-attack.html.

[39] Wikipedia. Ransomware-wikipedia. 2020. Available from, https://en.wikipedia.org/wiki/Ransomware.

[40] Jowitt T. Boots suspends payments after cyber-attack \textbar silicon UK tech news. 2020. Available from, https://www.silicon.co.uk/security/cyberwar/boots-suspends-advantage-cyber-attack-334837.

[41] Wikipedia. Denial-of-service attack-wikipedia. 2021. Available from, https://en.wikipedia.org/wiki/Distributed_denial_of_service_attack.

[42] Sukkar E. Large pharmacy chains to set up 'crisis team' following cyber attack on NHS-the Pharmaceutical Journal. 2017. Available from, https://pharmaceutical-journal.com/article/news/large-pharmacy-chains-to-set-up-crisis-team-following-cyber-attack-on-nhs.

[43] Short, J.E., S. Todd, M.I. of Technology. What's your data worth?. 2017. Available from, https://sloanreview.mit.edu/article/whats-your-data-worth/.

CHAPTER 15

The molecular gastronomy of digital therapeutics*

Timothy Dy Aungst

Department of Pharmacy Practice, MCPHS University, Worcester, MA, United States

Synergy and serendipity often play a big part in medical and scientific advances.

Julie Bishop

The fast-growing digital therapeutic (DTx) applications often propagate the drive to create a symbiosis with traditional well-immersed pharmaceutical interventions. This symbiosis is similar to molecular gastronomy, which focuses on the physical and chemical transformations that occur during cooking. DTx may develop a symbiotic relationship with medication treatments as well during the course of providing health care.

DTx use clinically evaluated software to deliver medical interventions across multiple conditions using varying mechanics. This can include a standalone app, a DTx with a drug, or in combination with a peripheral device such as a wearable or VR headset. In addition to managing disease, many DTx companies aim to decrease the dosage of drugs or even eventually eliminate the need to take medications. DTx can serve as an adjunctive or standalone treatment option for patients bypassing or limiting medication use.

Technology

DTx, a subset of digital health and often a combination of the digital techniques described in previous chapters, is a health discipline and treatment option that utilizes digital and often online health technology to treat, manage, and prevent a medical condition. This approach engages patients and can lead to clinically relevant outcomes. DTx relies on behavioral and lifestyle changes that are usually spurred by a collection of

---

*In this chapter, you will read about DTx that can be used as autonomous treatments or may augment the effects of drugs. Pharmaceutical care providers may consult future digital health management teams on the synergy between drug and DTx use.

QR Code 15.1
What are digital therapeutics?

digital impetuses. Because of the digital nature of this methodology, data can be collected and analyzed both as a progress report and as a preventative measure (QR Code 15.1) [1].

DTx solutions consist of a variety of different technological interventions. DTx products can generally be split into three categories: those that deliver software directly through an app have a DTx combined with medication or have a DTx combined with hardware. Some of the standalone DTx provided a digitalized intervention that may traditionally be offered in person, such as cognitive behavioral therapy (CBT) or self-directed interventions with controlled feedback loops. This may encompass digitalizing the talk therapy involved with CBT or even educational prompts traditionally explored in person. DTx may also be combined with medications, especially combination products (e.g., injector, inhaler), to track medication utilization and make adjustments to dosing or timing. Lastly, other hardware, such as wearables or worn peripheral devices, may be used to provide an intervention, such as VR headsets.

Once a DTx product is chosen and recommended for patient use, it is essential to track whether the intervention works as intended. Compared to traditional medications, DTx provides real-time feedback and assessment of impact, allowing remote changes to be made to the DTx intervention as needed. Data is collected and processed through the app interface or via peripheral devices used by the patient in conjunction with the DTx software. Many products include clinical assessment, outcome tracking, and improvement tools, with data feeding into clinician monitoring dashboards. When these capabilities are integrated into clinical practice, physicians and other healthcare providers may prescribe these products just as they do with any other medication or intervention.

DTx may have applications on mobile platforms, and some require additional sensors or technologies to function. We will see examples of these DTx products in this chapter.

Clinically evaluated DTx products, which promise a true clinical intervention, are supposed to undergo rigorous clinical testing through randomized clinical trials and real-world pilots to demonstrate their safety, efficacy, and economic benefit. These DTx solutions are positioned as medical devices depending on the region, and to distinguish them from "wellness" gadgets, they undergo a thorough review and regulatory clearance process by federal agencies such as the U.S. Food and Drug Administration (FDA) and European Medicines Agency (EMA) (DTX Alliance, 2017). The regulatory compliance conditions for DTx can be found in Chapter 17.

DTx treatments are being developed to prevent and manage a wide variety of diseases and conditions, including Type II diabetes, congestive heart failure, obesity, Alzheimer's disease, dementia, asthma, COPD, substance abuse, ADHD, anxiety, and depression. DTx often employs strategies rooted in CBT or digitalized care pathway traditionally done in person.

DTx are also evolving as they are initiated and managed with patients. For example, some DTx products may be available based on an initial referral to a program supplying it, while a provider must prescribe others. These prescribed DTx products are now being called "PDTs" to differentiate their model toward patient distribution from other DTx products.

Impact on core responsibilities in pharmaceutical care

DTx, as do individual apps or other technologies, may significantly affect the activities that take place in a pharmaceutical care pathway. Additionally, with many DTx now being combined with medications or may impact how a medication is utilized, there is a greater need to understand how a patient's pharmaceutical care plan may be impacted.

Thus pharmaceutical care providers should be aware of the fact that a patient is supported by a DTx and that, as a consequence, drug dosages, and patterns may need to be changed over time. This can include data regarding how well a medication is working for a patient or direct changes to the dosing of medication. In addition, the differeint factors of access can complicate the pharmaceutical care process. For example, some DTx products may be something pharmacists need to know about based on how they impact pharmaceutical care, while others may directly come from the pharmacy since it is a PDT.

Here is the general impact that DTx is expected to have on the five domains of pharmaceutical care provision (refer to Chapter 6 for a more detailed discussion).

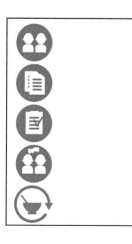

A. **Professional relationship between PCP and patients**: This relationship goes beyond medication and considers DTx as an optional treatment

B. **Adequate collection and recording of health data**: DTx devices and data are considered in PC plans

C. **Review health data and provide adequate PC proposal**: If required, care that blends DTx and medication is considered

D. **Patient alignment and facilitate execution of PC plan**: Offer the possibility of using DTx if feasible, and align it with informed consent for data sharing

E. **Circular management of PC plan**: Use DTx data to measure outcomes and adjust the plan, if required

Implementation in daily practice

A number of DTx interventions have been introduced that patients, pharmaceutical care providers, and doctors can utilize.

Digital therapeutics to enhance or replace medication

Digital therapies tend to fall into two categories, which are often called "medication augmentation" and "medication replacement." The therapies either optimize the effect of the drug intervention chosen or are so effective that medication can be tapered or stopped completely at a certain point in time. Fig. 15.1 shows a potential process flow for choosing a DTx in a pharmaceutical care chain.

The agreed outcome of the treatment should be a collaborative process between the patient, doctor, pharmacist, and other relevant care providers and should be driven by the patient's personal preferences. For example, a patient's digital health management team can decide which DTx technology will best enhance the treatment plan and who needs to see what kind of data to augment the disease's management. It is, however, the patient who subsequently gives authority to share certain data with respective providers depending on the type of intervention and condition being managed.

The role of the pharmacist in a digital health management team

In Chapter 6, we note that a pharmacist's role can be considered an optimizer of medication treatments. Thus, pharmacists acquire the knowledge needed to determine which DTx can augment and affect medication outcomes directly or indirectly. This may be due to a DTx changing the dose of medication or a DTx serving as adjunctive therapy, which may alleviate the need for certain medications to be taken by the patient. This will necessitate that pharmacists have an understanding of the mechanism of action for DTx products and provide education to patients when providing a DTx that may impact the medications they are on or if it is combined with the medication itself.

In addition to knowing what kind of tools are available and understanding certain technical details, in the future, pharmacists will work in a domain that requires them to understand which patients will benefit most from a synergy between DTx and medication. Making such a determination will also require setting up structured pilot studies in pharmaceutical environments, in which pharmacy software data is linked to DTx outcome data, as

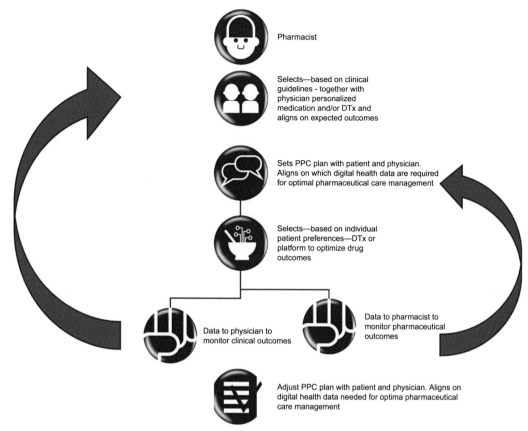

Figure 15.1
Choosing a digital therapeutic in a pharmaceutical pathway.

explained in Chapter 8. Creating these pilots and sources of data holds significant importance in implementing DTx in practice but is very costly. As DTx and practice evolve together, the pilots and trials of DTx will have to deal with the significant costs associated with these early studies.

With these networks in place and a scientifically sound pilot study format, statistics, including integrated trend analyses, can predict which DTx provides value for which category of patients.

Next, we review a number of DTx interventions that may fit well in pharmaceutical care pathways. The interventions discussed are not all-inclusive but are representative of those relevant to pharmaceutical care.

An examination of the increasing number of DTxs and the difficulty in understanding their differences indicates the future need for a "comparison and overview database system," as discussed in Chapter 10.

Diabetes

A number of interesting DTx examples can be found in the cardiometabolic space, with diabetes being at the forefront of innovation. Evidence shows that certain lifestyle changes give people with diabetes better control of their disease (and prevent most people with prediabetes from developing the disease), so this created an opening for digital lifestyle support services focused on the prevention of disease and reduction or enhancement of medication use. In addition, newer sensors and integrated devices are increasing the ability to augment and automate patient insulin delivery.

 In the past decade, there has been a growing interest in the creation of an "artificial pancreas" or closed-loop insulin delivery system. Toward the end of the 2010s, the expansion of continuous glucose monitoring (CGM) devices, DTx that can calculate insulin dosing, and the creation of connected insulin pens and novel insulin pumps led toward the ability to have an automated system. This can be accomplished by CGM collecting patient data that is then handled by the DTx platform, informing a patient to inject a certain amount of insulin themselves or handled automatically by a pump. The healthcare team can then see if the appropriate medical outcomes (e.g., A1c or blood glucose levels) are being met and what adjustments are required, whether changing insulin type or dose.

A diabetes DTx platform

Dario is a DTx platform designed to treat both Type 1 and Type 2 Diabetes. The platform works by having the patient track their blood glucose with a smart meter connecting to a user's smartphone. The data collected from the patient's blood glucose and other health information input allows the DTx to provide lifestyle modification advice to the patient. The Dario Dtx has shown a reduction of hypoglycemia and blood glucose variability for patients. Essentially, it helps ensure that pharmaceutical care has less variation and serves as an adjunctive treatment for diabetes. It has undergone regulatory clearance in the US, Europe, Canada, Australia, and Israel. Dario is an example of a DTx product that patients can buy on their own and then continue to use on a subscription model, offering a coaching service to help guide them. In 2022, Dario and Sanofi entered a strategic collaboration to use the Dario platform to engage more patients and give Sanofi an area to offer its own platform to users. The interwork between DTx companies, drug manufacturers, and others demonstrate how the DTx market will navigate with many stakeholders to help leverage products and services in the future.

 Another DTx platform is Insulia, which aims to support insulin dose titration for basal insulins in people with Type 2 Diabetes. Similar to other diabetes-focused

DTx software, education and coaching are key aspects, but the platform is meant to serve as a PDT whereby a provider assigns target blood glucose ranges that Insulia will follow. Based on collected blood glucose ranges, Insulia will then adjust the basal insulin dose to achieve target ranges, and the provider can monitor via a portal to see how therapy is working.

Substance use disorder (SUD)

Pear Therapeutics, was a company that integrates clinically validated software applications with previously approved pharmaceuticals and treatment paradigms to provide better patient outcomes, smarter engagement and tracking tools for clinicians, and cost-effective solutions for payers. Pear's lead product, reSET, is an FDA-cleared PDT, 90-day intervention using CBT for substance use disorders to be used as an adjunct to standard outpatient treatment. reSET has been shown to increase abstinence from abused substances during treatment and also when used as part of an outpatient treatment program. The product uses a patient-facing smartphone application (providing behavioral support tools for the patient) linked with a clinician-facing web interface. After reSET was cleared in 2017, reSET-O was cleared in 2018 for opioid use disorder (OUD). reSET-O is a PDT that patients follow for 84 days using CBT techniques as an adjunct to outpatient OUD treatments with buprenorphine. Neither reSET or reSET-O are standalone treatments but adjunctive treatments to encourage treatment for SUD or OUD.

Migraine treatment

Nerivio is a DTx to treat migraines with an app and hardware system. Made by Theranica, Nerivio works as a combination of software via an app and a piece of hardware worn by the patient. The hardware is a device worn on the patient's upper arm that provides remote electrical neuromodulation controlled and regulated by the app. The neuromodulation helps stimulate a nerve that can help relieve migraines. For some patients, this may be preferable to the use of medications that may have side effects they do not like. The app can share data with the patient's provider to see how therapy is going and if any changes need to be made.

Virtual reality (VR, as described in Chapter 13) is also used as a DTx in disease management. This includes tackling mental health, serious mental illness (SMI), and pain management. In addition to medical management, counseling in mental disorders can be effective to a degree, but the most powerful changes happen when individuals are presented with situations that cause them distress and are forced to learn directly how to think, feel, and behave more constructively. That often means getting out of the consulting room and into the real world, with the therapist acting much more like a personal trainer or leadership coach, but available time is the limiting factor.

Here, virtual reality may offer digital therapeutic help as it can immediately create powerful simulations of the scenarios in which psychological difficulties occur. Suddenly, there's no need for a therapist to accompany a client on a trip to a crowded shopping center or up a tall building, and the patient can focus on getting the therapy where and when they want.

Situations that are more or less impossible to build into a course of therapy—flying, for example, or the shocking events that often lie behind posttraumatic stress disorder, or the potential frightening side effects of a drug—can be conjured at the click of a mouse. The in situ coaching that's so effective for so many disorders is now delivered in the consulting room or even in the pharmacy environment, with the simulations graded in difficulty and repeated as often as necessary.

Education and self-guided training can also be delivered to help patients better understand sensations and how to manage them. This has opened new options for pain management therapy using VR as a means to reduce the need for analgesics or at a reduced dose.

Having this opportunity available means that psychologists, psychiatrists, and other providers may decide less often to initiate medical treatment directly or that they have tools available that may help reduce drug dosages, leading to a better tolerance profile for the patient. Moreover, when medical treatment is chosen, explanations for what to expect when a drug is first used can be better guided through VR training, potentially resulting in better compliance and acceptance profiles.

Pain management

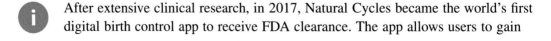 RelieveVRx is an example of a VR DTx for at-home adjunctive treatment of chronic lower back pain. The patient engages in a self-directed program using VR sessions. Each session lasts around 7 minutes and continues over the length of the program for 8 weeks. RelieveVRx provides patients with mindful escapes, relaxation techniques, and education on their pain. After the patient is done with the system, they mail it back. As a PDT, RelieveVRx is an example of a prescribed virtual therapy that may change a patient's pain management and could impact pharmaceutical care regarding what analgesics a patient may use and how they address their pain.

Digital contraceptives and womens health

After extensive clinical research, in 2017, Natural Cycles became the world's first digital birth control app to receive FDA clearance. The app allows users to gain knowledge about their bodies and supports them in truly understanding how individual menstrual cycles work. The app is positioned as providing protection with more sexual freedom, minus the side effects of contraceptives.

The app stores information on every cycle, as every cycle can be different, and determines when a woman ovulates and is most likely to get pregnant, with pregnancy generally possible 6 days (5 days before ovulation and about 24 h after ovulation). The woman takes her temperature in the morning and enters the information into the app; the app then emits a red light (fertile days) or a green light (nonfertile days), indicating when the woman needs to use protection or abstain from sexual intercourse.

Other similar products also received clearance for use, like Clue, which uses menstrual cycle data and its algorithm to help determine the risk of pregnancy.

 Urinary incontinence is a condition many women struggle with, and they can often rely on medications to help manage multiple side effects. Leva is a DTx product that combines an app and a device to help train pelvic floor muscles to help reduce urinary leakage. The device is inserted intravaginally, and the built-in sensor can detect muscle movement. The patient is then guided through coaching sessions that last 5 minutes to practice pelvic floor exercises. These exercises may help lead to a reduction of urinary leakage for the patient.

Mental health and psychological conditions

With a large rise in mental health and SMI, there has been a growing concern regarding providing interventions with a limited healthcare workforce. Using digital health to help provide remote counseling and interventions is being greatly increased, but a limited number of providers to conduct sessions is a rate-limiting step.

A growing emphasis on detaching interventions from synchronous live sessions has been under consideration, and the use of DTx solutions that address psychological conditions is gaining reception. While there has been a growth in health apps focused on anxiety and mindfulness training, tackling SMI is still difficult. Several DTx products are now FDA-cleared to provide treatment for generalized anxiety disorder, depression, PTSD, and others are under investigation into schizophrenia. Additional DTx is being developed focused on providing mental health support to patients with other conditions, like diabetes or cancer.

Depression

Deprexis is a DTx developed by Orexo to provide treatment for depressive symptoms. It works by having a live therapist serve as support and using data collected through sessions to provide CBT techniques and education to help adjunctively treat depression symptoms. In comparison, SparkRx by Limbix also helps manage depression symptoms in adolescents by using coping skills deployed via CBT. They engage in coping exercises through a 7-week program, which works adjunctively to their current care.

ADHD

Another interesting example is Akili's video game, which fosters compliance and has a therapeutic effect on ADHD; the game is delivered through a creative and immersive action gaming experience. Treatments leverage art, music, storytelling, and reward cycles that keep patients engaged and immersed in the delivery of therapeutic activity. The company is known as a prescription digital medicine company, combining scientific and clinical rigor with the ingenuity of the technology industry to reinvent medicine for a number of indications in the neuroscience field.

Their DTx product, EndeavorRx, was FDA cleared in 2019 to provide treatment for children between 8 and 12 years of age with ADHD. By engaging with the DTx through a video game, it can help improve the child's attentional control. It is delivered alongside other treatments the child may be receiving for ADHD. Each session can last around 25 min, and treatment can be prescribed for several months.

Considerations

Defining exactly what a DTx actually remains a fluid space that many small and large companies alike are trying to categorize. The general consensus among researchers in the field of DTx is that the discipline of DTx is a form of software that requires clinical evidence to support its use. Subsets of analyses are done on individual tools used as DTx, for instance, research on the effectiveness of wearables or virtual reality. Information on those results can be found in the respective chapters.

The number of products as well as regulatory developments in the DTx sector is expected to expand in the near future. Further delineation of how a DTx is provided or prescribed leads to further classifications like PDTs. DTx systems will be tested for their efficacy and for their added value from both the perspective of their benefits to patients and their cost-effectiveness in the healthcare system and by payers and regulators.

Regulatory and reimbursement framework

Software development is not a linear, one-and-done process. Instead, it is an iterative process that goes much faster than the timelines known for developing innovative medication (>12 years).

Not all DTx need to satisfy the rigors of regulatory review and approval. For example, as noted in Chapter 10, noninvasive devices that are intended for general wellness use hardly ever undergo strict certification, whereas medical wearables with a clear clinical purpose do because if they are not used properly, a user's health can decline.

Currently, the business of DTx is still in the early stages, including matters of reimbursement. Many authorities and healthcare payers still mainly reimburse only the cost of drugs and traditional interventions and are still in the process of getting used to compensating for DTx. Varying organizations are offering coverage to DTx and PDT products. Overall, there has been no set pathway to achieve payer coverage; this is an area of focus for many stakeholders. Payers and related national organizations will conduct strategic plays in therapeutic areas where the benefits of DTx may help alleviate the total cost of care or lead to downstream benefits currently not achievable by current health models and practices.

This approach plays into the hands of payers, who may encourage their customers to use digital interventions (that are shown to be effective in clinical studies) in the early stage of treatment and move to pharmaceutical products only at the second stage (or in parallel with adjusted dosing). The approach may completely disrupt therapeutic guidelines in days to come.

It is essential that governments develop structured health technology assessments on what is considered appropriate cost-effectiveness for DTx in order to achieve reliable reimbursement for both pharmaceutical and digital interventions.

One organization that is pushing the ecosystem's progress in this respect is the DTx Alliance, a global nonprofit trade association with the mission of broadening the understanding, adoption, and integration of clinically validated DTx into healthcare through education, advocacy, and research.

Owner of the prescription of digital therapeutics

It is still unclear how pharmaceutical providers will perform their future role in digitally managed healthcare. Therefore, a structured approach will be necessary to define who is the key responsible healthcare provider in the patient journey to prescribe and integrate DTx interventions in individual treatment programs, including medication.

Many commercial providers currently develop their own DTx platforms, and in that roll-out, differences in approaches are evolving between hospitals, regions, and countries.

It may be very confusing for patients to be prescribed a digital lifestyle support program 1 day by a physician and the next day by a pharmacist. Communication and building upon data interoperability will be key to providing patients with a clear understanding of whom is monitoring any digital interventions like a DTx. Thus working in one data-and-prescription ecosystem with close alignment between all care providers is essential.

In this respect, the patient's responsibility also comes into play, as DTx asks for a secure and updated virtual environment, retention, and user accuracy to bring them to their full potential.

Another interesting aspect here is that many adverse events are known only to the patient, as they are often not formally communicated. With the quantified-self era having DTx at hand, these events become known to the entire virtual disease management team the minute they happen. This requires a completely different business setup in order to adequately and timely follow up on events and comply with prevailing pharmacovigilance regulations.

Thus, in the next couple of years, it is expected that the combination of DTx with medications will be further entangled and that strong contributions from pharmaceutical care providers are required to valorize DTx systems to support adequate and appropriate use of drugs.

In the next Chapter 16, we will look at digital health technologies that promise great patient outcome improvements, but concrete and validated use will most probably only be globally seen some 5 years from now.

 This means for blended pharmaceutical care:

- DTx is a fast-growing health niche focused on evidence-based software that is often delivered through an app.
- DTx can exist as standalone technologies or as integrated platforms and are sometimes provided in a synergistic combinatory package with drugs.
- DTx products have undergone rigorous clinical testing through randomized clinical trials and real-world pilot projects to demonstrate their safety and efficacy.
- Reimbursement structures for DTx are in their early stages, and further regulation should ensure that a comparison of health technology with traditional medication is done appropriately and that the value of DTx is quantified.
- Pharmaceutical care stakeholders are recommended to become knowledgeable about which DTx can augment the impact of drugs and how they do so in order to contribute optimally to a digital health management team.

Reference

[1] Dahlberg LE, et al. A web-based platform for patients with osteoarthritis of the hip and knee: a pilot study. JMIR Res Protoc 2016;5(2):e115.

CHAPTER 16

What's cooking beyond 2028*

Ardalan Mirzaei[1], Claudia Rijcken[2]
[1]*School of Pharmacy, Faculty of Medicine and Health, The University of Sydney, Australia;* [2]*Pharmi, Maastricht, The Netherlands*

What is coming, is better than what is gone.

Arabic proverb

Thus far, this book has dealt with digital innovations expected to disrupt the pharmaceutical ecosystem between 2023 and 2028 significantly.

Predicting the future can be compared to cooking a meal without a recipe. Just as a chef may have to use intuition, experience, and taste to create a dish without a written recipe, predicting the future requires us to use past patterns, current trends, and our own judgment to make informed guesses about what may happen in the future. Although looking into an open cooking pot or a crystal ball is always tricky, it is to some extent possible to envision which other innovations will further change how we organize pharmaceutical care.

The content of this chapter is not meant to be all-conclusive but is meant as an inspiring view of what lies ahead. We focus on five technologies under significant development that are expected to grow further in the next decade and will create paradigm shifts in future health care.

- Precision medicine
- Pharmacogenetic self testing
- 3D printed drugs
- Social robots in every home
- Blockchain

---

*In this chapter, you will read about digital health technology already showing great promise and some early 2023 examples. However, technologies such as full precision medicine, 3D printing of drugs, social robots, and blockchain are not expected to reach their full potential until 2028 and beyond.

Pharmaceutical Care in Digital Revolution. https://doi.org/10.1016/B978-0-443-13360-2.00008-3

Precision medicine

QR Code 16.1
What is precision
medicine?

Precision medicine, as also discussed in Chapter 5 and visualized in QR Code 16.1, is an emerging model that aims to customize therapy to subpopulations of patients, categorized by shared molecular and cellular biomarkers, to improve patient outcomes. Precision medicine differs from *personalized medicine* in that the latter refers more to tailoring procedures and therapeutic interventions at an individual patient level.

Computational pharmacotherapy is supportive of precision medicine and incorporates multiple sources of raw data (e.g., clinical electronic medical records, laboratory data, pharmacogenomics, metabolomics, imaging, microbiome, nutrigenomics, personal health application (PHA) data, and digital health data). Furthermore, computational pharmacotherapy extracts biologically and clinically relevant information from those data and subsequently uses mathematical models at the levels of molecules, individuals, and populations to generate diagnostic inferences and predictions.

The methods used in precision medicine and computational pharmacotherapy technology are driven largely by AI (refer to Chapter 11).

Computational pharmacotherapy technology can present clinically actionable and relevant knowledge to users through dynamic and integrated reports and interfaces, enabling pharmacists, physicians, patients, and other healthcare system stakeholders to make the best possible medical and pharmaceutical decisions.

The output of such technology will help providers select the most appropriate and efficient laboratory tests, run a multidimensional diagnosis, drive faster and more accurate preventive management, and target therapeutic intervention and follow-up for individual patients.

Pharmaceutical care providers are experts in applied therapeutics and are uniquely positioned to understand, integrate, and utilize diverse experimental approaches to realizing precision medicine.

The historical one-size-fits-all approach is no longer valid, and patients and healthcare systems greatly need and will benefit from research and implementation of precision medicine.

Considerations

In many countries, having a patient's DNA profile scanned and integrated into medical information systems is still prone to regulatory, ethical, and procedural challenges. Data privacy requirements and complex informed consent procedures can limit access to a precision medicine approach.

Cost is also considered as a major hurdle. Precision medicine initiatives, such as those President Obama introduced in the United States in 2015, have cost many millions of dollars over the years. Using technologies such as sequencing large amounts of DNA is also expensive (although the cost of sequencing is decreasing quickly), and that doesn't include the costs related to effectively linking these data into electronic health records, electronic pharmacy records, or PHAs.

Nevertheless, implementing precision medicine may be a worthwhile investment because of the prevalence of and, therefore, costs for adverse events, nonresponding users, and disease deterioration are expected to decrease significantly when precision medicine is adopted.

It is expected that, with the integration of current population-based data sets with the broader genotypic and phenotypic data sets, precision medicine will be gradually further implemented toward 2028 and beyond.

Pharmacogenetic self testing

Pharmacogenetics (PGx) studies how a person's genes affect their response to a drug. These genetic variations can influence drug metabolism, drug efficacy, and drug toxicity. By analyzing a person's genetic makeup, healthcare professionals can gain insight into how a patient is likely to respond to a particular medication or dosage, which can help them tailor treatment to the individual's needs [1].

Every person's genetic makeup is unique, and these genetic differences can affect how a person responds to drugs. PGx seeks to identify these genetic differences and use this information to optimize drug therapy. For example, a person's genetic makeup may affect how quickly they metabolize a drug, which in turn can affect the drug's efficacy and toxicity.

PGx testing can help identify genetic variations that affect drug metabolism and other drug-related functions. For example, testing can identify genetic variations in enzymes that are responsible for drug metabolism, such as cytochrome P450 enzymes. These enzymes play a critical role in breaking down drugs in the body, and genetic variations in these enzymes can affect how quickly or slowly a drug is metabolized.

PGx testing can also identify genetic variations in drug receptors and transporters, which can affect a drug's efficacy and toxicity. For example, variations in the gene that codes for the drug receptor may affect how strongly a drug binds to the receptor, which can affect its efficacy. Similarly, variations in the gene that codes for the transporter protein may affect how well a drug is transported into or out of cells, which can affect its toxicity.

By combining PGx testing with other clinical information, healthcare providers can personalize drug therapy to improve patient outcomes. For example, pharmacogenetic testing can help identify patients who may be at higher risk of drug toxicity or who may require lower doses of a particular drug. This can help reduce the risk of adverse drug reactions and improve patient safety.

PGx testing can be done in the care provider's environment, however, it is increasingly also provided as a self-management tool and executed in a person's home situation. PGx testing at home involves collecting a DNA sample, usually through a saliva or cheek swab, and sending it to a laboratory for analysis.

Several at-home PGx testing kits are available on the market and can be ordered online or purchased at some pharmacies. Patients get the test results on phone applications and can send that information to their pharmacist. This can support the pharmacist in making choices toward the correct drug and dosing for the patient and/or discuss the results with the general practitioner and/or specialist to improve shared decision-making.

Considerations

Although the PGx information can be very useful, healthcare professionals should also be conscious of the limitations of PGx home testing kits and their potential implications for patient care.

While some PGx testing kits are accurate and reliable, others may provide incomplete or inaccurate results. Healthcare professionals should therefore understand whether their patients use reputable and reliable testing kits and that the testing process is properly validated.

Also, while PGx testing can provide valuable information, it should not be used as the sole basis for treatment decisions. Instead, healthcare professionals should consider the test results in the context of a patient's overall medical history, symptoms, beliefs, and behaviors toward various therapies.

PGx testing results can be complex, and patients may need guidance in understanding what the results mean for their treatment. Therefore, healthcare professionals should be prepared to explain the significance of test results and provide guidance on how to interpret them.

Healthcare professionals should also be aware of ethical and legal considerations related to PGx testing, including issues related to privacy, informed consent, and the use of genetic information in treatment decisions.

In conclusion, pharmacists can largely benefit from having the data from a patient but also need to be aware of the current limitations in accuracy and reliability as this between home testing kits can vary. Also, testing can provide valuable information for treatment planning but is not a substitute for clinical judgment.

3D-printed drugs

Once computational pharmacotherapy becomes a reality, personalized 3D printing is the logical next step toward precision medicine. 3D printing drugs is not a fantasy anymore. Unbelievable shapes and any kind of drug can be fabricated with groundbreaking technology [2].

To envision the potential of 3D-printed drugs, think about the fact that most people get a "general" drug dosage that is, however, not aligned with their personal profile, which can lead to a number of the previously mentioned issues. Or think, on another level, about the aggravation of standing in line at a pharmacy. Would not it be more convenient for people to make their particular medicines safely at home, have a dose that is calculated exactly for them and never have to queue up again? That future will be here once 3D printers become mainstream in pharmacies and maybe even home environments and enable local synthetization of pharmaceuticals and other chemicals from widely available compounds and feed these products directly into smart reactors.

Multiple techniques for 3D printing are now being developed and tested, for example, layer-to-layer printing by combining powdered medications and liquid droplets; or by applying heat and pressure to melt a polymer and print drugs into different geometric shapes, which due to the reduced surface area may help to fasten the release of the active ingredient; or via organic vapor jet printing, which deposits nanostructured films of small molecular pharmaceutical ingredients with accuracy on the scale of micrograms per square centimeter onto different drug carriers, such as tabs, needles, and adhesives.

QR Code 16.2 exemplifies how 3D printing can work for the manufacturing of theophylline. Another drug, Spritam, the first 3D-printed drug to treat epilepsy, received FDA approval in 2015. The manufacturing technique allows rapid dispersion of the tablet, high drug loading, and modified release.

QR Code 16.2
Example of 3D printing.

As another example, the University of Glasgow plans to follow the tactics Spotify did with music (and Uber did with transportation) for the discovery and distribution of prescription drugs in which a prototype 3D printer capable of assembling chemical compounds at the molecular level is used. The device is designed and constructed using a chemical-to-computer—automated design that can translate traditional synthesis into platform-independent digital code. They demonstrate the system's potential by producing Baclofen, establishing a concept that could pave the way for the local manufacture of drugs outside specialist institutions [3].

3D printing toward individualized dosing

Spritam is now printed commercially in a number of fixed doses. The ultimate result would be to print tablets customized according to a given patient's genetic profile and other factors influencing optimal individual doses (e.g., concomitant medication, food preferences that influence the drug's metabolism, and environmental circumstances like allergen load). Such opportunities are particularly promising for drugs with a narrow therapeutic dose, as personalized 3D printing may prevent overdosing and the occurrence of adverse events. Also, a 3D-printed drug can be tailored to patients in terms of its size, appearance, and delivery, all of which can make the drug safer and more effective.

After receiving a digital prescription from a doctor, patients will go to an online drugstore, buy the blueprint and the chemical ink materials needed, and then print the drug at home in the prescribed dose; or go to their local pharmacy, where a pharmacist will take their physical measurements, perform a finger-prick blood test, and input the data online on the pharmacy's 3D printing medicines portal. Instead of storing and distributing packets of tablets, pharmacists will have reels of filaments of the base product (the prescribed drug) and will customize the dose and shape of a tablet to individual needs.

New techniques in printing may also make it possible to print multiple drugs in one pill [4]. Although there are still many hurdles to overcome, like the potential impact of drug—drug interactions within a pill and the shelf life of combined compounds, the technique could reduce the number of pills that poly-pharmacy patients have to use every day and thus improve their quality of life and the likelihood they will adhere to taking the drugs.

Added value of 3D printing

 Compared with the way drugs are manufactured and distributed now, 3D printing may solve a number of issues:

- The cost of drug development may be reduced by allowing faster customization of trial material in the research and development phases.
- Faster disintegration of a drug may make it easier for patients to swallow it.

- No longer will large stocking quantities of nonpatient-specific pills be needed.
- Personalizing the dose, size, appearance, and smell will make it possible to tailor a drug to a patient's (pharmacogenomics) profile.
- Printing customized pills 24/7 in a home setting will be possible.
- Counterfeit drugs will be reduced, as drugs will be printed from digital databases (however, the raw chemical materials are prone to fraud).
- Waste of medications will be reduced, as necessary adjustments of dosing can be made in a more agile way. Thus, fewer fixed-dose drugs must be destroyed if patient dose changes (provided that chemical ink cartridges can be redistributed or delivered in small quantities of drug packages).
- Pharmacy waiting times will be reduced, potentially saving lives in time-sensitive situations.

Considerations

Before 3D printing can take off in consumer markets, a real challenge is fully digitizing the chemistry so that a digital blueprint exists for all molecules and so that computers can build drugs from scratch. Those blueprints should be encrypted to ensure that drugs are always produced according to a validated blueprint and to eliminate the use of counterfeit chemicals as much as possible.

With respect to the encryption of blueprint and further security, both pharmacy-delivered and home-printed 3-D drugs need to be strictly governed and controlled. Only login codes with a complexity similar to those for bank accounts or biometric access techniques should allow access to domestic 3-D printing machines used for medication. In addition, integrating transactions done with a device (e.g., a doctor's prescriptions being directly referred to a domestic 3D printer) into, for instance, a blockchain environment may provide better patient safety.

Also, 3D printers may be hacked, and securing them from unauthorized access will be important. In a world where even cruise ships' navigation systems can be hacked, it is clear that 3D printers can be threatened to disrupt individual lives, to steal personalized data, or to disrupt larger operational systems where networked 3D printers are used.

Drug regulation authorities will need to establish strict and guaranteed guidelines to ensure that future mass marketing of 3D-printed drugs is safe, reliable, secure, and safeguarded against human error. Risks need to be adequately mapped, requirements for safety and security settled, and guidelines made to prevent all cybersecurity-related risks.

As with more digital health technologies described in previous chapters, in the case of technical errors or malfunctions that result in physical harm to patients, legal authorities will need to determine whether the 3D printer's manufacturer, a drug company, or another party is liable. It may still take years of trial and error or case-by-case studies before satisfying solutions are found.

An additional complexity of the technology is its global, decentralized distribution. It will be difficult for drug companies and pharmacists to ensure that the right packaging and user instructions are made accessible to patients promptly. Virtual assistants, like those noted in Chapter 12 and augmented reality, as noted in Chapter 13, may offer connected digital pharmaceutical solutions that provide holistic care that includes both the product and the service.

Big opportunities ahead

Assuming that the conditions for safe and reliable use of 3D printing are in place, providing patients with the exact amount of the drug they need, supporting them with continuous digital and human care services, and subsequently enabling them to measure outcomes with customized digital health technologies are the panacea for pharmaceutical care.

In the field of 3D-printed drugs, several innovations are expected to impact in the near future significantly. Some of these include:

- **Multi-Material Printing**: The ability to 3D print with multiple materials in a single process, creating more complex and sophisticated drug delivery systems.
- **Improved Drug Formulations**: The use of 3D printing technology to create new drug formulations with improved properties, such as improved solubility, bioavailability, and stability.
- **Complex Drug Delivery Systems**: The creation of more complex drug delivery systems, including combination products incorporating multiple active ingredients, using 3D printing technology.
- **Expansion into Bioprinting**: The use of 3D printing technology to create living tissues and organs could significantly impact the development of new treatments for a range of diseases and conditions.

The future of 3D-printed drugs is expected to be marked by continued innovation and advancement, creating more personalized and effective treatments for patients. Printing drugs via 3D printing is likely to increase in the future, but true integration in healthcare systems and printing mass-marketed drugs may still be years away.

Social robots in every home

 The principle definition of a robot is a machine—especially one programmable by a computer—capable of automatically carrying out a complex series of actions. An external control device can guide robots, or the control may be embedded within, mainly driven by AI algorithms [5]. Robots increasingly substitute human tasks in predominantly repetitive situations. Gradually, as more algorithms like machine learning and deep learning (see Chapter 11) are added, their value will spread to broader services and care tasks as well.

A large percentage of current robots are still industrial step-and-repeat machines designed to perform a task in industry or at home with no or limited regard to how they look or interact with humans.

For decades, integrated pharmacy automation systems that automate partial or entire processes for delivering packages or dispensing unit-dose medications have existed in the pharmaceutical industry. Those pharmacies using dispensing robots are augmented in such a way that the robots' increased speed and efficiency allow the human labor force to spend more time with patients or other healthcare professionals and to focus on better patient outcomes. Also, robots help to decrease medication errors, as the variability of robots' preciseness is usually less than that of humans.

Some special forms of robots are microscopic and nanorobots (10^{-9}) robots. Microscopic robots were inspired by insects such as spiders and could 1 day be capable of migrating through and performing delicate medical tasks inside the body. Nanorobots can be swallowed and assist in, for example, targeted drug delivery. An example is origami robots built into medication capsules. The robot's capsule dissolves in a patient's stomach and unfolds itself when swallowed. An external technician most often controls these robots, and with the help of magnetic fields, they, for example, patch up wounds in the stomach lining or safely remove foreign items such as swallowed toys.

Attitudes toward robots

Initial attitudes toward social robots are only *slightly* positive, indicating people's lack of understanding and limited exposure to social robots [6]. One factor that influences a person's attitude toward robots is prior experiences with technology [7]. For example, robots in Japanese culture are more common and with repeated exposure to robots. Furthermore, different cultures have various attitudes toward robots and artificial intelligence, which can assist or hinder the progress of robots in healthcare. Japan is the world leader in robotics, and demand is high for robots, which could help fill the huge shortfall in nursing care due to the country's aging population. The country is, for example, home to Erica, one of the first realistic female humanoids in existence, and (as shown in QR Code 16.3), Azuma, a holographic girl in a jar that combines virtual personal assistant functionality with a

QR Code 16.3
Example of a social robot.

cute look and a simulated, submissive personality. In addition, Japan's labor shortage will hit service industry jobs like eldercare with ferocity; therefore, future caretakers may currently be under development in a Japanese factory [8].

In the United States, the view on robots is mixed, with 50% saying robots are bad for society and 41% saying it is good [9]. However, this question was asked about people's thoughts on using robots to *automate jobs*. There still is some resentment toward using robotics, as some still perceive "robots taking over our jobs." Nonetheless, people's attitudes toward robots can be complex and multifaceted, influenced by various individual and societal factors. As robotic technologies advance and integrate into daily life, attitudes toward robots will likely continue to evolve and change.

Robots in hospital care

During a hospital stay, many patients prefer to interact frequently with human nurses. Nurses draw blood, check your vital signs, check on your condition, and take care of your hygiene if needed. Unfortunately, they are often exhausted by physically and mentally daunting tasks, and the result of people being overworked is often an unpleasant experience for everyone involved, including the patient.

Robotic nurses can help carry this burden in the future, as certain robots can, for example, take blood samples or support with dressing or grooming. Also, social companion robots may entertain and reassure people, where possible. Supported by these robots, the staff may conserve the energy needed to deal with issues that require human decision-making skills and empathy.

A few countries have already established themselves as "robotic" societies, with Japan, China, the United States, South Korea, and Germany in the lead.

Social companion robots in healthcare

Alongside industrial robots, the number of aesthetically appealing and even adorable social robots is growing.

A social robot is a specific kind of AI system designed to interact with humans and possibly with other robots (QR Code 16.4).

Social (companion) robots come in different forms:

- Monolithic voice-user interfaces like the ones noted in Chapter 12

QR Code 16.4
Example of a
humanoid robot.

- Anthropomorphic devices with tangible body frameworks, holograms, or avatars that exhibit adorability and that excite human empathy
- Humanoids or androids with faces resembling humans (see QR Code 16.4)

Robots may solve many issues in home-situated or hospital healthcare in light of an aging population combined with a smaller workforce available to meet the increasing need for care.

Social companion robots may act as a jack of all trades, thus freeing up time for care providers to focus on the human touch in the (health) care system. Social robots may entertain, perform small household tasks, remind people of drug-related activities, and motivate physical activity.

In hospital or community care situations where the amount of attention given to patients is driven by restricted resources, the results may be unnecessary disease deterioration or unnoticed adverse events. In such cases, social robots can play a caring and alerting role, making sure patients feel comfortable and cared for as much as possible.

Additionally, in homecare settings, social isolation and loneliness can be soothed by certain forms of companion robots. Many home healthcare environments are already equipped with an increasing number of smart robotics, and these machines may simultaneously and in real-time analyze large sets of data, using a combination of deep learning, machine reading, and data augmentation to identify trends and that create a holistic vision of a patient's status. Based on these data, the robots are able to anticipate a patient's needs, signal alerts in case of medical abnormalities, and provide companionship when asked for. Thus they help to ensure safe environments where patients can feel comforted.

Social robots are often made to look adorable in order to increase the level of trust and the likelihood that people will follow the advice offered by the robots. Humanlike robots tend to increase a person's comfort level, and they may be perceived as easier to communicate with than another person. A potential disadvantage is an expectation that a robot can do a broad set of human activities, which is still not the case. Moreover, if robots are too humanlike, people may "forget" the difference between a human and a machine, which may be experienced as scary by some.

Social robots in pharmaceutical care

Within a pharmacy, tasks like those a receptionist performs (with smart AI integration) may be conducted by social robots. In fact, Chinese hospitals already have hospitality robots at the entrance to the hospitals. Robots also may be a combination of an anthropomorphic device and personal assistant technology that, in the future, can perform triage activities, for example, helping patients with straightforward, over-the-counter medication questions.

Robot technology is also increasingly used to help in homecare settings with medication adherence programs (like Mabu in QR Code 16.5), using drugs according to prescription, and providing educational support when part of a domestic environment. Some robots are able to learn the interactions specific to a household and adapt to offer more personalized support.

QR Code 16.5
Mabu.

Considerations

In–home virtual care assistants will never replace human interaction or the human touch, but they are programmed to reduce many of the inefficiencies associated with healthcare today, which may contribute to an increase in value-driven healthcare.

As with 3D printers, with robots safety and security are essential, and it must be nearly impossible for unauthorized people to access a robot's infrastructure. Also, biometric patient recognition and fully secure encryption of data sharing with external care providers are still big challenges; however, solutions for them are expected in the future.

Ethics in the time of robotics

Other important considerations are the ethical aspects behind using robots in general. Ethical judgment involves systematically reflecting on normative issues (see Chapter 18). There are many definitions of digital ethics, but basically, the term refers to the values and moral principles for the conduct of digital interactions.

In his 1942 short story, *Runaround*, science fiction writer Isaac Asimov introduced the Three Laws of Robotics, engineering safeguards, and built-in ethical principles that he would go on to use in dozens of stories and novels.

The laws of Asimov are

- a robot may not injure a human being or, through inaction, allow a human being to come to harm;
- a robot must obey the orders given to it by human beings, except where such orders would conflict with the First Law, and
- a robot must protect its own existence as long as such protection does not conflict with the First or Second Laws.

Using robots in health care may raise fundamental questions regarding the responsible use of digital technology, such as the unintentional discovery of confidential information in medical scans, database searches, or algorithms supporting clinical decision-making without transparency of validity and evidence.

As such digital technology, including robots, is not neutral. Rather, they enshrine a vision and reflect a worldview, as they are programmed by humans living in a certain ecosystem. For instance, social robot technology from Japan may not land in other contingents, as cultural backgrounds and beliefs may imprint the actions that social robots execute.

Thus, when using social robot technology in pharmaceutical care, it is recommended that providers understand the way the algorithms are programmed and ask for transparency in machine learning mechanisms and how they are connected to what is considered "good care" by individual patients (as discussed in Chapter 5).

The profession's principles (see Chapter 19) and the moral values linked to the pharmacist's role may serve as guides at the current time, as digital ethics standards are not yet sufficiently developed.

The value of humans

Additionally, the more basic question should be posed: Will human beings be allowed to choose to be treated by a human professional rather than a robot? Although it promises tremendous societal and economic benefits, as this technology is implemented, it may become more and more difficult for people to act in a self-determined way, and thus their freedom of choice and action may be put at considerable risk.

Human compassion is central to the welfare of people, and in fact, the human touch is considered to be vital in the practice of medicine. It is an integral part of the patient–pharmacist relationship, in which patients feel that they are cared for by fellow human beings and are not alone in their time of need.

Even if ethical frameworks are built such that future robotic applications are empathic, they will never be able to relate as humans do. As in the movie *Ex Machina,* the question is asked: Would you believe it if a robot could show authentic emotion?

Artificial intelligence and robots may outpace human intelligence from a hardware perspective, but humans, definitely the ones who are ill, may want to choose on the side of human judgment; a caring, warm arm; an empathic ear; or a calming, soft hug. Moreover, there is also the phenomenon of trust, in which humans are not sure robots can make the right choices for human healthcare, despite the fact that human choice is itself not always infallible.

A good way forward will be to develop people's trust in robots, which can be done by creating a transparent understanding of how the algorithms are fed with data, how the robots are programmed, how they analyze, and how they provide reasons for actions.

However, even if an adorable-looking social robot displays full transparency through adequate data and structures and consistent decision-making trees, some real-life situations ask for intuitive human consideration and judgment that will never be programmable. Thus it becomes our challenge to develop models fitting for a synergistic society in which robots and humans live in creative cooperation.

Full integration of social robots within the pharmaceutical care journey is not expected to take place prior to 2028.

Blockchain technology

A blockchain (originally blockchain) is a decentralized digital ledger that records transactions across a network of computers securely and transparently, without the need for a central authority or intermediary. In a blockchain, transactions are grouped together in blocks and each block is linked to the previous block, forming a chain of blocks (hence the name blockchain). Once a block is added to the blockchain, the information it contains cannot be altered or deleted, creating an immutable record of all transactions [10].

Records or blocks can contain any form of data, such as digital money, real estate (ownership), and healthcare data. Each block typically contains a hash pointer (digital fingerprint) as a link to a previous block, a timestamp, and transaction data.

As a digital ledger, a blockchain is typically shared by all the computers in a decentralized peer-to-peer network, collectively adhering to a protocol for adding and validating new blocks. Once recorded, the data in any given block cannot be altered retrospectively without the alteration of all subsequent blocks, which would require collusion or compromise of the majority of computers in the network (QR Code 16.6).

QR Code 16.6
Blockchain
explained.

Blockchains are secure by design, and the decentralized consensus is a main characteristic. In addition, blockchains use cryptographic techniques to ensure the security and integrity of the data stored on the network, making it extremely difficult for malicious actors to alter or manipulate the data. This makes blockchains suitable for recording transactions of events, medical data, and other record management activities [11].

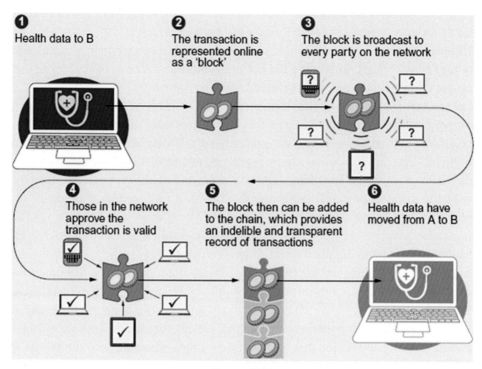

Figure 16.1
How the blockchain works?

Fig. 16.1 shows what a transaction on a blockchain network looks like.

It is important to mention that every transaction (a smart contract) in a regular blockchain is open, although transactions are not allowed to be made public in Europe. In a permissioned or private blockchain, users (in health care, this may be the patient) are in the lead and determine who sees which type of information in their blockchain.

Blockchain implementation for healthcare

Blockchain technology is being increasingly adopted in the healthcare industry to improve healthcare data security, transparency, and efficiency. Some of the ways blockchain can be used in healthcare include:

- **Electronic Medical Records (EMRs)**: Blockchain technology can be used to securely store and manage electronic medical records, ensuring that sensitive patient data is protected from unauthorized access. An example of EMRs is Medicalchain, a decentralized platform for exchanging and using medical data through blockchain technology. As a result, patients are in control of their data and can provide access to their physicians to manage their condition remotely. The platform also rewards patients for providing access to their data for medical research [12].

- **Clinical Trials**: Blockchain can be used to securely store and manage data generated during clinical trials, improving the accuracy and transparency of trial results. It is estimated that nearly half of all clinical trials go unreported, and investigators often fail to share their study results (e.g., nearly 90% of trials on ClinicalTrials.gov lack reported results). This may create safety issues and knowledge gaps for patients, healthcare stakeholders, and health policymakers. Blockchain-enabled, timestamped, immutable records of clinical trials, protocols, and results could potentially address the issues of outcome switching, data snooping, and selective reporting, thereby also reducing the incidence of fraud and error in clinical trial records. Further, blockchain-based data witnessing systems could help drive collaboration between participants and researchers around innovation in medical research in fields like precision medicine and population health management [13,14].

- **Supply Chain Management**: Blockchain can be used to track the movement of drugs and medical supplies through the supply chain, improving the visibility and accountability of the supply chain and reducing the risk of counterfeiting and fraud. Based on global industry estimates, pharmaceutical companies incur an estimated annual loss of $200 billion due to counterfeit drugs. About 30% of drugs sold in LIMC countries are considered to be counterfeited. A blockchain-based system could ensure a chain-of-custody log, tracking each supply chain step at the individual drug or product level. Furthermore, add-on functionalities could help build in proof of ownership of the drug at any point in the supply chain

- **Claims Adjudication**: Blockchain can be used to securely and transparently manage the adjudication of insurance claims, improving the claims process's efficiency and accuracy. Blockchain-enabled solutions streamline the exchange of data among and between contractual parties in pharmaceutical care contracts would increase efficiency. For example, rather than independently collecting and reconciling data related to contractual terms and obligations, insurance companies and pharmaceutical care providers could share contractual updates via a private, shared transactional ledger jointly operated by the network of players in the value chain. This will promote real-time transparency in health claims transactions, reduce the need for clearing houses, and improve currency flow after the transaction has taken place, meaning that PCPs or patients are paid in nearly real time after the prescription transaction.

- **Research Data Sharing**: Blockchain can be used to securely store and manage data generated during research studies, enabling researchers to securely and transparently share data. The process of delivering medication to a patient is a complex process for almost all prescriptions, and certainly for specialty medications. Multiple parties, including the payer, the dispensing pharmacy, and the manufacturer, engage in repetitive information exchanges to determine the suitability and sustainability of a given drug therapy. These steps include but are not limited to clinical guidelines benchmarking, step therapy requirements, patient support assessment, patient education, medication therapy management, and prescription adherence tracking.

Considerations

The challenge of identity and privacy

The big challenge to using blockchain in future pharmaceutical care chains is probably to secure the identity and privacy of the user (patient), as public ledgers currently do not afford this privacy by default. Therefore in healthcare environments, only private blockchains seem to be feasible. In this context, identity on the blockchain is how one can make "claims" to rights, membership, and ownership of healthcare and pharmaceutical data. In addition, biometric authentication increasingly secures identity, uniquely identifying you within a given set of users.

Several companies are actively working on identity solutions independent of a central authority, such as a governmental body, enterprise, or physical representation. These solutions involve identity claims on a blockchain to achieve decentralization, executable contracts, secure encryption, and consensus.

Uncertainty in regulation

The amount of regulatory uncertainty on blockchain legislation hinders blockchain uptake to a certain extent. National and Global regulations that support the use of blockchain for business purposes, such as contracts and financial audits, will likely tip the scales in favor of mass adoption. The legislation will need to answer several questions, for example: Does private blockchain activity represent an inherently reliable confirmation? Can a smart contract represent the execution of a legal contract in law? Who are the responsible persons when the blockchain is used for illegal practices? [15] Providing clarity in those questions will require changes in regulations, laws, practices, and protocols; however, with these answers, scaling blockchain will be quicker and easier to facilitate.

In the next part of this book, we will describe the conditions to drive combinatoric pharma-digital innovation and to make adequate and ethically sound digital pharmaceutical care implementation happen.

This means for blended pharmaceutical care:

- Computational pharmacotherapy will help healthcare providers drive precision medicine, leading to optimal individualized treatment patterns.
- Pharmacogenetic testing will guide users to informed choices about their medicines.
- Multiple techniques for 3D printing can offer tailored drugs to patients in terms of dosage, size, appearance, and delivery system.
- Social companion robots come in different forms, that is, monolithic voice-user interfaces, anthropomorphic devices, and humanoids.
- Social companion robots may act as a sort of jack of all trades and, for example, may entertain, may perform small household tasks, and may remind people of activities and motivate physical action.
- Robots free up time for healthcare providers so that they can focus more on the human touch, an empathic touch that cannot be simulated by robots.
- To warrant ethical use of social robotic technology in pharmaceutical care, it is recommended that we understand how the algorithms are programmed, how machine learning mechanisms work, and how the connection is made to what individual patients consider to be "good care."
- Both 3D printing and robotics are prone to privacy and security challenges, and the future challenge is to provide safe systems that can be trusted by both providers and patients.
- Blockchain offers great opportunities for health care, but the conditions to succeed are still in the development phase.

References

[1] Hansen JM, Nørgaard JD, Sporrong SK. A systematic review of pharmacogenetic testing in primary care: attitudes of patients, general practitioners, and pharmacists. Res Soc Adm Pharm 2022;18(8):3230—8.
[2] The Medical Futurist. The future of 3D printing drugs in pharmacies is closer than you think. 2022 [cited 2023 16/02/2023]. Available from: https://medicalfuturist.com/future-3d-printing-drugs-pharmacies-closer-think/.
[3] Kitson PJ, et al. Digitization of multistep organic synthesis in reactionware for on-demand pharmaceuticals. Science 2018;359(6373):314—9.
[4] Brown KV. The future of pharmaceuticals is custom-printing drugs. 2017 [cited 2023 04/02/2023]. Available from: https://gizmodo.com/the-future-of-pharmaceuticals-is-printing-custom-drugs-1818846684.
[5] robot n.2. Oxford English dictionary. 2023.
[6] Naneva S, et al. A systematic review of attitudes, anxiety, acceptance, and trust towards social robots. Int J Social Robot 2020;12(6):1179—201.
[7] Leite I, Martinho C, Paiva A. Social robots for long-term interaction: a survey. Int J Social Robot 2013;5(2):291—308.

[8] Ross A. The industries of the future. New York, NY: Simon & Schuster; 2016.

[9] Pew Research Center. Public views about science in the United States. 2020 [cited 2023 16/02/2023]. Available from: https://www.pewresearch.org/science/fact-sheet/public-views-about-science-in-the-united-states/.

[10] Chelladurai U, Pandian S. A novel blockchain based electronic health record automation system for healthcare. J Ambient Intell Hum Comput 2022;13(1):693−703.

[11] Engelhardt MA. Hitching healthcare to the chain: an introduction to blockchain technology in the healthcare sector. Technol Innov Manage Rev 2017;7(10).

[12] MedicalChain. Medicalchain Whitepaper 2.1. 2018.

[13] Hang L, et al. Blockchain for applications of clinical trials: taxonomy, challenges, and future directions. IET Commun 2022;16(20):2371−93.

[14] Maslove DM, et al. Using blockchain technology to manage clinical trials data: a proof-of-concept study. JMIR Med Informatics 2018;6(4):e11949.

[15] Oderkirk J, Slawomirski L. Opportunities and challenges of blockchain technologies in health care. OECD Blockchain Policy Ser 2020;12.

PART 3

How: conditions to drive combinatoric pharma-digital innovation

CHAPTER 17

Whisking the digital health compliance*

Anne Sophie Dil, Amy Eikelenboom
NAALA B.V., Rotterdam, The Netherlands

If you think being compliant is expensive, try noncompliance.

Paul McNulty

Digital health solutions have the potential to monitor medical adherence, measure medical conditions, determine medical diagnoses, analyze anomalies during treatments, and produce big (health) data for scientific research purposes. A few examples of how digital pharmaceutical care can improve future care pathways are discussed in depth in previous chapters. Innovations are necessary to face the increasing demand for (pharmaceutical) care and exploding costs in the (near) future.

Although many believe in the potential of game-changing digital health solutions, patients and medical specialists sometimes seem reluctant to use and adopt the innovations [1]. This is partly due to concerns related to the unfamiliarity and uncertainty of reliability, security, and liability surrounding digital innovations in health care.

In the whisking the innovation adoption, many rules and regulations prevail that may seem overwhelming. This chapter aims to provide a practical overview of the requirements and principles relevant to the development of digital innovations for pharmaceutical care and explain how to create an integrated management system for regulatory compliance that is feasible for all.

At the base, the definition of your compliance blueprint is essential. A compliance blueprint is a risk-based overview of the requirements that must be considered for your digital health solution and organization.

From the standpoint of the principles of risk management, a compliance blueprint consists of one or more of the following most common aspects:

---

*In this chapter, you will read about risk management principles, data protection, quality, and information security. By implementing an integrated management system throughout the design and development of your product, you may find that adherence to requirements becomes a true business enabler.

Pharmaceutical Care in Digital Revolution. https://doi.org/10.1016/B978-0-443-13360-2.00010-1

- laws and legislation on data protection;
- regulations and quality standards for medical devices;
- guidelines and best practices for information security and cyber security; and
- internal organizational rules.

At the end of this chapter, you will find a structured approach to constructing an integrated management system using your compliance blueprint.

Managing risks

Successful digital health solutions in pharmaceutical care journeys are built upon the pillars of data protection, quality, and information security. These pillars contribute to what is most important for digital health solution acceptance: trust. Trust in the correct functioning of medical devices (e.g., "Will I not get injured or sick if I follow the algorithms' advice?"), in security (e.g., "Will my data be safe?"), and in data protection (e.g., "Will my personal data not be used for any other purposes?").

Compliance is not a one-time activity. The combination of advancing technology and changing regulations results in the constant emergence of new risks. To ensure the quality, security, and data protection of digital solutions, continuously managing such risks is essential.

Continuous compliance starts with a thorough risk analysis.

 Risk is the combination of:
- the probability of occurrence of harm; and
- the severity of such harm.

Each resource (i.e., assets, organizational resources, and processes) carries its risks. For example, consider an office, electronics, human resources, and development processes. Before risks can be analyzed and mitigated, they should be mapped using an overview of the organization's resources and situations that potentially pose risks to the quality, information security, or data protection of the product or organization.

Evaluating risks is often difficult and subjective by nature. Stakeholders may place different values on the risk probability and potential severity. Involving all stakeholders (including patients where relevant) is, therefore, recommended when analyzing the probability of any harm occurring and the severity thereof.

Following a thorough risk analysis, effective mitigation must be implemented. All three pillars (data protection, quality, and information security) propose their safeguards. For example, when the risk is breaking into the office, the quality control would be to make sure the implemented alarm system meets all initial requirements of such a system, the security control would be to provide a limited amount people with a key to the office, and the data protection control would be to store no physical information at the office. To ensure the office is protected tomorrow as well as today, a continuous system for risk management is required.

A management system allows the assignment of all controls to internal roles responsible for the performance of the corresponding tasks. This way, all employees contribute daily to the digital solution's quality, security, and data protection. However, before a management system can be implemented, all applicable legal and regulatory requirements must be mapped. The following paragraphs will present an overview of quality, information security, and data protection requirements.

Data protection: patient in control of data

Health data are considered the new gold in healthcare. As these data accumulate and data analysis techniques become increasingly better (as discussed, e.g., in Chapters 8 and 11), the ability to create a holistic view of individuals is becoming easier. This trend offers many advantages; however, safeguarding the data protection of individuals is under increasing pressure.

Data protection case 1: Nike + Running app

The Dutch Data Protection Authority concluded in 2015 that the Nike + Running app violated the Data Protection Act. The app, which was downloaded 10—50 million times worldwide on Android devices, helped people track their running activities. The app allowed Nike to collect various types of personal data, including health data. Nike was accused of failing to adequately inform app users about processing their health data for Nike's analysis and research purposes. Moreover, Nike had not obtained lawful consent nor established retention periods for the data.

Nike has taken steps to update the app to comply with applicable regulations [2].

Almost all countries have some form of data protection regulation, specifically concerning health data. One may be familiar with the European General Data Protection Regulation (GDPR), the Health Insurance Portability and Accountability Act (HIPAA) of the United States or the Australian Privacy Act (Australian Privacy Principles). QR Code 17.1 shows a video on data protection for the future. The GDPR has often served as a reference point for third countries developing legislation in this field. This chapter will therefore focus on requirements stemming from the GDPR to highlight generally accepted data protection

QR Code 17.1
Data protection.

measures. In general, the following principles provide essential protection for data processing wherever the processing may take place:

- **Lawfulness, fairness, and transparency:** To be able to process personal data, the data subject must be able to trust that the organization processing the data. This may be realized by communicating to the data subject for what reasons which categories of personal data are processed, with whom the data is shared, and how long the data will be retained. This allows data subjects to make an informed decision about whether or not it wishes to let the organization process their personal data. Furthermore, data must be processed lawfully. This means that personal data may only be processed when an organization has a lawful basis to do so. Such a legal basis may be (explicit) consent, a contractual agreement (e.g., when a sales agreement is when you buy a product in order for the supplying party to deliver the product to your home address), or a legitimate interest.
- **Purpose limitation:** Personal data must only be processed for specified, explicit and legitimate purposes. This means that it must be clearly communicated (as discussed in the previous principle) for what purpose(s) the personal data will be processed. Personal data may then not be further processed for another purpose than originally communicated. If one desires to do so, a (new) legal basis is required to allow for such (further) processing.
- **Data Minimization:** Nowadays, many organizations collect all kinds of data from the perspective that data may be useful in the future. However, the aforementioned data protection laws place limits on this practice. Both the principle of data minimization and purpose limitation raises specific challenges for such unlimited data collection. Data minimization means that organizations responsible for the data processing determine the minimum amount of personal data necessary to achieve the purpose of the data processing (e.g., data necessary for the correct operation of the app). The organization is only allowed to process that amount of data.
- **Accuracy:** It must be ensured that the correct and up-to-date information is processed from an individual. This means an up-to-date version of a dataset must be obtained prior to starting the analysis activities. Additionally, safeguards such as a four-eye principle may be required to ensure no data are tampered or corrupted.
- **Storage limitation:** The period for which personal data will be retained must be clearly and transparently communicated to the individual. In some cases, it is required to store personal data for a minimum amount of time, for example, when it concerns a clinical investigation or when personal data is part of the medical device file. In general, personal data must not be retained for longer than necessary for the purpose

for which the personal data are processed. This means that following the determination of the specified and explicit purpose, it must be determined for how long it is necessary to retain the personal data.

- **Integrity and confidentiality:** The final principle is essential to safeguarding the processing of personal data in general. Personal data itself and the processing thereof must be appropriately protected against unauthorized or unlawful processing and against accidental loss, destruction, or damage. This must be done by implementing so-called "technical and organizational" measures. Data protection regulations do not state these measures in much detail. International standards may therefore be used to give substance to these measures. More specifically, ISO 27701 provides a comprehensive framework that may be used to adequately and continuously protect (the processing of) personal data. ISO 27701 combines both technical and organizational measures referencing ISO 27001 and ISO 27002 information security controls.

In addition to the principles related to the processing, the natural person or organization determining the means and purposes of the processing shall be responsible for ensuring these principles are complied with.

International personal data transfers

It depends on local regulations whether personal data may be shared with other parties and with other countries. Operating in an international market may therefore challenge the data sharing among collaborating parties or larger organizations. The European approach is to ensure that the protection of data travels along with the data itself. This means that data may only be shared with countries that provide a similar level of protection as the originating country (in this case, a European country). How can this be ensured? The GDPR provides a so-called toolkit with mechanisms that may be used to allow for international personal data transfers. In addition to that, the European Commission may adopt adequacy decisions with certain third countries. Via these adequacy decisions, the European Commission assesses the third country's data protection mechanisms, oversight, and available redress mechanisms. As a result of such an adequacy decision, personal data may flow to that third country without requiring additional safeguards. In the absence of such an adequacy decision, the following toolkit mechanisms may be used:

- standard contractual clauses,
- binding corporate rules,
- certification mechanisms, and
- codes of conduct

The aim of any "tool" is to provide an adequate level of data protection. Before using a tool, this level of data protection must be (continuously) assessed. To this end another tool has been provided, a Transfer Impact Assessment (TIA). A TIA provides a structured approach to analyzing the level of protection of any third country as opposed to your own as well as the assessment of the effectiveness of any mechanisms implemented. The European Data Protection Board has provided a useful recommendation to deploy a TIA [3].

Secondary use of personal data

According to data processing principles, personal data must be collected for a specified purpose. However, if the purpose changes and the original data is wanted to be used for another goal, a "compatibility test" must be performed. This test is required when the original data was not collected on the basis of consent nor was it collected following any law requiring the data to be processed for national or international safeguards. The compatibility test takes the following into account[1]:

- the purpose of processing the data must be related to the original purpose of collecting the data;
- the context in which the personal data was originally collected, e.g., the relationship between the person who controls the data (the data controller) and the data subject, needs to align with the new (intended) processing purpose;
- the type and nature of the data, i.e., the sensitivity, must also be taken into account. As health-related personal data concerns sensitive data, it is generally not allowed to process these without an exemption from this prohibition;
- the possible consequences of the intended further processing, i.e., the impact on the data subject;
- the existence of appropriate safeguards, i.e., encryption or pseudonymization.

When processing the data for another purpose, the data controller should inform the data subject about the new purpose and any other important information (as defined in art. 14(2), GDPR) before the data is processed for the new purpose. General information should be provided when the individual can not be identified because data originates from multiple sources.[2]

European Health Data Space (EHDS)

To facilitate the exchange and use of health data among various stakeholders in the European Union, the European Health Data Space is being developed by the European Commission. The EHDS aims to build on regulations currently regulating the use and re-use of personal health data, such as the GDPR and the Clinical Trials Regulation. In addition, newly proposed regulations, such as the Data Governance Act and the Data Act,

---

[1]   Article 6(4) (e), GDPR.
[2]   Article 14(4), GDPR.

aim to strengthen further opportunities to share and re-use general and sector-specific personal data while ensuring an individual's rights.

Quality: trust in patient safety

Securing (personal) data and organizational processes is part of a broader set of quality requirements. Quality requirements for digital health solutions and medical devices specifically aim to ensure the continuous quality, safety, and effectiveness of the medical devices placed on international markets. A consumer must be certain that every product offers the same level of quality, despite the batch it is produced in or the version released.

Poor-quality digital health solutions potentially have a significant effect on the health and safety of patients. It can result in physical injury or even death.

A blood collection device

Theranos, a once-successful startup in Silicon Valley with a value of over $9 billion, set out to revolutionize the blood testing industry. With a capillary tube nanotainer, the company claimed that it could run over 200 tests with just one finger prick and a few drops of blood. After an investigation by the FDA, it appeared that, in addition to analysis accuracy questions, the blood collection device was sold as a class I device but in fact was a higher classified medical device. The FDA concluded that Theranos did not adequately document risk or hazard analysis for its products, which resulted in an immediate risk to the health and safety of patients. Theranos' founder and CEO, Elizabeth Holmes, was sentenced to 135 months (11 years, 3 months) in federal prison for defrauding investors in Theranos of hundreds of millions of dollars [4].

Following a series of incidences where the quality of medical devices was not adequately ensured, regulations around the world were updated to provide a stricter regulatory framework. Some well-known regulatory frameworks that allow market access for the respective jurisdictions are:

- Title 21 Code of Federal Regulations (CFR) Parts 800-1299. This contains most of the FDA's (United States) medical device and radiation-emitting product regulations.
- Medical Devices Regulation and In-Vitro Diagnostic Regulation. These recently revised requirements regulate medical devices, in-vitro diagnostic medical devices, active implantable medical devices, and certain devices without an intended medical purpose on the European market.

To support an international approach to unified medical device regulatory systems, the Global Harmonization Task Force (GHTF) was conceived in 1992 and succeeded by the International Medical Device Regulators Forum (IMDRF) in 2012. The IMDRF publishes guidances and frameworks that are used by national legislators to align legislative frameworks.

MDSAP

Supporting uniformity, a single audit was designed to allow companies to be assessed on meeting quality management system requirements for multiple regulatory agencies by the performance of a single audit by an authorized Auditing Organization. Currently, regulatory agencies from Canada, Brazil, Japan, Australia, and the United States participate in MDSAP. The requirements audited follow the international standard on quality management systems for medical devices (ISO 13485:2016) and country-specific requirements.

More detailed information on the regulatory frameworks can be found in the Appendix.

ISO 13485 specifies the requirements for a quality management system for medical devices. The standard applies to organizations regardless of their size and type and provides detailed requirements for the design, production, installation, and delivery of medical devices and related services.

International standards

Not only ISO 13485:2016 is generally referenced by legislators to detail quality management system requirements, but other international standards may also be used to give substance to medical devices. Some examples of medical device software are:

- ISO 14971:2019 Medical devices—application of risk management to medical devices
- IEC 62304:2006 Medical device software—Software life cycle processes
- IEC 80001-1: Safety, effectiveness, and security in the implementation and use of connected medical devices or connected health software - Part 1: Application of risk management,
- IEC 81001-5-1 (not published): Health Software and health IT systems safety, effectiveness, and security—Part 5-1: Security—Activities in the product lifecycle.

Medical device conformity assessments

Conformity assessment involves evaluating evidence produced by the manufacturer through their internal processes to ensure that they meet regulatory standards and that the medical device being examined is safe and functions as intended by the manufacturer.

To sell medical devices, manufacturers must show that they meet the minimum requirements for safety and effectiveness. This conformity assessment includes the following components:

- a quality management system,
- a postmarket surveillance system,
- technical documentation,
- a declaration of conformity, and
- registration with the relevant regulatory authority.

While these elements are typically required for all types of medical devices, manufacturers may need to provide additional documentation based on the specific requirements of each country's regulatory authority.

An insulin pump

In 2016 Johnson & Johnson informed doctors and about 114,000 patients in the United States and Canada about a security vulnerability in one of its insulin pumps. It was possible to hack this device, which could allow a hacker to exploit it to overdose diabetic patients with insulin. Although the probability of unauthorized access was extremely low, the risks associated with a cyberattack are huge. J&J appropriately informed patients on how to diminish the risks to the bare minimum [5].

Security: data protection as the foundation for building trust

In recent years, theft of personal (including medical) records increased as the digital revolution increased access to more data. The website https://haveibeenpwned.com, which allows users to check if their email and password had been comprised from a data breach, had reported a total of 12,462,926,409 accounts had been leaked worldwide as of the beginning of February 2023.

Due to the increasing amount of data breaches, patients and medical specialists have growing concerns about the protection of their data. Information security is a set of processes and tools designed and deployed to protect sensitive business information (including, but not limited to personal data) from alteration, disruption, destruction, and inspection. These processes together produce a system for information security management (information security management system; ISMS). Information security is part of the broader concept of "cybersecurity," which indicates the protection of systems, networks, and programs from digital attacks.

In addition to individual harm, cybersecurity incidents can impact digital solutions' availability, continuity, and correct functioning. Should someone gain unauthorized access to a digital solution, data can be altered, critical algorithms changed, or devices disabled. All of which can lead to widespread damage.

(Inter)national legislation on information and cyber security is limited. Currently, data protection and quality legislation refer to obligations to take appropriate security measures, as this affects the extent to which quality and data protection can be assured. However, it is not clear from this legislation, nor from recently developed security legislation (such as the NIS Directive and the Cybersecurity Act at a European level) what is considered appropriate when it comes to security safeguards.

Various bodies support organizations in defining and implementing appropriate security safeguards based on globally accepted standards, guidelines, and best practices such as:

- ISO/IEC 27001 Information security management system (ISMS);
- Open Web Application Security Project (OWASP);
- Service Organization Controls (SOC) 2; and
- National Institute of Standards and Technology (NIST) guidelines.

These security standards, guidelines, and best practices are often based on globally recognized standard models. One of the most widely accepted models, which is used in ISO standards such as ISO 27001, is the confidentiality, integrity, and availability (CIA) triad:

- **Confidentiality:** Prevents unauthorized disclosure of sensitive information. Confidentiality is the ability to ensure that information remains hidden from unauthorized users.
- **Integrity:** Prevents unauthorized modification of data, systems, and information. Integrity is the ability to prevent unauthorized or accidental alteration, loss, or other contamination of information to ensure that information is reliable and actual at all times.
- **Availability:** Prevents loss of access to resources and information. Availability is the ability to provide access to the information in question to those who have the right and authority to access it when needed.

> **Connected pacemakers**
>
> The FDA recalled about 500,000 internet-connected pacemakers manufactured by Abbott Health, formerly St. Jude Medical, due to hacking fears in 2017. The security vulnerability of the pacemakers could allow an unauthorized user to access a patient's implanted, connected pacemaker remotely, and could result in patient harm and, in the worst case, death from rapid battery depletion or administration of inappropriate pacing or shocks.
>
> Rather than having patients remove or replace the device, the manufacturer released a firmware update. During the update, the device ran in backup mode, and loss of diagnostic data or settings was possible. Patients were requested to talk to their doctors about the risks and benefits of updating their pacemakers [6].

QR Code 17.2 and the Abbott example underline the necessity for the adequate design of medical devices' security, including digital solutions.

Security-by-design is a structured approach to making digital solutions as free of vulnerabilities and impervious to attack as possible by applying measures such as continuous testing, authentication safeguards, and adherence to best programming practices.

OWASP contains many guidelines for implementing security-by-design principles [7]. They contain, for example, the use of nondefault passwords and best-encrypted USB devices and involve intensive vulnerability testing on servers.

Humans are still considered a weak link in any system that contains risks, and this also applies to the security chain. Therefore, security awareness is considered to be the knowledge and attitude that members of an organization possess regarding the protection of the physical and, especially, the informational assets of the organization.

In a world where all devices are connected to the internet, there is always the possibility of a cyber-attack. Seamless security may never be possible, so you may assume you will be hacked to be as secure as possible.

Preventing cybersecurity incidents begins with awareness, both upfront during design and when security breaches are identified. Awareness can be created and maintained through an awareness program that suits the organization. Such a program includes all

QR Code 17.2
Cybersecurity.

necessary information, such as everyone's responsibilities and theoretical security policies, as well as what this means practically for each role involved.

Finally, during the development of digital tools, best practices, and guidance advice need to be used, as described in the Appendix (including for encryption methods). These best practices are published by various security parties and communities.

Organizational rules

In addition to laws and regulations, internal organization rules may also apply. These rules are typically included in documents like standard operating procedures (SOPs), contracts, codes of conduct, and mission and value statements. To construct an effective and sustainable management system within the organization, all requirements, including self-defined organizational rules, are essential. Implementing this set of rules requires an internal role- and responsibility-based training program and general awareness training. Everyone working for the company must be aware of their contribution to the quality of the medical device produced and be regularly informed on the appropriate way of performing daily tasks to ensure this.

Compliance blueprint: what to do tomorrow

At this point, we want to provide an overview of what will be required shortly to remain compliant on all aspects of data protection, quality, and security. Taking a structured approach may be best called making a "compliance blueprint."

Before starting, one should always beware that laws and legislation exist on global, regional, and local levels. Before executing a digital pharmaceutical care initiative, identify the applicable laws and regulations (your compliance blueprint starting point) that must be complied with.

Table 17.1 shows some of the key considerations for making an adequate compliance blueprint.

Compliance within the context of your organization

Laws and regulations generally allow for interpretation, which often depends on the context of the organization or the innovation.

For example, a company or institution's economic situation (the types of investments justified to ensure the continuity of the organization) and the state of its technology (the types of technology which are effective and affordable) are considerations that need to be taken into account once products are audited or inspected [8]. Compliance framework

Table 17.1: Some of the key considerations for making a compliance blueprint.

Make a proper risk assessment (based on ISO14971 methodology)			
🔒 Privacy	◎ Quality aspects	📑 Information security	🔀 Organizational rules
Take a compliance-by-design approach for all four elements into account			
Document privacy impact analysis with template of HIPAA/GDPR	Identify whether the quality standards are applicable; for example, is my solution a medical device and if so which class of medical device?	Encrypt all data connections	Determine which organizational rules you need to comply with
Consider privacy-by-design approach	Determine intended use (wellness or health) and classification	Run periodic security tests	
Document how transparency is provided	Follow quality management system rules (ISO 13485)	Secure and encrypt data storage	
Obtain consent on what will be tracked and analyzed (processed)	Prepare documentation on operational, technical, and legal controls (technical file)	Use best practices as mentioned earlier in the chapter	
Minimize data to the essentials	Implement processes and specific requirements	Create a high level of security awareness in the organization	
Create a high level of privacy awareness in the organization			
Automate where possible and efficient Remain compliant-aware on all four levels and adjust where required			

requirements for a small pharmacy software developer differ from those for a multinational pharmaceutical company. The data protection, safety, and patient security requirements are essentially the same; the implementation of safeguards to this end may differ.

Fig. 17.1 can be used to assess whether an organization's compliance lies in the immediate stage or a future stage. This information enables organizations to set goals and understand expectations when a digital health solution becomes a commercial success.

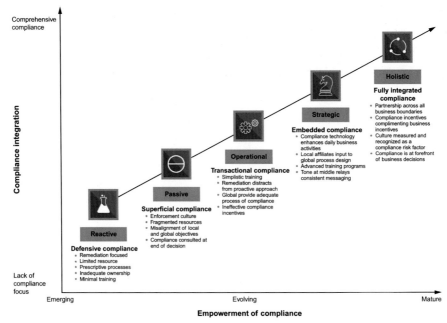

Figure 17.1
Compliance maturity model [9].

The model also shows that potential compliance risks are defined in the context of the organization (a small organization has different types of risks than a larger organization would have and therefore implements alternative safeguards).

Definition of the applicable legal framework

The applicable legal field depends on an organization's context and the proposed digital innovation. A thorough risk analysis is useful to determine the compliance approach and, consequently, appropriate safeguards.

An organization's main risk is having insufficient knowledge of the applicable legal framework. Therefore, the starting point for managing risks related to data protection, information security, and quality is establishing this legal framework. This involves assessing whether an organization or innovation processes personal data, whether other types of information need to be protected and whether the innovation can be considered a medical device. In addition, the jurisdictions in which the organization operates are important to determine which laws and regulations must be taken into account to be compliant.

Digital innovations in pharmaceutical care, data protection, information security, and quality will be the triptych for the material scope of the management system:

- digital solutions usually process users' personal data, for example when registering contact details and device data;
- information security is relevant to any organization that holds proprietary information, stores customer information, and/or otherwise processes (business-sensitive) data; and
- as described above, digital innovations in pharmaceutical care may be considered medical devices and the organization must implement processes and quality safeguards to this end.

The territorial scope of laws and regulations, due to digitization, is becoming increasingly wide. In this context, it is important to understand in which countries the organization has establishments, but also in which countries the organization operates and where the end users of the innovation are located. This all affects the applicability of laws and regulations, thus the scope of the management system.

Reduce compliance costs and work

This book provides examples that strongly suggest the disruptive adoption of technology in the next decade. As indicated previously, this fast uptake will drive the need to have newer types of rules and regulations.

The fast and ongoing innovations require large investments from stakeholders willing to develop and use digital health tools in a compliant way. Depending on the size of the organization, this means investment in (dedicated) compliance factors such as privacy officers, security officers, and data protection officers. It may include investment in processes and controls to mitigate noncompliance's (security, data protection, and quality) risks. Also, technology is required to protect the confidentiality, availability, and integrity of health data.

The risk of immediate loss of revenue, delayed product launches, costly remediation programs, fines, and long-term damage to your reputation is not just theoretical threats, as examples in this chapter have indicated.

There are positive triggers for compliance. Compliance "inside" refers to a situation in which compliance is experienced as a strategic asset rather than a liability. It means that by smart working and with the right mindset, compliance is experienced as a natural competence that enables a business. Because of this embedded insight, the organization can focus on client-facing processes and R&D, and it might even develop into a competitive advantage based on the ability to respond more quickly to regulation and build trust with clients and other stakeholders.

Management system

To ensure that an organization has effective control over the implementation of applicable laws and regulations, it is important to design processes in a way that supports rather than thwarts the organization. In this context, an appropriate and effective management system is what sets things apart. The field—as well as this chapter—mentions several management systems: risk, data protection, information security, quality, postmarket surveillance, and so on.

To avoid duplication of effort, an integrated management system provides the solution. Such a management system contains recurring tasks related to the processes for controlling risks for data protection, information security, and quality. The tasks are linked to the safeguards following laws, regulations, standards, and organizational rules, ensuring that the effectiveness of the safeguards is reviewed on a sufficiently regular basis. When a management system works well, the organization barely has to put effort into performing these processes, if at all, and their operation is recorded virtually automatically.

In the next Chapter 18, the ethical considerations for implementing digital pharmaceutical care will be given.

 This means for blended pharmaceutical care:

- Following regulations is crucial in generating trust among pharmaceutical care stakeholders in a world full of disruptive healthcare innovations.
- Digital health compliance always starts with a thorough risk analysis, integrated into a structured data protection, quality, security, and organizational assessment.
- A compliance blueprint means placing the digital solution within the context of an organization and helps to define a competitive compliance strategy that fits the developer's profile.
- Integrating various applicable requirements and standards into one management system can allow organizations to continue to improve products while minimizing disruption to daily operations.

References

[1] Deloitte. Personalized Health: preparing for tomorrow's healthcare. 2017. Available from: https://www2. deloitte.com/content/dam/Deloitte/nl/Documents/life-sciences-health-care/deloitte-nl-personalized-health-uk-version.pdf.

[2] DPA. Selection from DPA investigation Nike + running app. Amsterdam, The Netherlands; 2015. Available from: https://autoriteitpersoonsgegevens.nl/sites/default/files/01_conclusions_dpa_investigation_nike_running_app.pdf.

[3] EDPB. Recommendations 01/2020 on measures that supplement transfer tools to ensure compliance with the EU level of protection of personal data. 2020. Available from: https://edpb.europa.eu/our-work-tools/our-documents/recommendations/recommendations-012020-measures-supplement-transfer_en.

[4] Department of Justice - Northern District of California. Elizabeth Holmes sentenced to more than 11 Years for defrauding Theranos investors of hundreds of millions. US Food and Drug Administration; 2022. Available from: https://www.fda.gov/inspections-compliance-enforcement-and-criminal-investigations/press-releases/elizabeth-holmes-sentenced-more-11-years-defrauding-theranos-investors-hundreds-millions.

[5] Finkle, J. J&J warns diabetic patients: insulin pump vulnerable to hacking. 2016 [cited 2023 04/02/2023]. Available from: https://www.reuters.com/article/us-johnsonjohnson-cyber-insulin-pumps-e/jj-warns-diabetic-patients-insulin-pump-vulnerable-tohacking-idUSKCN12411L.

[6] Hamlyn-Harris JH. Three reasons why pacemakers are vulnerable to hacking. The Conversation; 2017.

[7] OWASP. Security by design principles. 2016 [cited 2023 04/02/2023]. Available from: https://wiki.owasp.org/index.php/Security_by_Design_Principles.

[8] EU. General data protection regulation. 2016/679. 2023 [cited 2023 04/02/2023]. Available from: https://eur-lex.europa.eu/legal-content/EN/TXT/?uri=celex:32016R0679.

[9] Deloitte. Deloitte enterprise compliance and life sciences compliance advisory. 2015. Available from: https://www2.deloitte.com/content/dam/Deloitte/ch/Documents/life-sciences-health-care/ch-en-lshc-challenge-of-compliance.pdf.

CHAPTER 18

The ingredients of ethical practice*

Jessica Pace

School of Pharmacy, Faculty of Medicine and Health, The University of Sydney, Australia

Educating the mind without educating the heart is no education at all.

Aristotle

Introduction

Ingredients are the foundation of any dish, and they play a crucial role in determining a recipe's flavor, texture, appearance, and overall success. Similarly, having the right foundations for ethical practice ensures better outcomes for patients and their practitioners. The digital revolution has a range of potential consequences for pharmacy practice—both beneficial and harmful. The corruption of scientific methodology by commercial interests can also weaken the evidence base available to inform care decisions. In this context, how, then, are we to provide good pharmaceutical care? Here, we argue for sustainable pharmaceutical care, combining knowledge translation with respectful communication with both prescribers and patients and optimal use of medications (which inevitably means accepting that, in some cases, medications are not the best option for our patients).

Ethics and moral theory in a technological culture

Ethics is the study of what we ought to do and is defined by questions such as "How should I live?" and "What would a good person do?" [1]. Importantly, ethics does not just rely on gut feeling or emotion. Rather, being able to justify our actions and rationally defend our actions, revise our decisions through reflection and debate, and as new information becomes available, treating similar cases in similar ways and specifying and

---

*In this chapter, we show how the core values of pharmaceutical care professionals are the fundament of providing care that patients consider as good and meaningful and delve into why appropriate use of data and integer scientific research supports ethical framing, what is considered a meaningful life, and why human rights may become more pivotal in the digital age.

Pharmaceutical Care in Digital Revolution. https://doi.org/10.1016/B978-0-443-13360-2.00018-6

weighting conflicting moral considerations as we answer these questions are defining features of ethical reasoning.

There are a number of different approaches to ethical reasoning. Table 18.1 provides a useful theoretical background, outlining some key ethical theories we will use in this chapter.

Clearly, there is a range of ethical theories and ways to use these to address the highly dynamic character of today's technological culture. However, this is complicated by a "technological blindness" caused by a complex interplay between technology, individuals, and society and a "normative deficit" and resistant attitude to ethics that has been demonstrated in science and technology studies [2].

 Additionally, we live in a morally pluralistic society, or one where there is a diverse range of reasonable views on what is morally or ethically correct, and people may reasonably disagree about the best way to resolve moral dilemmas [3]. This is partly because we think about ethical issues in ways that reflect our own experiences, attitudes and culture. People may therefore rely on different ethical approaches—such as deontology or consequentialism—each of which can lead to different outcomes or resolutions to the same moral dilemma. Moreover, every individual is unique (see QR Code 18.1), and worldviews are open to change—as they do under the influence of digitization—meaning that views on ethical frameworks also change. Thus, there is no static description of "a good life". Practitioners must therefore embrace the concepts of professional, social, and scientific integrity to align views on what is a good life with changing paradigms.

QR Code 18.1
The human game.

Meanwhile, it is increasingly accepted that principles alone may be insufficient to resolve ethical dilemmas in healthcare and alternative approaches—such as feminist ethics and virtue ethics—are being sought. Therefore, in this chapter, we argue not for the use of a specific ethical theory or set of ethical principles but rather for the ethical perspective of digital pharmaceutical care as a professional practice. Here, finding the right ethical framework and determining the right action in a particular situation requires pragmatic wisdom based on ongoing education, professional expertise, and meaningful life experiences. This is underpinned by a philosophy of practice, or a set of values that guides a practitioners' behavior to be ethically appropriate, clinically accurate, and legal, by defining the rules, roles, relationships, and responsibilities of the practitioner [4].

Table 18.1: Key approaches to moral-ethical reasoning.

Approach	Description
Deontology/duty-based ethics	Duties are expressed as universal statements or action guides (e.g., "do not kill" or "respect one's elders") A relevant universal statement is applied to the specific situation to determine what is morally acceptable Assessment of moral acceptability of action is separate from consequences or outcomes—if fundamental moral principles are violated, then the action is ethically wrong, even if it has good consequences
Consequentialism and utilitarianism	Judges the rightness or wrongness of an action based solely on the consequences of performing it, regardless of the nature of the action or the underlying motives or intentions of the person performing it The right act is the one with the best consequences, and no action is intrinsically right or wrong *Utilitarianism* prioritizes the principle of utility, which states that the morally correct action is one that produces the best possible outcomes as determined from a perspective that gives equal weight to the interests of each party *Utility* can be measured in different ways, including maximizing pleasure and minimizing pain, maximizing other values such as friendship, knowledge, health, autonomy, and understanding and maximizing individual preferences and desires
Principlism	Principles are specified to guide moral actions Most well-known is *Beauchamp and Childress' 4 principles of biomedical ethics:* Autonomy (people should be allowed to be self-governing and make decisions for themselves); beneficence (healthcare workers should be actively altruistic or act for the benefit of their patients); nonmaleficence (avoid doing harm); and justice (a fair division of benefits and burdens) Each principle is prima facie: There is no predetermined hierarchy of principles, and need to consider and balance principles in a specific context to determine the morally correct action
Virtue ethics	Rightness or wrongness of an action is derived from the underlying motives and attributes of the person taking action (as opposed to accepting that person who follows a set of predetermined rules or principles or acts in a way that has favorable consequences has acted morally) *Virtue* refers to competence in pursuit of moral excellence and the presence of character traits that are morally valuable, such as honesty, gentleness, integrity, and discernment

Continued

Table 18.1: Key approaches to moral-ethical reasoning.—cont'd

Approach	Description
Feminist ethics and ethics of care	*Feminist ethics*: Approaches reformulating aspects of contemporary ethics that devalue women's experiences, highlighting differences between men and women and providing strategies for dealing with ethical issues in a manner that counters the subordination of women Defining characteristics include rejection of emphasis on individual rights, autonomy, and rationality; denial of the requirement for value-neutral philosophies and abstract ethical principles; and emphasizing the significance of interdependence, caring, and empathy; shared responsibility of all members of society to each other; and importance of context and politics and power to understand ethics and healthcare *Ethics of care*: Based on psychological research that suggests the primary moral consideration of girls and women is care, as opposed to the justice orientation of boys and men, and therefore, rejects the philosophical emphasis on universal moral rules, impartiality, individual rights, law, objectivity and autonomy in favor of personal responsibility, love, trust, and caring Argue dominance of justice orientation and priority given to autonomy has obscured the significance of the special commitment healthcare professionals have to care for their patients
Capabilities approach	First, establish what it means to live well, then ask how well social and political institutions are addressing this Model of what is required to live and live well is termed *Thick vague theory of the good* The first level outlines *capabilities required for human life* (e.g., capacity to feel pleasure and pain, cognitive ability, and affiliation with other human beings) The second level includes *functional capabilities necessary for good human life* (e.g., live to end of complete human life; have good health; avoid unnecessary and nonbeneficial pain; have attachments to things and persons outside ourselves; laugh, play and enjoy recreational activities; and live for and with others)
Human rights approaches, liberalism, and communitarianism	*Rights* are justifiable claims that individuals or groups can make upon society or upon other individuals and often come with associated *obligations* on others to ensure the right is upheld *Positive right* is a right to be provided with a particular good or service by others; *negative right* constrains others from interfering with an individual's exercise of the right *Liberalism: the* belief that individual liberty or autonomy has moral primacy and should be respected and protected by the state *Communitarianism*: Social and moral rules are grounded in community standards of the common good, not individual rights; all individuals within the community are expected to conform to and promote the common good

Adapted from Kerridge I, Lowe M, Stewart C. Ethics and law for the health professions (4th ed.). The Federation Press; 2013.

In the next section, we outline these core values, or what is important to us and our patients as pharmacy care professionals when carrying out this virtue-based practice of pharmaceutical care.

Core values and virtue-based pharmaceutical care providers

Like any other well-established cultural practice, science has an inherent normative structure or a set of values—both epistemic (or knowledge-related) and ethical—that guide and govern its practice [5]. Many medical science professions have a specific value set based on a mandatory code of conduct or code of ethics. It is important to note that these professional codes are not of themselves ethics, as they miss a key part of ethical behavior—namely, an internal conviction by the practitioner of how to behave. However, they are still useful in that they clearly set out the values that both members of the profession and other stakeholders, such as patients and the general public, expect to govern the profession.

Codes of conduct for many medical sciences are similar or strongly related to the **Hippocratic Oath**. This Oath—one of the most widely-known Green medical texts—was historically taken by physicians. In its original form, it required a new physician to swear and uphold specific ethical standards. The Oath was the earliest expression of medical ethics in the Western world, establishing several principles of medical ethics that are still important today, including the principles of medical confidentiality and nonmaleficence [1]. Interestingly, the often used "first-do-no-harm" principle was actually not part of the initial text of the Hippocratic Oath. However, its current use reminds us that we need high-quality research to help better understand the balance of risks and benefits for the tests and treatments healthcare professionals recommend. In a similar vein, a Hippocratic Oath for scientists has been developed and addresses potential concerns with the ethical implications of scientific advances.

The pharmacy profession is currently transitioning in many countries as it moves from a supply-oriented practice to a more patient-care-oriented one. As such, topics of ethical practice and professional autonomy are now especially important to pharmacy practice. In this context, the International Pharmaceutical Federation (FIP) has acknowledged that a pharmacy cannot achieve its full potential, and patients will not benefit unless pharmacists are committed to the highest standards of professional conduct and have sufficient autonomy to serve patients' best interests [6].

Published codes of ethics or codes of conduct for pharmaceutical care professionals outline the expectations of professional virtue-based practice. These describe the professional standards on how care practitioners are expected to set priorities for the expectations and needs of both individual patients and the broader community. Some examples are shown in Box 18.1.

Box 18.1 Global examples of pharmaceutical codes of conduct and codes of ethics

- FIP Statement of Professional Standards Code of Ethics for Pharmacists https://www.fip.org/file/1586
- Australia
    - Australian Health Practitioner Regulation Agency (Ahpra) and National Boards Shared Code of Conduct https://www.ahpra.gov.au/Resources/Code-of-conduct/Shared-Code-of-conduct.aspx
    - Pharmaceutical Society of Australia (PSA) Code of Ethics for Pharmacists https://www.psa.org.au/wp-content/uploads/2018/07/PSA-Code-of-Ethics-2017.pdf
    - Society of Hospital Pharmacists of Australia (SHPA) Code of Ethics https://www.shpa.org.au/publicassets/0835179a-de53-ec11-80dd-005056be03d0/6._shpa_code_of_ethics.pdf
- New Zealand
    - Pharmacy Council of New Zealand Code of Ethics https://pharmacycouncil.org.nz/wp-content/uploads/2021/03/Code-of-Ethics-web.pdf
- United Kingdom
    - The Code of Ethics of the Royal Pharmaceutical Society of Great Britain (RPS) https://onlinelibrary.wiley.com/doi/pdf/10.1002/9780470690642.app7#:~:text=Pharmacists%20must%20ensure%20that%20they,public%20confidence%20in%20the%20profession.
- United States of America:
    - American Pharmacists Association Code of Ethics https://pharmacist.com/Code-of-Ethics
    - American Society of Health-System Pharmacists (ASHP) Code of Ethics for Pharmacists https://www.ashp.org/-/media/assets/policy-guidelines/docs/endorsed-documents/code-of-ethics-for-pharmacists.ashx

---

Pharmaceutical care providers are expected to contribute toward the efficiency of care and pharmacotherapy (treatment with medicines) and are facilitated in this role with information and knowledge about medicines, conditions, and patients. With the aid of knowledge systems, the pharmacist translates this complex data set into appropriate care for individual patients.

However, our ability to do this is completed by a range of factors. Health technology innovations mean that the knowledge within these systems as well as the data they generate have grown exponentially over time. This leads to uncertainty in and sometimes limited theoretical and empirical proof of the true value of these innovations due to the incompleteness of data. There is also a lack of clarity on how these digital health tools influence outcomes with regard to good care. This requires pharmaceutical care practitioners to assess daily whether an innovation is sufficiently aligned with ethical practice. We, therefore, need to think critically about and challenge the idea that interventions based on these new technologies are always the best option for our patients.

There are also significant challenges to healthcare practitioner autonomy. Economic matters and regulatory frameworks can dominate professional care matters, making healthcare situations even more complex for practitioners. Additionally, pharmaceutical care practitioners work within a broader setting that includes other care practitioners, healthcare insurers, and patients who have a right to self-determination. This is well-illustrated by the subsidy of and access to expensive, new technologies, which are often expensive and may have low-quality evidence to support their effectiveness. Here, the practitioner and individual patient may believe that providing subsidized access to this is the best treatment option for that patient. However, this may not be the most socially responsible course of action, as the money spent on this treatment may be better used, providing access to more cost-effective treatments with better evidence to support their use. This further emphasizes the need for an awareness of ethical considerations and the competency to make professionally responsible decisions autonomously. Each pharmaceutical care professional is responsible for their decisions and for adhering to the frameworks established by society. They ensure good pharmaceutical judgment while balancing their commitment to patients and a socially responsible course of action.

In finding a responsible course of action when faced with ethical dilemmas, pharmaceutical care providers need to be aware of and act according to the core values of their profession. Box 18.2 provides an example of how these values were formulated for Dutch pharmacists by the Royal Dutch Pharmacists Association (KNMP). Together, these values form the foundation of professional practice [7].

Box 18.2 Core values of the pharmacist as described by the Royal Dutch Pharmacists Association [7]

- Commitment to the patient's well-being
- Pharmaceutical expertise
- Social responsibility
- Reliability and care
- Professional autonomy

However, while the expressed values of professional practice differ semantically among countries, their contents are generally similar. Core pharmaceutical values are usually developed at a country level and cover both individual pharmaceutical care practitioners and professional associations. The professional codes of ethics and standards are based on the philosophy of practice and the profession's core values. For practitioners, these values act as beacons in the open-ended journey of ethical decision-making and support a professional, virtue-based practice that delivers good patient care.

We will now turn our attention to digital ethics and the unique ethical issues that are raised by the increasing use of and developments in digital technology.

Digital ethics

Digital ethics can be defined in many ways. However, all definitions emphasize that this is a framework in which to work ethically with digital technology by understanding the background, methods, principles, procedures, regulations, and institutions that determine the responsible use of digital technology. Digital ethics includes concepts such as confidentiality, risk, privacy, and responsibility. It also examines issues raised by the distinction between causality and correlation when determining how to use the output of (scientific) data analyses.

Digital ethics is receiving significant attention for a number of reasons. Firstly, an increase in the global amount of data creates a range of ethical concerns, as illustrated in box 18.3.

Box 18.3 Ethical concerns related to big data analysis [8]

Meta-analysis of the literature on big data has identified the following five key ethical concerns related to big data analysis.

- Informed consent, obtained in a timely manner
- Privacy, including anonymity and data protection
- Ownership of data
- Epistemology and objectivity of data used
- "Big data divides" between those who have and those which lack the necessary resources to analyze and use increasingly large data sets

---

Additionally, as technology like artificial intelligence (AI) grows and develops, so too does its effect on society. Noted in previous chapters, all industries—including healthcare—increasingly use algorithms to assist, augment or replace human decision-making. However, this raises questions about the appropriateness of data processing, the adequacy of artificial intelligence systems that interact (e.g., chatbots), and the support of automated decision-making. Consider the following example. A new algorithm identifies a correlation between two data groups—such as gender and the fatality rate among individuals with a certain symptom—which is later proven unfounded. Without adequate scientific background checks and analysis, such digital findings might lead to inaccurate, potentially fatal recommendations, like advising patients to proceed with a surgical intervention when it is unnecessary.

It does not take much imagination to consider where AI in pharmaceutical care can achieve great health benefits and financial and social gains. Large groups of patients will be able to be diagnosed more efficiently and treated more effectively. Care can be used more reliably, carefully, socially justly, and sustainably.

In this approach to reality, logic is based on rationality. Here, AI can adjust human decisions based on well-researched and up-to-date hard facts. Efforts can then be made to strive for pharmaceutical care aimed at the efficient, effective, and safe use of medicines.

Habermas and Schön discussions on logic express that people's lives are often very complex and face physical, mental, social, and financial challenges, which are often related. Therefore, finding a suitable answer to people's complex care questions is often not easy [9,10].

Not least because pharmaceutical care always occurs in a web of relationships of care recipients and pharmacists, relatives, prescribers, allied health practitioners, and health insurers. In addition, when providing pharmaceutical care, attention must be paid to the patient's vulnerability when being prescribed and using medicines.

The vulnerability defined here relates to reduced health literacy and limitations that make taking and administering medication difficult. Also, for example, a degree of understanding and trust in the pharmaceutical treatment plan is relevant. The patient's questions and arguments are not always considered rational, but the patient experiences a sense of discomfort.

The type of pharmaceutical care needed in these situations takes into account the patient's vulnerability. This requires pharmaceutical care that answers that individual's care needs and contributes to what Machteld Huber calls "positive health, as reflected in Chapter 3" [11].

The meaning and relevance of care are of the utmost importance for the care recipient and for the care provider to be able to provide good care. Responsive communication is so essential for giving and receiving care. Not only saying what is going well but also certainly discussing together what has not gone well is of great value.

It would be very promising if the use of AI in pharmaceutical care makes it possible to strengthen professionality and signal the alert of good versus not good. It also allows space and time for attentive involvement and the mutual discussion between caregiver and patient. This interaction deeply affects who we are as human beings in a relationship, in connection with each other. It strengthens the treatment relationship the patient has with the pharmacist.

AI algorithms should be regarded primarily as complementary mechanisms that augment human cognitive intelligence and require meticulous human judgment before being used, rather than a substitute for human care. Additionally, for algorithmic support to gain trust, full transparency of the quality of the data analyzed and how an algorithm's decision-making tree is built are required. Algorithmic output must also be synergized with human competency in order to understand both the context of the treatment situation and the scientific methods used (to distinguish causality from correlation) and thus provide personalized treatment advice that upholds key professional values.

We will now further explore the importance of humanity in providing appropriate pharmaceutical care in the digital age, including care that addresses the various sources of vulnerability discussed above.

Technology versus humanity

As mentioned in the preceding sections, digital health technology has an intrinsic moral significance, as its use has clear moral impacts. However, technology in and of itself is amoral and is not associated with the human experience of empathy and compassion. For example, when a computer first became the best AlphaGO player in the world, it did not cry, scream, or get goosebumps. This may have advantages in situations where human emotions may lead to subjective, suboptimal choices and a "neutral" decision-making support system is valued.

Saying that, technology is never value-neutral. It often depends on historical data that may be biased, skewed, or outdated. Humans also create algorithms with particular worldviews. Extrapolating the output of such algorithms will always require an educated human to understand the context and support a patient's perception of what constitutes good care. Additionally, technology such as chatbots and digital humans may challenge the distinction we have long made between the human and the nonhuman and bring us to the boundaries of what we understand as humanity, of what is humankind and what is machine-kind. As a result, patients may increasingly feel uncertain about what or whom to trust and how to consider their treatment options carefully.

While digital tools can support pharmaceutical care practice, it is the ethical responsibility of each autonomous healthcare practitioner to enable a patient to guard the boundaries of digital treatment and issue a timely alert for human care when needed. This is where the human part of the STEM + education of pharmaceutical care practitioners comes into play as described in Chapter 19. This refers to the social competency needed to contextualize technical knowledge so as to provide a safeguard for patients' pharmaceutical care pathways. This requires human skills like translating knowledge at different literacy levels, reading social cues, showing empathy and compassion, and balancing broader societal challenges toward the best-accepted solution. This human touch is key to practicing medicine or pharmacy and is integral to the patient-doctor and patient-pharmacist relationship.

Importantly, making a balanced care decision means more than complying with regulatory conditions and communicating them. Digital compliance mechanisms are being developed worldwide, and at first glance, this is a positive move. After all, increasing the number of rules designed to curtail unethical or damaging behavior is an obvious, straightforward way to prevent it. However, an unsettling and unintended consequence of viewing ethics-as-compliance is a checkbox mentality that gives the illusion of reducing risk without really doing so [12].

Instead, making a balanced care decision means internalizing pharmaceutical care values, acting with integrity, and taking a virtue-based approach. Human integrity is characterized by consistency in attitude, actions, expectations, principles, and values. Consistent alignment of professional integrity with individual *and* societal needs is central to the development and sustainability of professional practice and can be experienced at different levels—in relation to oneself, with patients and peers, and with society at large. For pharmacy as a value- *and* science-based practice, it comes as no surprise that the principles and values of research are well aligned with the core values of pharmacists. Moreover, a "good" pharmacist knows how to find his way in difficult decisions, balancing the values of patients, peers, and society while maintaining the profession's core values. This reflects the pharmacist's historical reputation as a trusted and well-recognized healthcare team member.

Acting with integrity in complex ethical situations requires continuous interaction and alignment with the needs of the patients and with the perspectives of peers, experts, and policymakers. The ability to do so is predominantly acquired in daily practice rather than through statements and proclamations. Therefore, global communities of deliberative practice should be stimulated to allow pharmaceutical care practitioners to share and discuss their concerns about ethical dilemmas due to the adoption of digital innovation.

This allows practitioners to develop new roles and relationships with corresponding responsibilities to adjust the standards of professional practice.

In the next section, we examine key questions raised by pharmaceutical care practitioners' increasing use of technology. These include how to ensure the appropriate use of patients' health data and that digital tools are adequately researched before adoption, as well as giving examples of everyday dilemmas raised by new uses of digital technology in pharmaceutical care.

Key ethical questions raised by increasing use of technology in pharmaceutical care

Responsible use of patient's health data

The International Data Corporation (IDC) forecasts that by 2026, the global data sphere will grow to 221 zettabytes [13]. We must digest all of this to make sense of information sources within a specific context. We treat data as the new gold, but in doing so, we tend to overlook how personal these are and that they relate to identified or identifiable living individuals. With the current use of social media, sensitivity to the ownership and privacy of data is a topic of increasing debate.

In the spectrum of global data, health data are considered sensitive data and expected to be handled with the greatest possible care. In other chapters, we have already explored some of the most prominent data privacy regulations, how they protect persons, and how they relate to informed consent. Importantly, many people are happy to share their healthcare data for research on better care options, provided appropriate safeguards are in place to protect their data and privacy. However, both patients and ethics committees prefer that steps are taken to ensure that patients provide informed consent when their health records or other data are used for clinical management or research. Because this may not always be possible (e.g., when dealing with historical data sets), methods based on analyzing only aggregated, anonymized data sets with no unique identifiers have been introduced.

However, individual health data are also increasingly shared in a type of unaware or "implied" consent. Big platforms like Google and Amazon, which have billions of users, tend to form partnerships with health technology vendors and create big data sets of pivotal health data by combining user databases. Big platforms generally do acknowledge that data may be used for research purposes; however, users often do not read these "fine prints."

Similarly, various tools—including attendance tracking via QR codes, proximity tracking through contract tracing apps, COVID vaccination, and test and recovery status certificates—were developed for public health purposes during the COVID-19 pandemic. As a result, governments now hold a large amount of personal data related to the pandemic and some of this is being used for purposes other than those for which it was collected. Many governments are now making this available for research purposes. For example, in Australia, the NSW government is making available its datasets for COVID-19 cases and tests to researchers [14]. This includes data on cases, tests, public transport routes, and flights. While this appears a worthy use of data that has already been collected, it is unlikely that consumers have given clear consent for this as they provided it for public health purposes and did not consider that it could also be used for research purposes. In a more sinister development, also in Australia, police officers from a number of states accessed QR code check-in data for criminal investigations unrelated to the COVID pandemic. Some states—such as NSW—have introduced laws banning police from accessing this data for the purpose of criminal investigations unrelated to the COVID pandemic [15].

⚠️ The combination of big data mining and big platforms' or governments' vast influence and increasing pharmaceutical interests is a global concern for both individual patients and policymakers. Even if the reasons behind selling or otherwise providing access to data to truly enhance patient care, inappropriate commercialization of data can result in profiling patients without their knowledge or proper informed consent. The next step might be that some doctors wind up using inadequately acquired data sets and may even recommend drugs based on such data. Merged data may result in the development of algorithms (called "profiling") that predict which healthcare professionals are most likely amenable to using such data to treat patients and to share patient data to improve care. While patients may not be opposed to this practice as long as their care is improved, both data privacy regulations and ethical considerations require that everyone knows how their data is used and should be able to make an informed decision about whether and with whom their data can be shared.

The number of dilemmas in this area is increasing. In this context, pharmaceutical care providers' professional autonomy and values can help patients, and big platforms responsibly use sensitive health data. Tools and systems have been established worldwide that help healthcare professionals determine that data are used ethically in projects and in the development of digital products. In addition to addressing the quality of data, they also address questions such as whether the data are adequately anonymized, whether results are appropriately visualized, whether data are easy to access and will be reused, and whether an expiry date is designated.

Additionally, the open sharing of health data for medical and pharmaceutical research, policymaking, and humanitarian purposes is increasingly recognized as a crucial means to improve private and public life in mature, data-driven societies. At the same time, competing tensions concerning data control and ownership, respect for individual rights and consent, and lack of appropriate frameworks for coordination and ethical governance pose serious challenges to what is called "the safe donation of data." In Europe, the Digital Ethics Lab at the University of Oxford has published an ethical code for data donations [16]. It aims to provide the necessary guidance to meet these challenges and shape data donation practices to ensure respect for users' individual rights and consent, foster transparency and trust, and harness data's value to spur scientific research, public debate, and private and public well-being. We can also look to the Global Alliance for Genomics and Health. It has developed a framework for the responsible sharing of genomic and health-related data [17] based on the "human right to science and culture,"—one of the economic, social, and cultural rights claimed in the Universal Declaration of Human Rights and related documents of international human rights law. The framework promotes responsible data sharing, indicating that data-intensive science may gradually come to be founded on a more communal ethos.

Responsible scientific research

The European Code of Conduct for Research Integrity [18] describes research as "the quest for knowledge obtained through systematic study and thinking, observation and experimentation." Principles illustrate fundamental values of integrity in research. They should guide individual researchers as well as other parties involved in research, such as the institutions where it is conducted, publishers, scientific editors, funding bodies, and scientific and scholarly societies—all of which, given their role and interest in responsible research practices, may be expected to foster integrity. Box 18.4 gives examples of key research from this code.

Box 18.4 Fundamental principles of research integrity as outlined in the European Code of Conduct for Research Integrity [18]

- Reliability in ensuring the quality of research, including design, methodology, analysis, and use of resources
- Honesty in developing, undertaking, reviewing, reporting, and communicating research in a transparent, fair, full, and unbiased manner
- Respect for colleagues, research participants, society, ecosystems, cultural heritage, and the environment
- Accountability for the research from conception to publication; for its management and organization; for training, supervision, and mentoring; and for the scope of its impact

Research is moving from empirical evidence-based to statistical data-driven concepts in data-driven societies. Establishing causality instead of correlation is probably the most difficult task in both models, as the probability of inadequate output is high. In big data analysis, correlations may be found more quickly due to the magnitude of data sets; however, proving causality is more complex as the boundaries of statistics are being sought. Here, the correlation suggests an association between two variables, while causality shows that one variable directly affects a change in the other. Although correlation may imply causality, it is different from a cause-and-effect relationship. For example, if a study reveals a positive correlation between happiness and liking digital health technology, this doesn't mean that an affinity for digital health technology causes happiness. In fact, a correlation may be entirely coincidental, such as a correlation between Napoleon being small in stature and his rise to power. Conversely, if an experiment shows that a predicted outcome unfailingly results from manipulating a particular variable, causality is more likely and denotes a correlation.

Scientific research in contemporary medicine is characterized by an evidence-based approach, meaning conscientious, explicit, and judicious use of the available evidence in making decisions about optimal care patterns. The evidence is based on observations that come from clinical studies of populations to establish cause-effect pairs. The gold standard is the double-blind, randomized clinical trial (RCT), where an adequate sample of patients is selected, some are given a particular treatment, and others are given either a different treatment or a placebo (and no one, neither the patients nor the researchers, knows who gets what). Subsequently, a predefined, measurable endpoint is analyzed.

Randomized controlled trials have high internal validity but can have limitations, such as those related to expense, speed, reproducibility, generalization to routine practice, selection bias, characterization of confounding factors, and ethical constraints. Additionally, "checklist" trials may limit the ability to choose the most appropriate trial design.

If running a randomized experiment is not possible (e.g., due to logistical reasons or ethical considerations), existing data sources may be used in an observational study design. The events compared in such studies happen without any control, and the selection process is most often not randomized. Big data analysis with observational event data presents resources and methodologies that can be incorporated into the design of RCTs in order to augment and extend them and address the RCT issues previously described.

Meanwhile, using supervised learning techniques may help improve accuracy in the analysis of big data (see Chapter 11). Classification and standardizations in, for example, the designation of key data elements or nomenclatures may reduce the complexity introduced by variability and increase the reliability of consistency checks on inputs and outputs. The use of standardization in routine clinical care and in trials facilitates the development of sharable automated curation algorithms to flag outliers or longitudinal variations in data entries that may signal errors [19].

An increasing number of digital health technologies, such as digital therapeutic solutions, are expected to undergo thorough scientific study in order to gain regulation-approved certification as medical devices. Understanding how these digital health technologies prove their value in clinical trials or big data analysis is an essential part of the professional expertise of pharmaceutical care practitioners. It is pivotal for analyzing ethical dilemmas related to data and science matters.

Managing everyday ethical dilemmas

As well as the bigger picture ethical issues discussed above, the increasing use of digital technology can raise smaller dilemmas that we, as pharmaceutical care professionals, need to be aware of and manage in our everyday practice. Changes to how pharmacy technology was used to dispense and provide pharmaceutical consultations during the COVID-19 pandemic are salient examples. A key change in Australia was the increasing use of telehealth to provide pharmacy services such as medication counseling, medication review, and disease state management, with many pharmacists using this approach almost exclusively. This benefitted both the broader community—including reducing the risk of viral transmission and associated morbidity, mortality, and healthcare system costs—and patients. However, it disadvantaged patients who lacked the financial and technological resources to obtain healthcare in this way or for whom face-to-face consultations were beneficial or preferred. This could include people from lower socioeconomic backgrounds, older people, people from culturally and linguistically diverse backgrounds, and people who are socially isolated and for whom a visit to the pharmacy provides much-needed social interactions. In this instance, an awareness of the uneven distribution of the benefits and burdens of digital technology and a firm commitment to justice on the part of the pharmaceutical care practitioner can help to mitigate these negative impacts. For example, face-to-face consultation options could be maintained for those patients for whom it will be of benefit, respecting patient autonomy if they feel that telehealth is not the best option for them to receive pharmaceutical care and utilizing other risk mitigation strategies (including mask-wearing, vaccination, and adequate airflow) to achieve the same aims as telehealth consultations.

Another change in Australia related to how prescriptions were transmitted between prescribers and pharmacists. To support the move to telehealth by prescribers such as medical and nurse practitioners, and reduce the risk of transmission through paper prescriptions, regulations were changed to allow image-based prescribing [20]. Here, pharmacists can dispense from a faxed or emailed copy of a prescription without the previous requirement of a paper script to be forwarded to the pharmacy to confirm this.

However, the electronic prescription must be sent directly to the pharmacy, and the patient cannot obtain any refills or additional supplies allowed on that script from an alternative pharmacy. Unfortunately, there was significant confusion surrounding this change, with prescriptions sent to patients instead of the dispensing pharmacy and therefore unable to be dispensed, sent to the incorrect pharmacy, or patients being inconvenienced if they had to move away from the pharmacy where their prescription was originally sent. These regulatory and practical constraints threatened the autonomy of pharmacy care providers and potentially undermined good pharmaceutical care. Focusing on values such as respect and collaboration, working in partnership with patients and other healthcare professionals, and using our sound knowledge of the legal and regulatory environment can help to overcome these challenges.

In the next section, we consider what constitutes a meaningful life and human flourishing in the digital age and how pharmaceutical care providers can help their patients to achieve this.

A meaningful life and human flourishing in the digital age

As Friedrich Nietzsche addressed, humankind has a commitment to instituting some set of higher values. The cost of not doing so is vitiating our deepest aims and precluding a central form of happiness. But what is happiness in the context of a meaningful life, and what constitutes human flourishing in the digital age?

A meaningful life

In philosophy, a **meaningful life** is a way of being that brings purpose, significance, fulfillment, and satisfaction, and the capabilities approach outlined in Table 18.1 is one way of measuring this. Definitions of meaning have focused on several components, two of which appear central: comprehension and purpose [21]. Comprehension encompasses people's ability to find patterns, consistency, and significance in the many events and experiences in their lives, and their synthesis and distillation of the most salient, important, and motivating factors. Purpose refers to highly motivating, long-term goals about which people are passionate and highly committed.

Meaning, in general, is mostly related to concepts like sense-making. A feeling of loss will occur when something that has meaning is gone. This is especially applicable to health experiences, where disease and disability are generally considered as a loss of life value. A main goal of all healthcare practitioners is to minimize this feeling of loss by taking care that interventions first will do no harm.

As noted in previous chapters, successful health interventions ideally target individual goals to which patients feel committed. This reflects the core pharmaceutical care value of "commitment to patients' well-being" that practitioners take when providing a personalized treatment that aligns with a patient's key beliefs. This approach means both identifying what matters most to the patient and determining which part of treatments can be done digitally and which part should be performed by humans.

Additionally, many of the 10 factors that patients consider to be essential for good healthcare reflect aspects that support either the comprehension or the purpose of a meaningful treatment pathway. For example, selecting effective treatment refers to a treatment that matters to the individual patient, ideally enabling them to continue their preferred lifestyle and achieve their personal goals (e.g., career and sports-related goals and as providers of care).

Digital health tools can support good care and individualized treatment pathways, as described elsewhere in this book. However, the merger between humans and technologies may affect how we perceive ourselves as humans, as it creates what is referred to as a techno-human condition. Electronic coaches like chatbots and social companion robots facilitate self-monitoring and treatment. However, their data may also be used to profile human beings in all kinds of ways with the explicit commercial goal of intervening in human processes. Also, virtual care approaches may blur the quality and intrinsic value of human relationships, essential to foster meaningful life experiences. This raises the question about how best to protect the rights of individuals in the digital age.

Human flourishing in the digital age

Much of the bioethical debate on health technology and related human rights has so far focused on technologies that work inside the body. The Oviedo Convention was shaped around this premise. The convention created common guiding principles—such as the protection of private life, respect for autonomy, and the right to information and informed consent—to preserve human dignity in the way humans apply innovations in biomedicine [22]. However, a broad range of technologies that work outside the body also exist and can similarly impact human beings' bodily, mental, and social performance.

With the fast convergence of nano and biological data and cognitive technologies in the Internet of Things, each type of interaction between humans and those "intelligent artifacts" can raise important human rights issues. The Rathenau Institute, in 2017, submitted a report to the Council of Europe with the recommendation to adopt two new tracks toward ensuring human rights in the digital age [23]. The first recommendation relates to the right not to be measured, including the need to protect the privacy of data by respecting private and family life and people's ability to refuse to be subjected to profiling, to refuse to have their location tracked, or to refuse to be manipulated or influenced by a "coach." The second proposed new right was to have the opportunity, within the context of care and assistance provided to older adults and people with disabilities, to choose to have human contact rather than a robot. Although these rights are not yet formalized, they may give healthcare providers clearer guidance on where patients' rights need to be safeguarded. Most of the information in this book aligns with these two fundamental perspectives, reflecting that digital pharmaceutical care is an option but should be considered only after patients provide their informed consent to do so.

Pharmaceutical care practitioners' professional standing and value-based work are essential here (see the example in QR Code 18.2). It allows us to support patients on moral choices, alert patients where rights are potentially infringed, help them stay self-determined in the digital revolution, and serve those patients who demand human care rather than digital help, even in an economically restricted environment.

QR Code 18.2
Moral choices of
driverless cars.

In the final section, we provide some concluding thoughts on ethically sound digital pharmaceutical care and call for all pharmaceutical care practitioners to be given time to interact with their patients and reflect on ethical pharmaceutical care practices—i.e. to have time to care.

Final thoughts on ethically sound pharmaceutical care

Unfortunately, space does not allow for a more comprehensive discussion of the ethical issues raised in the digital age. However, you can find more comprehensive and detailed information online and most probably in your direct environment, where ethical communities debate the constantly emerging ethics of the exponential growth in technology (including AI and robotic technologies), and offer new insights, frameworks, and thought patterns. Additionally, in many countries, biomedical research is controlled by national consultative ethics committees. Similar bodies may be put into place either nationally or regionally to govern the ethics of digital health technology. Although these bodies may not monitor the regulatory compliance blueprint, they often address ethical boundaries such as those described in this chapter. Meanwhile, initiatives like the Partnership on AI [24] and the Future of Life Institute [25] are a result of societal concerns about how to keep our digital revolution benevolent, how to warrant unified digital literacy, and how to protect individuals in a fully connected ecosystem and aim to maximize the positive results from and minimize risks of new technologies.

Organizations and humans who want to proceed ethically must further scrutinize their actions. We must look beyond compliance and aim for the highest ethical standards instead. More institutions are drafting extensive codes of conduct, but it is questionable if these efforts will be a panacea for ethical difficulties. However, cultural factors such as feeling confident enough to speak up, balancing care with commercial pressures, identifying conflicting goals, or improving role modeling may create an intrinsic understanding of ethical standards. During their academic studies, most healthcare professionals internalize ethical standards such as those based on the principles in the Hippocratic Oath. Healthcare practitioners should be granted time to focus on this important aspect of care and be rewarded for investing time to facilitate making the right decisions together with our patients.

In many of today's healthcare systems, patients are viewed as numbers and symptoms in overcrowded waiting rooms. Doctors sometimes allow only a few minutes for a patient, and at times patients do not see a pharmacist. In addition, many healthcare practitioners are overwhelmed by administrative burdens, the lack of collegial consultations, and the number of repetitive tasks they perform, all of which can lead patients to think that these practitioners do not really care about them. However, when asked, many healthcare practitioners say that they chose their profession primarily to care for and give time to people in need of healthcare. These practitioners would like to have more time to make the ethical considerations needed in healthcare systems and to support personalized treatment of patients based on professional knowledge and values.

In our mind, the core values of pharmaceutical professionals and adequate time to care are the key ingredients of a system of ethical, well-grounded human care. Here, providers are fully embedded in society and possess the tools they need to determine the boundaries of good healthcare, take care for their fellow creatures, and prevent sabotage of these human-inspired roles by digital interventions, even while using them to patients' advantage.

We realize that one chapter in a broad-spectrum book such as this does not allow us to address all of the major topics of digital ethics adequately. Therefore, we have set ourselves the goal to continue working in and studying this field and in the future contribute to the specific, research-based literature on the evolving digital ethics in pharmaceutical care.

In the next Chapter 19 we will further elaborate on education, required to be prepared for the digital revolution.

 This means for blended pharmaceutical care

- Every pharmaceutical care practitioner is expected to responsibly balance the expectations and needs of individual patients with those of society.
- Pharmaceutical care practitioners' core values are meant to act as beacons in the open-ended journey of ethical decision-making.

This means for blended pharmaceutical care—cont'd

- Digital ethics provide the concepts to work ethically with digital technology through an understanding of the background, methods, principles, procedures, regulations, and institutions that govern the appropriate use of the technology.
- The human touch, potentially augmented by digital technology, is a key part of practicing medicine and pharmacy and an integral part of the patient—pharmacist relationship.
- Helping patients protect their data is a core task of all professional caregivers.
- The combination of consecutive data mining and the big platforms' vast influence and increasing pharmaceutical interests are a global ethical concern for professionals, policymakers, and patients.
- Successful health interventions ideally target individual goals that patients feel committed to and that support a meaningful life.
- Healthcare practitioners should be facilitated, rewarded, and granted time to solve ethical dilemmas that come with the digital revolution.

References

[1] Kerridge I, Lowe M, Stewart C. Ethics and law for the health professions. 4th ed. The Federation Press; 2013.

[2] Keulartz J, Schermer M, Korthals M, Swierstra T. Ethics in technological culture: a programmatic proposal for a pragmatist approach. Sci Technol Hum Val 2004;29(1):3–29.

[3] Weinstock D. Moral pluralism. In: The routledge encyclopedia of philosophy. Taylor and Francis; 1998. https://doi.org/10.4324/9780415249126-L058-1. Retrieved 1 Feb. 2023, from, https://www.rep.routledge.com/articles/thematic/moral-pluralism/v-1.

[4] Cipolle RJ, Strand LM, Morley PC. Chapter 3. Toward a philosophy of pharmaceutical care practice. In: Cipolle RJ, Strand LM, Morley PC, editors. Pharmaceutical care practice: the patient-centered approach to medication management services. 3e. McGraw Hill; 2012.. https://accesspharmacy.mhmedical.com/content.aspx?bookid=491&sectionid=39674903.

[5] Douglas HE. Science, policy and the value-free ideal. University of Pittsburgh Press; 2009. https://doi.org/10.2307/j.ctt6wrc78.

[6] International Pharmaceutical Federation. Reference document pharmacist ethics and professional autonomy: imperatives for keeping pharmacy aligned with the public interest. 2013. Retrieved 1 Feb 2023, from, https://www.fip.org/file/1368.

[7] Royal Dutch Pharmacists Association. Charter professionalism of the pharmacist foundation for acting professionally and ethically. 2018. Retrieved 1 Feb 2023, from, https://www.knmp.nl/sites/default/files/2021-12/Charter%20Professionalism%20of%20the%20Pharmacist.pdf.

[8] Mittelstadt BD, Floridi L. The ethics of biomedical big data. Springer International Publishing; 2016.

[9] Habermas J. Theorie des kommunikativen Handelns. Frankfurta.M.:Suhrkamp; 1981.

[10] Schön D. The reflective practitioner. New York: Taylor and Francis; 1986. see also Harry Kunneman, Amor Complexitatis (Amsterdam, SWP, 2017).

[11] Huber M, van Vliet M, Boer I. Heroverweeg uw opvatting van het begrip 'gezondheid'. Ned Tijdschr Geneeskd 2016;160:A7720.

[12] Rea P, Kolp A, Ritz W, Steward MD. Corporate ethics can't Be reduced to compliance. Harvard business review. 2016. Retrieved 1 Feb 2023, from, https://hbr.org/2016/04/corporate-ethics-cant-be-reduced-to-compliance.

[13] Burgener E, Rydning J. HighData growth and modern applications drive new storage requirements in digitally transformed enterprises. 2022. Retrieved 1 Feb 2023, from, https://www.delltechnologies.com/asset/en-us/products/storage/industry-market/h19267-wp-idc-storage-reqs-digital-enterprise.pdf.

[14] NSW Government. NSW COVID-19 data. 2022. Retrieved 1 Feb 2023, from, https://data.nsw.gov.au/nsw-covid-19-data.

[15] Hendry J. NSW bans police from accessing QR code check-in data. 2021. from, https://www.itnews.com.au/news/nsw-bans-police-from-accessing-qr-code-check-in-data-573015. [Accessed 1 February 2023].

[16] Krutzinna J, Taddeo M, Floridi L. An ethical code for posthumous medical data donation. In: Krutzinna J, Floridi L, editors. The ethics of medical data donation. Springer; 2019. https://doi.org/10.1007/978-3-030-04363-6_12.

[17] Global Alliance for Genomics and Health. Framework for responsible sharing of genomic and health-related data. 2019. Retrieved 1 Feb 2023, from, https://www.ga4gh.org/genomic-data-toolkit/regulatory-ethics-toolkit/framework-for-responsible-sharing-of-genomic-and-health-related-data/.

[18] All European Academies. The European code of conduct for research integrity revised edition. 2017. Retrieved 1 Feb 2023, from, https://www.allea.org/wp-content/uploads/2017/05/ALLEA-European-Code-of-Conduct-for-Research-Integrity-2017.pdf.

[19] Mayo C, Kessler ML, Eisbruch A, Weyburne G, Feng M, Hayman JA, et al. The big data effort in radiation oncology: data mining or data farming? Advances in Radiation Oncology 2016;1(4):260−71. https://doi.org/10.1016/j.adro.2016.10.001.

[20] Liotta M. Image-based prescribing has "served its purpose" for general practice. 2022. Retrieved 1 Feb 2023, from, https://www1.racgp.org.au/newsgp/professional/image-based-prescribing-has-served-its-purpose-for.

[21] Shin JY, Steger MF. Chapter 5 promoting meaning and purpose in life. In: Parks AC, Schueller SM, editors. The Wiley Blackwell handbook of positive psychological interventions. Wiley Blackwell; 2014. https://doi.org/10.1002/9781118315927.ch5.

[22] Council of Europe. Oveido convention and its protocols. 2023. Retrieved 1 Feb 2023, from, https://www.coe.int/en/web/bioethics/oviedo-convention.

[23] Van Est R, Gerritsen J. Human rights in the robot age. 2017. Retrieved 1 Feb. 2023, from, https://www.rathenau.nl/sites/default/files/2018-02/Human%20Rights%20in%20the%20Robot%20Age-Rathenau%20Instituut-2017.pdf.

[24] Partnership on AI. Homepage on the internet. 2023. Retrieved 1 Feb 2023, from, https://partnershiponai.org/.

[25] Future of Life. Homepage on the internet. 2023. Retrieved 1 Feb 2023, from, https://futureoflife.org/.

CHAPTER 19

Nourishing education to digitally enable pharmacists*

Nilhan Uzman[1], Aysu Selçuk[1,2], Aukje Mantel-Teeuwisse[3]

[1]International Pharmacutical Federation (FIP), The Hague, The Netherlands; [2]Department of Clinical Pharmacy, Faculty of Pharmacy, Ankara University, Ankara, Turkey; [3]Department of Pharmaceutical Sciences, Faculty of Science, Utrecht University, Utrecht, The Netherlands

Learning never exhausts the mind.

Leonardo da Vinci

Introduction

What is on the menu? Is it nourishing? The menu includes various types of dishes, from starters to desserts. They contain different ingredients which nourish the dishes. Consumers can pick and choose from the menu, according to their liking—which ingredients are their favorites and appetite—just a small snack or a full-course dinner.

Similarly, digital health education includes various digital tools as ingredients together with knowledge, competencies, and skills. Together, they become dishes to be served on the menu called the provision of pharmaceutical care. Patients may receive better treatment based on how ingredients nourish the educational dish consumed by healthcare professionals.

The digital revolution transforms the way we live, the way we work, and the way we learn. We know that some jobs will disappear due to artificial intelligence (AI), that others will grow, and that many jobs that do not exist today will become commonplace. We also know that the future workforce will need to align its skillset with these changes to keep pace. Moreover, we know that the winners would not be those who can run the fastest but those who are the most agile and can adjust their journey successfully.

---

*In this chapter, you will read about the competencies and skills of pharmaceutical care providers, how they are expected to change in the digital epoch, and which ones are required to lead pharmaceutical care. You will also find examples of educational changes in undergraduate and lifelong learning programs.

Pharmaceutical Care in Digital Revolution. https://doi.org/10.1016/B978-0-443-13360-2.00004-6

The recent outbreak of the COVID-19 pandemic affected the digital revolution significantly by accelerating the acceptance and adaptability of digital health tools by healthcare providers and patients [1,2]. New competencies and skills to utilize digital health in pharmaceutical care practice also emerged [3].

These are revolutionary topics for pharmacy and pharmaceutical sciences education, which must be placed in the curricula to enable the future-ready pharmacy workforce.

In response to the fast-shifting health landscape, pharmacists will be able to assume new roles in health and digital technologies to navigate toward a future of health care that is relevant, sustainable, and people-centered. Therefore, pharmacists, educators, regulators, and managers should prioritize digitally enabling the pharmaceutical workforce, which is the aim of the International Pharmaceutical Federation (FIP) Development Goal 20 (digital health) [4].

FIP Development Goal 20 (digital health) specifically focuses on enablers of digital transformation, including the pharmaceutical workforce, and on effective processes to facilitate the development of a digitally literate workforce by the following mechanisms.

- Development of courses, training material, and experiential learning opportunities in initial education and early career training to prepare a digitally literate workforce;
- Incorporation of digital health and literacy competencies and skills in pharmaceutical competency, advanced, and specialist frameworks;
- Development of multidisciplinary learning strategies for digital health literacy that include interprofessional education;
- Provision of opportunities for continuous education and development to ensure that the workforce remains up to date with digital health changes and innovations; and
- Incorporation of digital health within workforce development policies, including employment policies such as employment opportunities in the digital health sector.

Later in this chapter, it will be explained how a digitally enabled pharmaceutical workforce can be developed through education. Without a digitally enabled pharmaceutical workforce, innovative advancements in healthcare will lag in implementation. Also, sustainable and responsive systems to improve pharmaceutical care and health outcomes will struggle to emerge without a clear purpose for innovative digital advancement [3].

Let us take a look at what this new environment means for pharmaceutical care. In the following sections, we will look at the future of jobs, knowledge domains, competencies, and emerging skills for pharmaceutical care providers.

The future of pharmaceutical care and new roles

Pharmacists are healthcare professionals whose professional responsibilities and accountabilities include seeking to ensure that people derive optimal therapeutic benefit from their treatments with medicines. This requires them to keep abreast of developments in pharmacy practice and pharmaceutical sciences, professional standards and requirements, the laws governing pharmacy and medicines, and advances in knowledge and technology relating to the use of medicines [5].

Pharmacists who intend to play a more active role in direct patient care shift their focus from fully product-oriented to more people-centered care, ensuring patients use their products in the most optimal way. Pharmaceutical care is becoming increasingly personalized as it is a service that starts with understanding patients' concerns, beliefs, and behaviors associated with their medication and beyond [6]. It is a service beyond the distribution of medicines. However, to date, care responsibility is not mainstream in many countries. This is mainly driven by the fact that responsibility for this service has not been institutionalized as a formal role of pharmacists globally. Significant overlap exists in knowledge, skills, and roles with other patient care providers. Thus, pharmacists are not remunerated appropriately.

Nevertheless, many studies on pharmacy practice have shown that in an integrated approach with all healthcare professionals, pharmacists are instrumental in improving patients' adherence and health outcomes through interventions such as counseling, following up with patients for adherence, driving medication surveillance, or running medication reviews to optimize treatment profiles.

In countries where pharmaceutical care is institutionalized in patients' treatment and treatment outcomes, such as the Nordic countries in Europe, the Netherlands, Australia, New Zealand, and Canada, pharmacists are allowed to and remunerated for intervening and discussing treatments with a patient and the patient's other healthcare providers. Therefore, skillsets related to understanding human behavior, like mastering effective human dialogue, understanding the psychology of interviewing, demonstrating empathy, active listening, and effectively anticipating patient and customer needs, are expected to become increasingly important skills, as we explain later in this chapter.

Understanding the ecosystem of digital health technology

Health strategists worldwide promote the adoption of digital health to support patient care through collaborative working. The adoption of digital health and standards of digital literacy are key themes of interest at the global level [3].

As outlined in previous chapters in this book, digital health is essential to augment pharmaceutical care providers and drive enhanced apothecary intelligence. Thus, digital health education is essential from undergraduate pharmacy years and throughout pharmacists' professional years and may aptly even be integrated as continuing professional development (CPD). This will support pharmacists in understanding, selecting, and adopting digital health tools to continuously augment pharmaceutical care and its provision.

Digital health technologies must be people-centered, high-quality, evidence-based, effective and efficient for both the provider and the user, and sustainable, inclusive, equitable, and trustworthy in order to be integrated into practice [3]. With misinformation flooding the virtual space, it will become pivotal to be able to determine the reliability of digital health content and/or tools. Trained pharmaceutical care providers can consult patients to make decisions for reliable and ethical digital tools and can thus augment the existing trust and reputation of pharmaceutical care providers globally.

In the business world, companies mastering digital excellence differ from less innovative ones in that the former's leadership is constantly investing in more digital tools and skills [7]. The difference in skills usually extends beyond technology, as digital transformation also requires changes in processes and thinking, as addressed in Part 4 of this book.

Thus, in order to master digital excellence, dedicated, ongoing education is imperative.

The future of the pharmaceutical care job

Every now and then, warnings pop up that automation and new technology will wipe out large numbers of jobs. However, these warnings have existed for many decades. When the agrimotor was developed, farmers were afraid they would become redundant; however, there are still farmers, and some farmers effectively shifted to positions that had not existed prior to the introduction of the agrimotor.

Inherent to this development process is the fact that with the automation of some roles and jobs, novel ones will be created. For example, driving a car may not be a major source of employment a decade from now, but there will be new or other things that logically cannot be automated. A certain workforce is expected to move into those categories, just as many moved from agriculture to factories to the service economy. Fig. 19.1 exemplifies how jobs are expected to be changed by AI.

In a healthcare system under pressure due to aging demographics and budget constraints (see Part 1 of this book), automating some tasks may provide more space for others (human, nonautomated). In addition, the digital revolution will offer new roles, and

How AI will affect the job market
Predicted net job creation by sector (2017–2037)

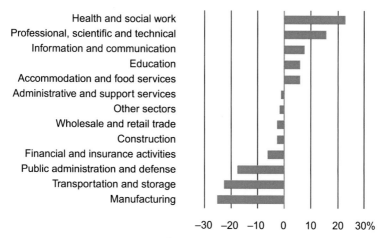

Figure 19.1
Job creation forecast in different industries. *Reproduced from PwC, 2018. AI will impact employers before it impacts employment. Available at: https://www.pwc.com/us/en/services/consulting/library/artificial-intelligence-predictions/employer-impact.html.*

existing healthcare professionals will be required to acquire new skills and competencies to work with digital health services.

Many digital health technologies strongly depend on their uptake and appropriate use by healthcare professionals. However, suppose digital health technologies are understood, designed, and implemented well. In that case, health professionals can coexist with them, which has the potential to ease some of the burdens to allow for more time with patients or carrying out lifesaving research. We expect a similar situation for the pharmaceutical workforce.

Analyze which tasks can be automated and which tasks cannot

Based on currently demonstrated technologies, almost half of the activities people are now paid to do in the global economy could feasibly be automated. However, in general, healthcare is not an industry where jobs can be easily automated. According to McKinsey, healthcare and social assistance have an automation potential of 30% based on demonstrated technology [8].

To understand the impact of the digital revolution on your own role, it makes sense to detail the tasks that belong to a certain competency framework and strive to identify which of those tasks are prone to automation versus which ones are much more difficult for machines to perform (the ones where the human factor is central).

Assessing the competencies listed in FIP's Global Competency Framework [9] can provide a pharmacy-specific perspective. Pharmaceutical public health competencies are one of the four knowledge domains of the framework. This domain includes behavioral competencies relevant to emergency response. While pharmacists' responses in public health emergencies cannot be automated due to the human factor needed, they can be complemented with, for example, AI strategies. These strategies could identify and develop possible pharmaceutical care scenarios based on available data from similar emergencies faced before. This way, pharmacists can be better prepared and respond promptly and effectively to emergencies. A similar analysis can also be undertaken for the other three domains in this competency framework.

Doing this analysis provides, first of all, insight into the areas where machines substitute some parts of certain functions, but it can also provide new perspectives on the actual value of a role and how to valorize the role in the future.

Even if the analysis ends up showing that your role can be automated in large part, another aspect must be considered. It is a Marxian concept [10,11] in which many roles will be obsolete due to automation, but as indicated earlier, the reality has been that machines also complement labor—raising output in ways that lead to higher or at least other demands for labor and that interact with adjustments in the workforce.

In conclusion, the half-life of knowledge is being reduced faster in the digital revolution, quickly changing the requirements of educational ingredients for pharmaceutical care providers. However, given the professional standards of pharmaceutical care providers, their competencies and skills, and the fact that it will still take quite some time before machines are capable of performing the valued roles that humans perform, pharmaceutical care providers will not be usurped any time soon but will evolve and adapt to adjusted and new role descriptions.

Be prepared for new roles

We keep calling it "digital health," but it is predicted that digital health will become ubiquitous and mainstream health care soon. Therefore, it has become essential for healthcare professionals to be equipped with digital skills to assume emerging roles in healthcare. Being intrinsically multidisciplinary and interdisciplinary, capacity-building for new roles entails instilling skills that may range from computer sciences, strategic planning, finance, and management to health sciences and care delivery, depending on the digital health tool or service and its context [12].

Pharmacists historically embraced information technologies. Therefore, they have the ideal predisposition and competencies to provide increasingly more digital health services to patients.

So, what could be the potential new roles in pharmaceutical care? It is easy to imagine that in the near future, both brick-and-mortar and online pharmacies will need a lead who will oversee the quality of wearables and may serve as a digital therapeutic associate or a pharmbot specialist.

In general, pharmaceutical care providers may need to obtain guidance from a digital apothecary intelligence leader or a virtual pharmacy reality officer. Moreover, roles like pharmacy data interoperability lead, digital health management team member, or adherence data expert will be the backbone of future pharmacy institutions. Because pharmaceutical care providers will be in an ideal position to answer questions such as what data we want and how do we work with that data. And how do we intervene in a workflow in a way that makes sense?

While the digital revolution changes the way pharmacists provide pharmaceutical care services, it also changes how people seek information or services on health and wellness, how they access these services, and how they respond to their health and wellness needs. These changes will also require people-centered pharmaceutical care providers to assume new roles. For example, pharmacists can become digital designers and developers of adherence, medication management, and/or disease prevention tools to achieve treatment success, adherence, or healthy patient behavior changes. Educating patients on how to use these tools will be an ongoing and inherited role that pharmacists will continue to lead.

The fast-paced changes in the digital sphere are disrupting the existing regulatory context. Data privacy challenges are causing ethical dilemmas as digital tools are processing patient data. Pharmaceutical care providers can be the custodians of patients' digital rights as digital health compliance officers.

The future of health is interesting, and the authors leave it up to the reader to imagine how these roles' job profiles will look, but trust in the fact that this way of thinking will spark our vision of how current pharmaceutical care roles can evolve to new ones.

In Part 4 of this book, we will deep-dive into activities to do today to be prepared for the digital future. But let us first focus on characteristics of professional practice, knowledge, skills, and competencies that will be required for the new roles described above for pharmacists.

Required knowledge, competencies and skills for future pharmaceutical care providers

As shown in Chapter 6, professional practice is the application of knowledge guided by a philosophy and purpose toward resolving specific problems. This precise knowledge held by a practitioner is applied according to a standard that is accepted by professional review. The FIP global competency framework provides global standards in the context of competencies and behaviors, and "pharmaceutical care" is one of the four main categories [9].

Pharmaceutical care providers become competent professionals through substantial academic training; they maintain their skills through CPD and commit to behaving ethically to protect the interests of both the individual and the public.

Knowledge domains in pharmaceutical care

According to FIP's Global Competency Framework [9], there are four knowledge domains.

1) Pharmaceutical public health competencies
2) Pharmaceutical care competencies
3) Professional/personal competencies
4) Organization and management competencies

Pharmacists' extensive understanding of the interactions among these domains adds value to the care continuum.

The study of pharmacy comprises knowledge of medicines in the broadest sense, both inside and outside the human body. The knowledge of medicines outside the human body includes the characteristics of products in terms of storage, use, development, production, quality control, and control of biopharmaceutical properties such as bioavailability and absorption.

Pharmaceutical knowledge also includes comprehension of the effects of medicines on the human body and the implications of their use and administration. This means that a clear understanding of the human body and human behavior in illness and in health are also included within the knowledge domain of pharmacy, which requires proficiency in anatomy, physiology, pathophysiology, and psychology. The tenets of this discipline enable the pharmacist to understand the actions and effects of medicines on the body.

In many countries, community and hospital pharmacies have evolved from a product-oriented profession to a more patient-centered profession. Thus, understanding human behavior is considered of growing importance in the provision of pharmacotherapy and the goal of achieving optimal patient outcomes [13].

Digital literacy competencies

To support existing competency frameworks for pharmacists in response to the emerging needs of pharmacists gaining digital literacy competencies, digital health guidelines and strategies are being developed [14].

Digital literacy as an individual competency is separately described by FIP in its global competency framework [9] in response to the expansion of the type of services that pharmacists may provide to their patients and the advances in technology and therapeutics.

As part of the professional/personal knowledge domain, digital literacy-related behavioral competencies are described as follows.

1. Identify, manage, organize, store, and share digital information
2. Critically appraise, analyze, evaluate, and/or interpret digital information and their sources
3. Where applicable, participate in digital health services that promote health outcomes and engage with digital technologies (e.g., social media platforms and mobile applications) to facilitate discussions with the patient and others
4. Maintain patient privacy and security of digital information related to the patient and workplace

Traditional skills required for pharmacists

In 1999 the WHO developed the concept of the "seven-star pharmacist," detailing the skills and attitudes required of pharmacists to be effective members of the healthcare team. In 2000, FIP adopted this concept in its policy on pharmacy education.

 The required skillsets of a pharmacist are described as

- caregiver;
- decision maker;
- communicator;
- manager;
- lifelong learner;
- teacher; and
- leader

The WHO and FIP later added the function of a researcher in their 2006 handbook, *Developing Pharmacy Practice: A Focus on Patient Care* [15].

After graduation, pharmacists can develop a generalist profile (as many community pharmacists are) or can specialize in a specific topic or range of skills (as seen more often in clinical pharmacies). The level of patient focus can vary significantly within these profiles.

FIP's global advanced specialist development framework supports the professional development and recognition of the pharmacy workforce everywhere. The framework primarily aims to identify broad areas for professional development and advancement for pharmacists and pharmaceutical scientists to develop their skills in a structured manner [16].

General skills required for pharmaceutical care in the digital revolution

QR Code 19.1
Future of jobs.

In 2016 the World Economic Forum (WEF) released an overview of skills considered as essential to thriving in the Fourth Industrial Revolution [17]. It was expected that over one-third of skills (35%) that were considered important in the 2015 workforce would have changed by 2020 (see QR Code 19.1). Even today, this picture previously sketched by the WEF provides useful insight into the fast-changing working environment we all face.

The skills listed by the WEF as remaining or becoming more important included, among others, complex problem-solving, creativity, and emotional intelligence. They are all fundamental for the changing pharmacy profession. So let us delve a bit further into several of these skills and their relevance for pharmaceutical care providers.

Complex problem-solving is expected to remain the most important asset that people can bring into a working environment. This is particularly relevant in the pharmaceutical care sector, as the academic fields of pharmacy and data science are becoming increasingly integrated, and the half-life of pharmaceutical science knowledge is reduced more than ever. The analytic and biochemical nature of undergraduate education enables a pharmacist to reduce a problem to its core elements and think critically and conceptually about the solution. In pharmaceutical care, this means being able to reflect on changing ecosystems, analyze the healthcare system needs, define the new role and skillsets of pharmaceutical care providers, and integrate analytic and predictive technology.

With the avalanche of new medicines, including the new advanced therapy medicinal products, *creativity* means new technologies and new ways of working, which is crucial for developing, staying abreast of, and benefiting from innovations. Although the algorithms and technologies described in Chapters 11 and 12 will enhance the work of pharmaceutical care providers, constructing these algorithms so that they are as creative and agile as humans will take a long time. In fact, it is still not clear whether robots will ever develop the creative and relational reasoning of humans, although progress has been made over the past years. Identifying the best digital pharmaceutical care solutions requires out-of-the-box thinking, and educational frameworks should encourage providers to develop this skill by, for example, periodically thinking and working outside of their own area, continuously learning about mechanisms, and developing cross-functional approaches.

Emotional intelligence, which was not one of the top 10 skills in 2016 identified by the WEF, will become a pivotal skill needed by pharmaceutical care providers [17]. Emotional intelligence (EI) is the ability of individuals to perceive, use, understand, and manage emotions: recognize their own and other people's emotions, discern between different feelings and label them appropriately, use emotional information to guide thinking and behavior, and manage and adjust emotions to adapt to environments or achieve one's goal [18].

EI is an essential skill that (at least at the time of this writing) separates humans from machines. Being able to read emotions, show empathy, understand feelings, and connect facts with emotions and react to them to guide interventions and solve issues are abilities that are, until nowadays, unique to humans. Although causality is difficult to establish, higher EI scores have among pharmacists been associated with increased work innovation, proactivity, and risk-taking levels [19] as well as lower levels of occupational stress, higher job performance, and higher psychological affective well-being [20]. In order for EI to thrive, qualities such as curiosity, empathy, adaptability, and emotional agility will need to be developed.

Judgment and decision-making will continue to be two of the most important skills enabling pharmaceutical care providers to adequately judge factors such as the value of digital tools, the ethical considerations of treatment choices, and the safety of AI. Whether it is the seasoning of apps, the infusion of wearables, or the taste of virtual reality, to truly make a balanced decision, digital health literacy needs to be augmented with discernment as to whether these data are unbiased, algorithms are programmed for benevolent outcomes, and last but not least how to synergize human factors with the results of big-data health analysis into something that is really meaningful for patients.

Connecting and coordinating with other healthcare system stakeholders was considered an essential skill in 2015. Although technology can facilitate connecting technically, it is the human connective skill that will reduce factors such as silo-thinking and drive a shift toward making integrated pharmaceutical care plans and developing joint pathways to improve patient outcomes. Healthcare systems are under severe pressure globally, and pharmaceutical stakeholders are a part of the puzzle that has to be solved. Only with a connected approach can sustainable and circular systems be developed, and in order to do so, coordination and human connectivity skills are crucial.

Pharmaceutical care providers often face the daunting task of communicating with patients, employees, insurers, and physician office staff under time and resource restraints. The providers' educational backgrounds, levels of understanding, and preferred learning modes vary. This is why effective communication skills should continue to get sufficient attention in educational programs, as they are considered the ultimate prerequisite for people working together, achieving synergy, and integrating the different stakeholder's perspectives [21].

Educating (future) pharmaceutical care providers in developing these skills requires a different approach to pharmacy education in many settings. Traditionally, the study of pharmacy includes Science, Technology, Engineering, and Mathematics, collectively known as STEM. To many, these four disciplines form the basis for the skills needed to be successful in the evolving jobs of the future, as can be seen in QR Code 19.1.

However, in light of the above, pharmacy education is expected to continue as an STEM + education with the plus referring to people-centric skills and the ability to care and interact in an uncertain environment, which is crucial for workforce preparedness. For future pharmacists, this encompasses developing empathy, a culture of care, and the ability to judge benefits and risks in a nonbinary way, among others. Technology should enable pharmacists to act cognitively in an efficient way [22].

Integrating the new fundamental competency

Taking into consideration the advances in health technology as described in the previous parts of this book, it can be argued that digital literacy as a new, fundamental competency relevant to pharmaceutical care should be strongly integrated into the existing competency frameworks of the pharmacist. This may need to go beyond the current digital literacy competency in FIP's Global Competency Framework as described above.

The new fundamental competency would link to all previously described knowledge and competency domains. Therefore, it can be defined as follows: *The pharmacist uses expertise in digital health care technologies to optimize patient outcomes of drug therapy and/or pharmaceutical interventions.*

 The competency translates into skills that enable the pharmacist to

- develop, review, judge, and use digital health technology and data to optimize the management of adequate and safe drugs;

- counsel patients on digital health technology that improves the impact of prevention, self-care, and medication use;
- analyze holistic data sets of both individual patients and broader populations to enable understanding of predictive analytics that support personalized care, prevention, and, if needed, population-based interventions; and
- translate analytic results into improved patient services.

As noted in Chapter 8, it will be beneficial for pharmaceutical care providers to gain an understanding of which (emerging) data and data sets will be important in a future pharmacy business; which digital tools are required to converge suitable patient services that track the required data; how to collect, analyze, and visualize data; and how to translate the outcomes into benefits for patients.

 Systematic integration of this new competency can produce three positive results.

- Pharmaceutical care providers will be more aware of how technology influences their profession, will be able to shape the design of digital health solutions and will have a basic understanding of how to implement this technology to optimize pharmaceutical care;
- Pharmaceutical care providers will be able to select and use patient data sets to tailor individualized pharmaceutical care; and
- Some providers will choose to specialize in digital health, e.g., in pharmaceutical informatics or data science. They may become experts in big data analysis for population-based risk monitoring, stratification, and intervention optimization.

Data consciousness

Being digital tool-savvy is one thing, but understanding how to use the data these tools produce is even more important. In the past few years, we have witnessed an upsurge in educational programmes in (applied) data science, data analytics, and AI, many of which have tracks related to healthcare or purely focus on this field. Nevertheless, in many countries, computer science, data management, and information technology educational tracks are siloed from traditional pharmacy educational tracks.

Thus, only pharmacy students with a clear affinity for technology and data topics will probably look for data science education during their academic education. They still tend to find themselves back in departments like bioinformatics, health informatics, epidemiology, or even econometrics; although examples from pharmacy schools are emerging, they are limited. In Box 19.1, an inspiration for pharmacy schools is described.

> **Box 19.1 Inspiration for Pharmacy Schools**
>
> Training programs are designed to meet the growing need for investigators trained in biomedical computing, data science, and related information fields. Many universities around the world increasingly offer these hybrid academic programs, which prepare students for valuable (new) positions in the medical and pharmaceutical arena.
>
> An example can be found at the University of Buffalo's Jacobs School of Medicine and Biomedical Sciences (New York). Its medical school's Department of Biomedical Informatics trains doctoral and postdoctoral researchers in three major areas: *clinical informatics*, including sociotechnical and human-centered design, workflow analysis and cybersecurity; *translational bioinformatics*, including database management, pharmacogenomics, and predictive modeling; and *clinical research informatics*, including a big-data science training program, statistical machine learning, and data mining.

On the other hand, although a number of universities have been introducing health data science master programs, many data scientists and (digital health) informatics students are educated with limited exposure to the professions that they will ultimately support once they join the labor market.

Thus, while many data scientists and data analysts tend to graduate with limited exposure to the true challenges in the pharmaceutical care journey, many data-savvy pharmacists tend to graduate with little access to information about the opportunities of healthcare technology, data analysis, and interpretation (for both individual patients and the broader population).

Once these graduates from different backgrounds enter the labor market, there is yet limited understanding of each other's competencies, so building effective combinatoric innovation (as in Chapter 2) will be a rather laggy process. The solution seems simple. Gradually, we bring the fields closer to allow cross-functional fertilization between digital and pharma knowledge early in the university track and in postgraduate curricula. There are already a number of examples where a hybrid approach could inspire pharmaceutical programs, as reflected in the example of Buffalo University in New York.

It will be important for both fields to become acquainted with continuous cross-functional approaches and to motivate interactions between personalities to bring together a variety of backgrounds, sparking comprehensive thinking patterns and building combined synergy. This synergy may drive creativity and better decision-making abilities, but above all, a shared understanding of how to optimize the pharmaceutical care pathway of the future.

It will not be necessary for practitioners in either field (pharmaceutical or data science and digital health informatics) to be experts in both fields to execute their role adequately. However, early awareness and understanding and engaging in dialogue about a digital solution in pharmacy will dramatically improve their position when they enter the labor market.

Specializing in pharmacy informatics

In some countries, a new academic track was formed to support candidates who intend to specialize in pharmacy informatics. The Healthcare Information and Management Systems Society (HIMSS) defines pharmacy informatics as "the scientific field that focuses on medication-related data and knowledge within the continuum of healthcare systems—including its acquisition, storage, analysis, use and dissemination—in the delivery of optimal medication-related patient care and health outcomes." Pharmacy informaticists take their knowledge of medication management and apply it to the design and development of discipline-specific systems and software. They can also be characterized as the interface between pharmacy and information technology (QR Code 19.2).

QR Code 19.2
Pharmacy informatics.

Pharmacy informatics specialists typically work in pharmacy chains or managed care organizations, hospitals, payer environments, academia, or startups. With access to a broad set of pharmaceutical care data, these specialists develop, for example, digital clinical decision support systems, digital pharmaceutical care tools, or software that analyzes patient outcomes.

Although not every pharmacist needs to be a pharmacy informatics expert, every pharmacist needs to be interested in the area, as many of us will work with zettabytes of data, as noted in Chapter 8.

In conclusion, we see many exciting developments in higher education to meet the needs of the future workforce and equip healthcare professionals with the competencies they need to fulfill future jobs. Let us now have a closer look at pharmacy education specifically.

An overview of digital health in pharmacy education

As outlined in previous chapters in this book, digital health technology is essential to augment pharmaceutical care providers and drive enhanced apothecary intelligence. Therefore, at both the undergraduate and postgraduate levels, understanding and selecting which digital (health) tools can contribute to supporting and augmenting professional pharmaceutical care is of increasing importance.

Digital health education aims to equip learners such as medical and pharmacy students to be part of a digitally enabled health workforce to work within a digitally literate healthcare environment [23]. However, digital health education is mostly shaped by experts outside the healthcare field. When provided by internal academic staff from the pharmacy school, the issue of lack of expertise often occurs. A confident, capable, agile, and digitally enabled pharmacy workforce is required to use digital health's full potential, and education must thus be given through interdisciplinary collaboration [3].

Previous research on a range of global pharmacist-led interventions reported that pharmacists lack confidence in their digital abilities. This perceived lack of preparedness was linked to a potential fear toward a responsibility shift, a slight tech-averseness in the profession, a strong preference for human interactions, and discomfort with new, ambiguous situations like the introduction of digital opportunities in the healthcare landscape [24].

However, the outbreak of the COVID-19 pandemic has changed the situation, and the use of digital health in pharmacy practice has become a crucial aspect of accessible, acceptable, and optimal pharmaceutical care [22]. For example, as a result of the restrictions imposed to combat the pandemic and the need for broad social isolation, pharmaceutical care via telehealth has significantly increased worldwide [22]. In this new era, pharmacy education should promote the development of specific competencies and skills for the cognitive, conscious, and effective use of digital health tools to provide pharmaceutical care [22].

Pharmacy education addresses the competencies and skills through programs that teach elements of medicinal product expertise, pharmaceutical patient care, medication policy, quality care and research, and innovation, both at the undergraduate and postgraduate levels [25].

But there was limited knowledge on whether the digital health element was integrated in pharmacy curricula or how pharmacy schools should teach digital health. Therefore, in 2020, FIP conducted a survey to determine "how the current and future pharmaceutical workforce should be educated and trained to embrace the impact of the technological revolution." The survey focused on two major areas: 1. the readiness and responsiveness of education programs to train the current and future pharmaceutical workforce on digital pharmaceutical care, and 2. knowledge and skill gaps in the pharmaceutical workforce on digital health.

Responses were collected from academic institutions, faculty members, students, practicing pharmacists, and pharmaceutical scientists. Academic institutions and faculty members responded to the readiness and responsiveness of education programs, while students, practicing pharmacists, and pharmaceutical scientists responded to the knowledge and skill gaps in the pharmaceutical workforce on digital health. In total, 1060 respondents from 91 countries participated in the survey.

According to the survey, a significant number of pharmacy schools were not offering digital health education in their curricula. Digital health education was mostly integrated into existing courses, and only a few schools offered it as a standalone course. Most of the pharmacy schools indicated a need for support, such as guidance, training, and resources, as experts on digital health did not give the education.

The top digital health tools covered in pharmacy curricula were online pharmacy,[1] mobile applications, and telemedicine, while students expected to learn more on AI technologies, bots, and blockchain technology.

E-Learning, active learning sessions, and access to digital care clinical platforms were the top three ways used to provide digital health education. Interprofessional collaboration, compliance, and knowledge of digital health tools were the top three skills taught to students. Similar to faculty members, students indicated the need for infrastructure and well-trained and qualified personnel to support them during digital health education [3].

According to the practicing pharmacists and pharmaceutical scientists, a few of them had received digital health education as part of CPD. Therefore, there is a low prevalence of digital health technology utilization among them. They expressed the need for greater support and guidance on how to apply digital health technologies in practice. The most commonly used digital health tools by practitioners were mobile applications, e-prescribing, and e-dispensing [3].

One of the identified ways forward is developing a FIP global curriculum and training resources for digital health education. To teach digital health, educators need these resources, support at all levels, and training themselves; the most common challenge related to digital health education reported by faculties was a lack of experts and resources. To respond to this need, targeted courses for educators are needed, such as the new train the trainer course for digital health educators developed by FIP [26].

There are several examples of digital health education in pharmacy. One of the first standalone courses about digital health for pharmacy students was developed by Utrecht University School of Pharmacy in the Netherlands. This digital pharmaceutical care course started as a pilot course involving five master Pharmacy students for a 5-week full-time commitment. It enabled students to work on both individual projects, which consisted of developing a digital solution for a daily practice pharmaceutical care challenge as well as

---

[1]An online pharmacy is an internet-based legal vendor which sells medicines and may operate as an independent internet-only site, an online branch of a "brick-and-mortar" pharmacy, or sites representing a partnership among pharmacies [36].

a group product, i.e., a framework for the elective course. The students highly appreciated this course, and the developed elective course is now offered in the pharmacy curriculum at the university [27]. Another digital pharmacy course was developed by the Faculty of Pharmacy Novi Sad, Serbia, where an elective course was introduced. The course included the basic principles of digital health and digital pharmacy and information such as digital therapeutics, digital pills, telepharmacy, wearables, AI, apps, and pharmabots. The course is provided not only by pharmacy staff but also by an interdisciplinary team including IT experts, representatives of digital health companies, and other relevant experts. The course received positive feedback from the students [28].

Another example of digital health education stems from The Association of Faculties of Pharmacy of Canada and Canada Health Infoway. They created a unique program to improve graduates' preparedness for work in technology-enabled environments by integrating digital health into curricula at the 10 Canadian pharmacy schools. During the program implementation, an informatics special interest group was formed to serve as a resource for pharmacy faculty members to facilitate the inclusion of health informatics in pharmacy curricula. After several phases and versions, which embedded students', instructors' and peer leaders' feedback, peer review, editorial oversight, significant revisions, and additional learning activity development, the program included content for not only pharmacy but for interprofessional students, community-based prescribers, and pharmacy professionals [29].

The healthcare field lacks a standardized program development for educational courses on digital health. Although there are a few courses offered by universities and schools, such as the examples described above, there is a great variation among them. Courses are unlikely to be taught by academic staff who have experience with and knowledge about digital health in pharmacy practice or—as would be even more preferential—by an interdisciplinary team that may possibly include a mathematician, behavioral scientist, and interface designer. Other issues are a need for hands-on practice to teach digital tools and a place or laboratory to practice and keep such technology [3]. While the implementation of digital health education has so far been highly heterogeneous, the potential of digital health in the healthcare workforce is enormous [30].

Due to emerging patient needs and the new digital health era after the COVID-19 outbreak, the pharmacy profession can no longer wait for the slow integration of digital health technologies into pharmaceutical care and pharmacy education [22]. There is no doubt that pharmacy students must receive enough competency and skills in digital health tools and be able to incorporate them into the pharmaceutical care practice.

Lifelong learning paradigm and adopting digital change

In 2022, experts convened at the WEF emphasized we have witnessed an acceleration in a shift to digital due to the COVID-19 pandemic, and they called for rapid action: by 2030, 77% of jobs will require digital skills [31]. Pharmaceutical care providers will be no exception.

While the fundamental competencies linked to the current knowledge domains will remain of vital importance, many, if not all, pharmacists worldwide acknowledge that after they entered the labor market, several additional competencies and skills did also become very relevant to grow fast in their professional leadership.

As in all professions, a lifelong learning attitude is essential, but it is particularly the case in the health field, where we must adapt to nearly constant innovations, such as new, advanced methods of administering medication, progress in cell and gene therapy, the demand for precision medicine, and changes in the dynamic relationship between patients and healthcare providers. In many countries CPD and continuing education (CE) is mandatory for licensed pharmacists, and CPD strategies is one of the FIP development goals (Goal 9) [32]. As mentioned previously in this chapter, the current workforce acknowledges that their training in digital pharmaceutical literacy has been limited or even absent, and they experience educational needs in this area.

Pharmacists may benefit from an initial broader set of skills related to understanding the (local) healthcare system, ethical scoping, and balanced communication, which are increasingly domains that become more important in the digital pharmaceutical care process. Additionally, as explained in Chapter 6, initial and ongoing education on digital abilities and digital health literacy may bridge potential gaps in the fast-developing digital global ecosystem.

Serious gaming to enhance skillsets

In their classification of digital health interventions, the World Health Organization describes interventions targeted at healthcare provider training [33]. An interesting way to enhance the previously mentioned skills of the future may be through gaming. Serious gaming can be defined as the use of game principles for the purposes of learning, skill acquisition, and training. Although learners typically enjoy serious games over traditional lectures, serious games are effective not because they are games but because of the cognitive and psychological processes involved when learners play them [34].

One distinct advantage of gaming is the ability to establish a hypothetical "real" environment for learning in which the consequences of mistakes are minimized. Thus,

QR Code 19.3
Gaming to train
communication skills.

when undergraduate and postgraduate pharmacists are exposed to digital advances such as virtual reality, wearables, or chatbots; or to real-world data analysis and interpretation; or to future moral dilemmas, they have the opportunity to recognize the potential real-world needs of their future patients and learn how to respond to those needs adequately. For instance, serious gaming can be used to train communication skills (QR code 19.3).

Game-based learning has increased in complexity with technologies being used at different levels, depending on the activity's purpose and intended learning outcomes [35]. Topics covered by game-based learning can be pharmacotherapy focused but also focus on other areas such as communication, pharmacy management, and leadership. Examples of high-technology activities incorporated in pharmacy education besides training communication skills include advanced software simulations in the areas of opioid use, immunology, cough therapy, herbal medicines, community pharmacy in general, and perspectives of patients in poverty. As a lower technology but high immersion option, escape rooms have been introduced [35].

Unlike the vast majority of traditional educational methods, in game-based learning environments, participants receive dynamic and immediate feedback on their skills, knowledge, and strategies. This adaptive feedback permits them to learn from their previous failures, which is a vital feature of game-based learning. Learning from mistakes can be extremely powerful, as shown in Chapter 2, as it can boost pharmacists' confidence and enable them to approach digital challenges with sureness in future endeavors.

In the last Part 4 of this book, we will deep-dive into activities to do today to be prepared for the digital day after tomorrow.

 This means for blended pharmaceutical care:

- Pharmaceutical education is expected to continue as an STEM + education.
- Digital literacy is a new competency added for pharmaceutical care providers
- Not every pharmacist needs to be a pharmacy informatics expert, but every pharmacist should be digitally literate to understand the digital revolution that healthcare is going through.
- Pharmaceutical care providers historically have embraced information technologies in their practice. Cross-fertilization between pharmacy and data science should start as early as possible in educational pathways to stimulate faster synergy in later working environments.

This means for blended pharmaceutical care:—cont'd

- General skills needed to excel in the digital revolution are expected to shift largely to human emotional intelligence, sound judgment, and excellent reasoning abilities; thus, these skills need to receive sufficient attention in future educational tracks.
- Based on the digital revolution, new pharmaceutical care roles will develop, and at this point, we can only guess what their formal titles will be.
- Pharmaceutical care providers will not be taken over by machines any time soon but will evolve and adapt to their adjusted and new role descriptions.
- Digital health education must develop competent and confident pharmacists to obtain a digitally enabled pharmaceutical workforce as well as to use the full potential of digital health in pharmaceutical care.
- There is a great variation in current digital health education. Therefore, it must be standardized and given by not only pharmacists or health care professionals but by an interdisciplinary team, which may include mathematicians, behavioral scientists, and interface designers.
- Lifelong learning is essential to keep up with the fast pace of developments and may include digital interventions targeted at healthcare professional training.

References

[1] Unni EJ, et al. Telepharmacy during COVID-19: a scoping review. Pharmacy 2021;9(4):183. https://doi.org/10.3390/pharmacy9040183.

[2] Fahy N, et al. Use of digital health tools in Europe: before, during and after COVID-19. 2022.

[3] International Pharmaceutical Federation (FIP). FIP Digital health in pharmacy education. 2021. Available from, https://www.fip.org/file/4958.

[4] International Pharmaceutical Federation (FIP). 20-digital health. FIP development goals. 2021 [cited 2023 09/02/2023]; Available from, https://developmentgoals.fip.org/dg20/.

[5] World Health Organization. Joint FIP/WHO guidelines on good pharmacy practice: standards for quality of pharmacy services [Annex 8]. 2011.

[6] Cipolle RJ, Strand LM, Morley PC. Pharmaceutical care practice: the patient-centered approach to medication management. McGraw Hill Professional; 2012.

[7] Westerman G, Bonnet D, McAfee A. Leading digital: Turning technology into business transformation. Harvard Business Press; 2014.

[7a] PwC, 2018. AI will impact employers before it impacts employment. Available at: https://www.pwc.com/us/en/services/consulting/library/artificial-intelligence-predictions/employer-impact.html.

[8] Carrus B, Chowdhary S, Whiteman R. Making healthcare more affordable through scalable automation. McKinsey Digit; 2020.

[9] International Pharmaceutical Federation (FIP). FIP global competency framework: supporting the development of foundation and early career pharmacists, version 2. 2020. Available from, https://www.fip.org/file/5127.

[10] Vertesi JA, et al. Pre-automation: insourcing and automating the gig economy. Sociologica 2020;14(3):167−93.

[11] Wikipedia contributors. Marx's theory of alienation. 2023. 18/02/2023]; Available from, https://en.wikipedia.org/w/index.php?title=Marx%27s_theory_of_alienation&oldid=1135431873.

[12] World Health Organization. Global strategy on digital health 2020-2025. 2021.

[13] Royal Dutch Pharmacists Association (KNMP). Pharmacist competency framework and domain-specific frame of reference for The Netherlands. 2016. Available from, https://www.knmp.nl/media/197.

[14] Pharmaceutical Society of Australia. Digital health guidelines for pharmacists. 2021. Available from, https://www.psa.org.au/resource/digital-health-guidelines-for-pharmacists/.

[15] International Pharmaceutical Federation (FIP). FIP community pharmacy section—vision 2020. 2009. Available from, https://www.fip.org/files/content/pharmacy-practice/community-pharmacy/CPS_Vision_2020.pdf.

[16] Galbraith K, et al. FIP global advanced development framework handbook version 1: supporting advancement of the profession. 2020. Available from, https://www.fip.org/file/4790.

[17] World Economic Forum. The 10 skills you need to thrive in the fourth industrial revolution. 2016 [cited 2023 09/02/2023]; Available from, https://www.weforum.org/agenda/2016/01/the-10-skills-you-need-to-thrive-in-the-fourth-industrial-revolution/.

[18] Colman AM. A dictionary of psychology. 2015 [Oxford quick reference].

[19] Senćanski D, Tadić I, Marinković V. Emotional intelligence and pharmaceutical care: a systematic review. J Am Pharmaceut Assoc 2022;62(4):1133−1141.e2.

[20] Ruble MJ, et al. The relationship between pharmacist emotional intelligence, occupational stress, job performance, and psychological affective well-being. J Am Pharmaceut Assoc 2022;62(1):120−4.

[21] Pharmahubng. 4 leadership skills every young pharmacist should master. 2020 [cited 2023 10/02/2023]; Available from, https://pharmahubng.medium.com/4-leadership-skills-every-young-pharmacist-should-master-cd28eb8e92a2.

[22] Silva RdOS, et al. Digital pharmacists: the new wave in pharmacy practice and education. Int J Clin Pharm 2022;44(3):775−80. https://doi.org/10.1007/s11096-021-01365-5.

[23] Brown TMH, Bewick M. Digital health education: the need for a digitally ready workforce. Archives of Disease in Childhood-Education and Practice; 2022.

[24] Rosenthal M, Austin Z, Tsuyuki RT. Are pharmacists the ultimate barrier to pharmacy practice change? Can Pharm J/Revue des Pharmaciens du Can 2010;143(1):37−42.

[25] Rug, et al. Pharmacy-specific frame of reference and competency standards framework for pharmacists [Dutch]. 2016. Available from, https://research.rug.nl/en/publications/domeinspecifiek-referentiekader-amp-raam-plan-farmacie-2016.

[26] International Pharmaceutical Federation (FIP). The FIP provision and partnerships programme. 2022 [cited 2023 10/02/2023]; Available from, https://www.fip.org/provision-and-partnerships-programme.

[27] Boughalab B, et al. Cursus digitale farmaceutische zorg bereidt voor op innovaties (Dutch). Pharm Weekbl 2019;37.

[28] Farmaceutski Fakultet Novi Sad. Become a master of pharmacy. 2023 [cited 2023 10/02/2023]; Available from, https://faculty-pharmacy.com/program/farmacija/.

[29] Association of Faculties of Pharmacy of Canada. E-learning for healthcare professional students. 2023 [cited 2023 10/02/2023]; Available from, https://elearnhcp.ca/.

[30] Makri A. Bridging the digital divide in health care. The Lancet Digit Health 2019;1(5):e204−5. https://doi.org/10.1016/s2589-7500(19)30111-6.

[31] World Economic Forum. Why are young people not prepared for the jobs of the future? workforce and employment. 2022 [cited 2023 10/02/2023]; Available from, https://www.weforum.org/agenda/2022/10/why-are-young-people-not-preparing-for-the-jobs-of-the-future/#:~:text=Even%20when%20the%20COVID%2D19,the%20jobs%20of%20the%20future.

[32] International Pharmaceutical Federation (FIP). 9-continuing professional development strategies FIP development goals. 2021 [cited 2023 10/02/2023]; Available from, https://developmentgoals.fip.org/dg9/.

[33] World Health Organization. Classification of digital health interventions v1. 0: a shared language to describe the uses of digital technology for health. World Health Organization; 2018. Available from, https://apps.who.int/iris/bitstream/handle/10665/260480/WHO-RHR-18.06-eng.pdf.

[34] Cain J, Piascik P. Are serious games a good strategy for pharmacy education? Am J Pharmaceut Educ 2015;79(4):47. https://doi.org/10.5688/ajpe79447.

[35] Oestreich JH, Guy JW. Game-based learning in pharmacy education. Pharmacy 2022;10(1):11. https://doi.org/10.3390/pharmacy10010011.

[36] Fittler A, et al. Consumers turning to the internet pharmacy market: cross-sectional study on the frequency and attitudes of Hungarian patients purchasing medications online. J Med Internet Res 2018;20(8):e11115. https://doi.org/10.2196/11115.

PART 4

How: what to do tomorrow as a pharmaceutical care leader

CHAPTER 20

Digital by design: recipes for success*

Claudia Rijcken
Pharmi, Maastricht, The Netherlands

You must be the change you want to see in the world

M. Gandhi

A recipe is a set of instructions for preparing a particular dish, including a list of the ingredients required. To make an excellent dish, one has to ensure the ingredients are of the highest quality and the process includes the elements necessary to provide a high culinary experience.

To create an optimal blended care environment in which digital pharmaceutical care (DPC) can thrive, one has to make sure to implement the principles in the design of the solution, to continuously identify areas that need improvement, areas that are open to change, assign adequate resources and tools, followed by seamless execution and agile adjustment.

In digital transformative processes, technological choices and strategies for their use are expected to match the results of up-front strategic analyses, as this information sets standards for how processes, products, and services are designed.

The Quality by Design principles are also helpful in pharmaceutical care systems. Joseph M. Juran, a quality expert, first outlined this concept.

Designing for quality is one of the three universal processes of the Juran Trilogy, in which Juran describes what is required to achieve breakthroughs in new products, services, and processes. Juran believes that quality can be planned and that most quality crises and problems relate to the way in which quality is planned in the design process. In this respect, the principles of Quality by Design were introduced in pharmaceutical

---

*In this chapter, you will read about Digital by Design (DbD), which is a structured framework meant as a guide to implement digital innovation into daily pharmaceutical care practices effectively. DbD is accomplished in several phases that address the domains why, who, what, and how, followed by the do (execution) and sustain phases.

development as a systematic approach to achieving quality in pharmaceutical manufacturing by implementing six well-defined steps [1].

The European Medicines Agency welcomes applications that include Quality by Design. Quality by Design is an approach that aims to ensure the quality of medicines by employing statistical, analytical, and risk-management methodology in the design, development, and manufacturing of medicines. Furthermore, it may be extrapolated to the care provision surrounding the supply of medicines.

 Indigital transformative processes in pharmaceutical care, this framework may be referred to DbD. " refers to a strategy in which digital technology is integrated into all aspects of an organization's operations, processes, and products from the very beginning of their design. It is a systematic approach to digital service development that begins with predefined objectives and emphasizes the target population and process understanding and control based on solid analysis and up-front risk management.

In DPC, this approach means that the likelihood of a digital solution's success is determined mainly by the attention paid to the digitization processes during the design phase. DbD is not a statistical method but an early structured framework to build digital perspectives into a service model (see also Part 3 of this book).

DbD is best depicted as six crucial steps:

The six steps shown in Fig. 20.1 are further explained in the following sections.

1. WHY: Identify true pharmaceutical care problem and the blue sky
2. WHO: Select the most relevant patient group
3. WHAT: Validate how the target population sees the blue sky
4. HOW: Choose the most suitable future solution (may be digital)
5. DO: Lead the (digital) transformation process
6. SUSTAIN: Check the new process and adjust, where required

Figure 20.1
Digital by design in pharmaceutical care.

WHY: identify the true pharmaceutical care problem, the why and the blue sky

As a first step, a defined priority problem and the desired result need to be made transparent by describing the Achilles heel (the fatal weakness in the overall strength of the system) and envisioning the best possible outcome (i.e., its future blue sky).

There is the impetus for change for example due to innovative product improvement goals or more to resource efficiency, improved patient satisfaction, or changing healthcare policies. The current pharmaceutical care pathway will in all cases have to be adequately analyzed and potential bottlenecks in that pathway transparently brought to the table, in order to improve future pathways and processes (QR Code 20.1).

QR Code 20.1
Power of why.

The outcome of this analysis needs to be mirrored toward the effect the intervention wil have on the quadruple aim goals of achieving healthier populations, better treatment for patients, more balanced costs, and happier care providers (Chapter 4).

As prioritization on what issue to solve first is needed in extreme resource-scarce healthcare systems (as we discuss in Chapters 1, 3, and 4), up-front researching and envisioning, where the most optimal outcomes can be created will be pivotal in order not to lose resources on nonpriority topics, After implementing a solution, it will become clear how a solid definition of the preferred and measurable outcome from the beginning positively affects the process and the role that WHY plays in the process.

For example, if pathway optimization for psoriasis is the focus, defining why all stakeholders see a PASI score of 100, which is above the more commonly used score of 90, as the preferred clinical outcome may be the first step. Or defining why a Quality of Life (QoL) improvement of 10 points on a Visual Analogue Scale is more clinically relevant than an improvement of five points in a certain disease. Or why choosing to track PREMS outcomes may prevail over PROMS in a given optimization project (see Chapter 3 for more on this topic).

Also, when defining the WHY, preferably consider aspects that may affect patients' needs, regulatory and legal boundaries, and potential corporate conditions. Furthermore, the internal execution team preferences and process optimization goals should be explicit.

WHY **Questions to ask in the WHY phase are, for example:** Why would we want to change a current pathway? Why are patient outcomes suboptimal in the current pathway? Why should we improve patient convenience? Why is the safety of patients in potential danger? Why is the process organized in an unsustainable way, leading to otherwise avoidable waste or harm? Why is a blended care approach most feasible? Why is an increase in cost-effectiveness a potential outcome?

Posing open-ended questions is preferred, and once analyzed in detail, they can lead to well-defined, demarcated topics that, if feasible, can be used in the next step: whom are we targeting?

The WHY phase often involves a labor-intensive, serious strategic management process that is analytical and requires formalized procedures to produce data and analyses that can then be used as input for strategic thinking.

One pitfall for many organizations is the time it takes to define a new strategy. An organization must align its goals and the pace of its strategic process in a timely way; otherwise, the solution it derives might be obsolete the moment it is presented. Because the process requires knowledge of and experience with current pharmaceutical care pathways and an analytical, curious, and structured mindset to identify bottlenecks, it is important to identify the right talent and skills required to do the job accurately and quickly.

The WHY process should lead, for instance, to a stated mission and a vision of how a blue-sky situation might look after the digital innovation project is completed and implemented.

WHO: select the most relevant patient group

Now that the mission and vision of a digital transformation are formulated, the next DbD step is to determine who will benefit most from the optimization of the process and whom to target in the first pilot. Every disease has its own type of treatment and determinants. Likewise, every drug optimization project has its own targets and complexities. The better those are understood up front, the easier it will be to select a category of patients that may benefit most from the outcome of the innovation pathway proposed. Is it the elderly population, who are slightly tech-averse but may have the highest likelihood of satisfaction after a social robot helps them with their medication? Or is it Generation Z, who are hesitant to visit physical pharmacies but instead want to manage their healthcare needs online and thus may be happy to have a chatbot provide answers to their questions?

WHO **Questions to ask in the WHO phase are, for example:** Who is most adversely affected by the current suboptimal process? Who is a stakeholder in the optimization process and, therefore, should be involved? For example, is it patients, physicians, payers, or governments? Who would be most happy with the improved outcomes, and should we define them as the target population? Who will benefit financially from a cost-effectiveness improvement? Who can work with digital tools, and who will not yet?

The WHO process should lead, for instance, to clearly segment the target population in scope and the relevant stakeholders to include in the digital service design.

WHAT: validate how the target population sees the blue sky

As noted in Chapter 5, the wishes and needs of patients should be addressed as early as possible in the DPC equation. Assumptions on why the mission and vision matter, whether envisioned outcomes make sense for patients, and which categories of patients will benefit most should be validated to develop a service that truly meets the final customer's needs.

A short proof-of-principle or proof-of-concept trial can be considered to gain better insight into the requirements and expectations of patients or healthcare system stakeholders. However, if that is not possible, validated survey techniques may be implemented to determine patients' needs. In addition, focus groups, structured polls, interviews, and broader analytic searches for expectations of customers may provide more insight into how to connect the professional's ideal world with the expectations of other pharmaceutical care stakeholders, such as patients and payers.

WHAT **Questions to ask in the WHAT phase are, for example:** What do we think of our mission, vision, and expected outcome improvement plan; are we tackling a real problem? What is the blue-sky outcome for patients (e.g., clinical value or changed process)? Will this principle work in our specific case? What value will the solution offer to the end consumer? What impact can we expect on quality of life? What determinants of health are most affected by the digital service concept? What advantages will it give other stakeholders? What is the balance between digital versus human care in this project?

The WHAT process should lead, for instance, to an aligned perspective on what matters most to the target population and the positive impact the new blended care concept will have on improving the lives of those taking medications.

HOW: *choose the most suitable future solution*

Once the reasons for the change are identified, the optimal outcomes are clearly defined and validated, and the target population is identified; thus, the basic strategies for selecting the innovation to be developed are almost complete. Because digital technology follows strategy in principle, now is the time to determine whether and how a digital solution can help relieve the identified problem.

As noted in other chapters in this book, digital technology does not always provide a solution. For example, if the target population sees its blue sky as an improvement of low-threshold verbal explanations, then adjustments to the current care pathway should start with solid communication planning (rather than a digital solution).

In other situations, an analysis may reveal that measuring digital biomarkers at home increases the likelihood of identifying adverse effects earlier than seeing patients in the community or hospital pharmacy, in which case digital therapeutic devices may be the most suitable option.

In the first case, the first three steps of the DdD model (WHY, WHO, WHAT) led to a nondigital solution that solved the problem; in the second case, digitalization provided the answer.

In the HOW phase, technology should be regarded as an enabler, may be supportive, may be an outcome measurement tool, or may even be the game changer in a program. Therefore, choosing the best equipment to provide optimal patient solutions requires a thorough analysis of the technologies proposed in Part 2 of this book and their conditions for success.

The current pharmaceutical care process needs to be viewed from a process-engineering perspective to redesign an implementation plan to offer a new paradigm. Business process reengineering is the complete overhaul of existing core business processes in order to improve outputs such as profits, product quality, costs, or speed [2].

Process redesign in healthcare

Kaiser Permanente (KP), a U.S.-based managed care organization (MCO), recognized in the early 2010s an opportunity to rethink how to deliver care specifically related to patient experience and affordability. Under the project name Reimaging Ambulatory Design (RAD), the organization explored how and where healthcare will be delivered in the future, how technology will be leveraged, how social trends influence health behavior, and how people will engage in their own care.

RAD consists of three design principles, six strategies, dozens of tactics, and five platform solutions. Each platform solution includes a detailed patient experience framework that recasts the entire network delivery strategy with aspecific service model, operations, facility design, and technology recommendations.

It completely changed the way new healthcare ecosystems at KP are currently being built [3].

In previous literature, pharmaceutical processes are typically described as networks of processes [4]. It is possible to take the full analytical approach and map the entire pharmaceutical process as a set of data points that experience transition into the next point and mathematically determine the efficiency or inefficiency of that transaction. This analysis offers insight into where the most time, money, patient satisfaction, or treatment outcomes are lost. To conduct an analysis like this requires data analyst expertise, as noted in Chapter 19.

However, if this capability is not available, simply sequentially mapping the stepwise process of the patient pathway, as explained in Chapter 6, will be sufficient.

HOW **Questions to ask in the HOW phase are, for example:** How does the current process look on a map? How could a digital solution lead to measurably improved outcomes? How much of a barrier is the literacy level of the target population that will use the digital solution, and what are the current adoption rates? How are the advantages and disadvantages of various digital solutions positioned? How should the maturity level of the proposed digital solution be considered, and which data regarding privacy, quality, and security are publicly available? How can we test the solution? How do we assure agility and flexibility? How developed is the chosen digital solution's interoperability with existing pharmacy applications? How much potential for scalability of the solution/platform is there? How much money do we need to make the pilot happen? How should the implementation team look and function? Finally, how do we set timelines?

This phase is also the time to run a digital health compliance blueprint, as described in Chapter 17, and to consider the ethical aspects, as proposed in Chapter 18. When deciding to work with privacy-sensitive data flows or artificial intelligent solutions, we need to consider potential ethical concerns and the prevailing moral values of good pharmaceutical care in the design phase.

The HOW phase is not only about technology but is also about resources, research, and timing. Although the end-stage benefits will be huge, innovation in smaller teams may require a significant number of people and a significant amount of time and money.

Another factor in the HOW phase is the scalability of the project. That is, consider whether the application will be used locally and whether it can be scaled up easily so that it can be used, for instance, in a regional pharmaceutical chain or even be scaled up to a global level. These factors determine the structure in which the digital tool must be developed, how the vendors work and the stakeholders involved in the development process.

The HOW process should lead, for instance, to a sound, well-thought-out project plan, including timing, tools, people, stakeholders, communication, and budget involved. Also, adequate project management expertise and support need to be considered in this and the DO phase, regardless of the organization's size.

How to lead digital transformation

The Philips Health Index 2022 reflected several critical factors determining the effectiveness of digital transformation in healthcare: technology infrastructure, data interoperability, data security, and policy and healthcare staff knowledge and mindset [5].

The relevance of these themes to pharmaceutical care has been reflected in different chapters within this book.

Pharmaceutical care providers, with their strong STEM and competency profile (see Chapter 19) combined with reinforced digital health literacy, are perfect leaders in the digital revolution.

While Mario Andretti's comment might seem unnerving initially, it is most appropriate for leaders who aim to navigate the digital world. No race—or transformation—is risk-free; thus, having the leadership and courage to make decisions that push the limits of an organization is necessary [6].

Here are a few tips that can help in the DO phase.

- Learn about digital health technologies that can optimize your pharmaceutical care pathways as much as possible. B. F. Skinner has been credited with saying, "Education is what survives when what has been learned has been forgotten." A vision based on this kind of knowledge can drive ongoing, innovative insights.
- Learn as much as you can about how people operate and leverage the wisdom of the crowd. Externally, it will help you understand patient behavior and achieve a smooth adoption process. Internally, it will help build a high-performing team that is willing, flexible, and resolute enough to implement innovation.
- Keep advocating the WHY mission and path. It will help you push forward when things become difficult (as they always do at a certain point in change processes). However, doing so will require reenvisioning the future again and again.
- In the execution phase, take time to see the bigger picture and identify new opportunities within the process. Strive to inspire teams, and let them propose adjustments and improvements. Doing so may motivate the team and ultimately create an iterative, innovative, self-learning environment.

DO **Questions to ask in the DO phase are, for example:** Does the digital solution truly support patient outcomes? Does the changed process meet target group expectations? Do we move according to plan? Do patients adopt the digital service according to expectations? Do we need to adjust strategy based on ongoing insights? Do we need to communicate first successes or failures, by whom and to whom? Do we need to involve additional stakeholders or team members?

The DO process should lead, for instance, to a proof-of-concept report showing the value of the (digital) service implementation, validation of the hypothesis of better patient outcomes, transparency in patient satisfaction, potential scalability, and financial sustainability.

DO: lead the (digital) transformation process

Now that the strategy, expected outcome, target population, and project plan are mapped, the project plan can be brought into seamless execution in the experimentation phase.

The well-known Chinese proverb, "A journey of a 1000 miles begins with a single step," is applicable here. Too many dreams and plans slip away simply because people are afraid to take the initial step. Courage begets the leadership needed to excite curiosity and the will to create new ideas. Chapter 21 expands on how to take on such a role and create a culture for success.

Another essential quality is being adaptive and open to change during the process. Mario Andretti, one of most successful racecar drivers in history, once said: "If everything seems under control, you're not going fast enough." Transformation is a volatile and unsettled phase. In this phase, the notion of brilliant failures (refer to Chapter 2) can help create a failure-and-risk-accepting attitude toward innovation, ensuring that failure is not seen as a demotivator but as a part of the process to succeed after all.

SUSTAIN: check the new process and adjust where required

This design phase sets the key performance indicators (KPI), and a disciplined pharmaceutical care professional follows up on the acquired KPI insights and adjusts the process where needed.

Experimentation in Step 5 in the DO process tends to lead to a wealth of new data, transformed into insights, that reflect either a strong improvement in a new blended care patient pathway or a potential need to adjust the primary digital innovation in order to achieve even better results in the second plan. Or it may lead to the conclusion that a blended care innovation was not beneficial, for instance, because of legal, adoption, quality, or other reasons.

A pilot that will not scale up can still be useful if the reasons for failure are shared to keep others from making the same errors. Thus, even if a pilot project is not successful yet for scaling, consider the value of learning from brilliant failures, as reflected in Chapter 1.

In cases of success, the new digital service can be scaled up to bigger or even different target populations. Additional stakeholders may be involved, more resources added, and new communication plans considered, including social media. A success is only a success once people become aware of it.

SUSTAIN **Questions to ask in the sustain phase are, for example:** Did we meet the prespecified KPIs and triple aim goals and do we wish to continue? Should we adjust parts of the services based on ongoing insights and target population expectations? Do tangible outcomes actually show improved patient satisfaction or treatment outcomes? For which populations could this digital tool offer a solution as well? Have projected outcomes been met within the expected time and budget frame? Which steps should be altered in order to produce even better outcomes? Can circularity or sustainability of the new blended care solution be made transparent, for example, by less medication waste, continued lower hospitalization rates, or sustainably improved quality of life? How can we share what we learned with other stakeholders?

The SUSTAIN process should lead, for instance, to a stop-or-continue decision, potential adjustment of the initial blended care innovation, views on optional scalability, vision on sustainability, communication of successes, or targeting of other benefiting populations.

Considerations

As much as there are many benefits to DbD approaches, it can be derived from the paragraphs above that there are hurdles as well. In summary, those hurdles entail.

- **Resistance to change:** One of the biggest hurdles to implementing DbD is resistance to change. Many organizations have established ways of doing things that are deeply ingrained, and introducing new digital technologies can be met with resistance from employees who are comfortable with the status quo.
- **Technical challenges**: Implementing DbD requires significant technical expertise, and organizations may struggle to find the right talent to lead the effort. In addition, integrating digital technologies into existing processes and systems can be complex and time-consuming, requiring significant investments in hardware, software, and training.
- **Data privacy and security concerns**: As organizations collect and store more data, there are increased concerns about data privacy and security. This can be especially challenging when integrating digital technologies into products and services that interact with customers or handle sensitive information. See Chapter 17 as well.
- **Regulatory and compliance issues**: Depending on the country or region, there may be regulations or compliance requirements that must be considered when implementing DbD. Organizations must ensure that they are in compliance with these requirements, which can add complexity and cost to the implementation process.
- **Cost**: Implementing DbD requires investments in hardware, software, and training. While the potential benefits of this approach can be significant, organizations must be willing to make these investments in order to reap the rewards.
- **Cultural issues**: DbD requires a culture of innovation and experimentation, and organizations that are not used to this way of thinking may struggle to adopt this approach.

FIP released 2023 a report which described the results of a global poll and round table discussion that—among other topics on digital care—entailed the barriers and challenges to implementing digital health in pharmaceutical care services [7].

In Fig. 20.2, the results of this roundtable are shown.

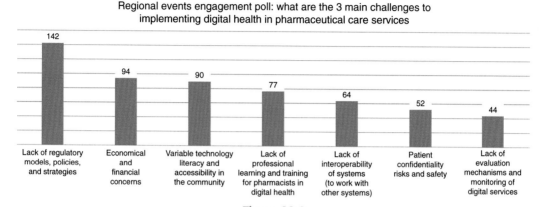

Figure 20.2

Main challenges in implementing digital health in pharmacy services.

Overall, implementing DbD requires careful planning, significant investments, and a willingness to embrace change. While there are hurdles to overcome, pharmaceutical care teams that are able to successfully implement this approach can benefit from increased efficiency, improved patient experience, and a competitive advantage for the future.

 This means for blended pharmaceutical care:

- DbD is a structured execution framework that facilitates leaders in effectively implementing digital innovation.
- WHY, WHO, WHAT, HOW, DO, and SUSTAIN are the six essential steps for transforming into blended care pathways in corporate and young business environments.
- "A journey of a 1000 miles begins with a single step." Just do it. With acquired digital literacy, a professional analytical and ethical mindset, and a structured DbD approach, the conditions are set for an optimal design process to start.
- Active sharing of DPC pilot experiences and insights will support the faster and more effective development of a sustainable pharmaceutical care future.

The next Chapter 21 explains how to build the optimal team culture in order to execute DbD frameworks successfully.

References

[1] DeFeo JA. The juran trilogy: quality planning. 2019 [cited 2023 16/02/2023]; Available from, https://www.juran.com/blog/the-juran-trilogy-quality-planning/.

[2] Laoyan S. How to start fresh with business process reengineering. 2022 [cited 2023 10/02/2023]; Available from, https://asana.com/nl/resources/business-process-reengineering-bpr.

[3] HDR. Kaiser permanente: Re-imagining ambulatory design. 2023 [cited 2023 21/01/2023]; Available from, https://www.hdrinc.com/portfolio/kaiser-permanente-re-imagining-ambulatory-design.

[4] Romero A. Managing medicines in the hospital pharmacy: logistics inefficiencies. In: Proceedings of the world congress on engineering and computer science; 2013.

[5] O'Reilly K. Philips' Future Health Index 2022 report shows healthcare leaders are rebooting priorities as they emerge from the pandemic. 2022. Available from, https://www.philips.com/a-w/about/news/archive/standard/news/press/2022/20220608-philips-future-health-index-2022-report-shows-healthcare-leaders-are-rebooting-priorities-as-they-emerge-from-the-pandemic.html.

[6] Arora A, et al. A CEO guide for avoiding the ten traps that derail digital transformations. Digital McKinsey; 2017. Available from, https://www.mckinsey.com/capabilities/mckinsey-digital/our-insights/a-ceo-guide-for-avoiding-the-ten-traps-that-derail-digital-transformations.

[7] International Pharmaceutical Federation (FIP). How can digital health interventions support national pharmaceutical care delivery. 2023. Available from, https://www.fip.org/file/5127.

CHAPTER 21

Broiling the high-performance culture*

Paul Rulkens

Agrippa Consulting International, Maastricht, The Netherlands

We shape our buildings; thereafter our buildings shape us

Winston Churchill

A high-performance team can be compared to a well-functioning kitchen, where each team member plays a specific role, similar to ingredients in a recipe. Each ingredient brings its unique flavor and characteristics to the dish, but when combined with other ingredients and broiled in an optimal way, it creates a delicious and harmonious meal.

The importance of various elements, such as having the right ingredients (skills and talents), having a clear structure and processes, having a good leader, and having good communication and collaboration within the team, is illustrated below, all of which are necessary for a high-performance team.

In recent panel discussions about the future of health care, one of the panelists mentioned that artificial intelligence (AI) currently has a better track record of interpreting MRI images than its human radiologist counterparts, which was noted in Chapter 11.

It was concluded that we would divide radiologists into two groups in the near future. The first group consists of radiologists who simply want their toys back and are doomed to defend an ever-shrinking turf of relevant expertise. The second group will consist of the radiologists who choose to expand their skills to be effective in those scenarios where human judgment, personal connection, and professional instinct trump AI.

This is an interesting example of *the approaching train dilemma:* Imagine a train coming at us at a predictable trajectory and speed, yet we find ourselves paralyzed, unable to react and rely on hope to avert imminent disaster. If we know change is coming, what can pharmacy leaders and professionals start doing today to build the right organizational high-performance culture for the future?

---

*In this chapter, you will read about an actionable pathway that describes how digital pharmaceutical care providers can immediately start role modeling the essential behaviors to build a high-performance organization.

Pharmaceutical Care in Digital Revolution. https://doi.org/10.1016/B978-0-443-13360-2.00017-4

Why culture drives results

In 1998, the struggling UK Olympic rowing team got a new coach. He quickly introduced a single rule for all athletes: Whenever you need to decide, ask yourself one question: *Will it make the boat go faster?* The athletes followed the coach's lead and applied this mindset enthusiastically to everything they did. Two years later, the team captured Olympic gold. By asking a simple question, the entire culture of the team changed. This example illustrates two things. First, organizational culture may drive exceptional performance or pose the biggest hurdle to future success. Second, the minimum effective behavior you show as a leader is A maximum behavior you can expect from others. Thus, by deliberately role modeling, a leader can influence the behaviors and culture of an entire organization.

The biggest myth about successfully preparing for the future is that availability of resources, understanding of cutting-edge technology, and fast application of new ideas are the main drivers of success. If this were the case, historically, big players in an industry or professional field would continue to maintain their dominant position when disruptive innovation enters their market. It is, however, very rare that established players make a successful transition to new business models or technologies. For example, Barnes and Noble, the bookselling giant, was quickly surpassed by the upstart Amazon when internet distribution of books took hold.

The same is true for the failed transition of Kodak to digital photography, or Nokia's inability to extend to the smartphone market. They had all the necessary resources available, yet they still failed. This will be no different for the pharmaceutical business. We may have full access to the newest insights, technology, and resources, yet success is far from guaranteed. The difference between the successful pharmaceutical care providers and the less successful ones will be cultural: a difference in mindsets, beliefs, and behaviors. Therefore the most important factor for maximizing chances of success as a pharmaceutical care provider is to focus on building a future-oriented, high-performance organizational culture where new ideas can bloom. Fertile grounds beat better seeds every time. The six keys to build this high-performance culture are creating clarity around goals, practical ways to measure progress, a mindset of playing to win, an attitude to fall in love with clients, using power laws, and understanding how to let go in order to reach out.

The need for clarity, connection, and goals

Organizational results are downstream from organizational culture; therefore, you will never get the new results you want from the existing behaviors you like. Only by changing the culture of an organization will you get different results.

Three elements are essential to start creating a future-oriented culture: vision, connection, and tangible goals. The most effective way to build a culture where innovation focus and future orientation are the norm is to deliberately build supportive language, metaphors, and stories to support your new goals clearly.

That's why a simple question such as, "Does it make the boat go faster," effectively improves performance. It creates a massive amount of clarity. It also provides the connection between individual decisions and the vision of a desirable future.

Next to having a vision and creating a connection, the third element of building a future-oriented organizational culture is translating a vision into tangible goals. It has been said that life is about goals and that all else is just commentary. Often, bright organizations simply fail because of vague, unrealistic, or missing goals. Criteria for good goals are.

- **A clear statement of where you are, to where you want to be**: For example, it's important to be very specific about the revenue of your current innovative products or services compared to the revenue of your future innovative products or services.
- **A feasibility check**: Has it been done before? If not, make your goal smaller. After all, often, the most successful organizations are not the first movers but those who enter the market shortly after the first movers. The latter tends to leverage the learnings of others: The iPod used existing technology in an attractive package to dominate the portable music market quickly.
- **A clear distinction between goals, alternatives, and boundaries**: For example, the goal can be to build a pharmacy business that is prepared for the future. Alternatives to achieve this goal may be the application of blockchain, AI, or wearables. A boundary can be to maintain positive cash flow. The simple rule is to keep your eyes on the ball and never confuse your actual goals with arbitrary alternatives to achieve your goals. If you do, you limit your options for success. Also, do not confuse goals and boundaries. A goal requires strategic initiatives to make it happen. A boundary condition does not.
- **Practical ways to frequently measure progress on a goal**: Which data tell you that you are on your way to achieving your goals and staying within your boundaries? Without checking your progress regularly, you will have no way to steer the ship and avoid shipwreck.
- **Incorporation of behavioral components**: If you picture future success, you need to realize that you will not see how to do it until you see yourself doing it. Which behaviors will help you most to support your goals? For example, if developing an AI solution is an important part of your goals, your organization must build trust and behave in such a way that more and more decision-making is delegated to a system or a process.

How distinctions build a culture focused on the future

Leaders who drive a cultural transformation make abundant use of behavioral distinctions to illustrate language, metaphors, and stories. A behavioral distinction describes the difference between good behavior and the best behavior. Two behavioral distinctions are essential for successful pharmaceutical care providers to lead the digital transformation.

The first important distinction is: are you playing to win, or are you playing not to lose

Imagine two companies. One is playing to win; the other is playing not to lose.

If you are playing to win, you're doing the following.

- **Always looking for ways to make your existing business obsolete** with new technology, products, or services.
- **You are focusing on dominating your marketplace niche.** You have developed a healthy allergy to average results and refuse just to hang on.
- **Willing to take controlled risks, quickly test ideas, embrace brilliant failures,** and aggressively expand on expected and unexpected successes.
- **You are having a structural process in place to prevent your best people from leaving.**
- **Spending more money, time, and energy on innovation,** and less on bending the rules in your favor, such as lobbying for preferential treatment with lawmakers.
- **You are building a business where your future services and products are very different from what you have today.**
- **Willing to confront your peers and invoke the ire of your competitors.** Attraction and repulsion are two sides of the same coin. When you move into uncharted territory, you will break current norms and standards often venerated deeply by existing players. This means that you will encounter a healthy share of both cheerleaders and detractors. This is why the majority is always wrong when it comes to high performance (see QR Code 21.1).
- **You are attracting the customers you serve best.** They typically value advanced products and new services over price. This enables you to step away from existing customers that are a poor fit for your new future business.

QR Code 21.1
Why the majority
is always wrong.

All of these behaviors will drive a culture of winning and enable your organization to incorporate new products and services quickly.

The second important distinction is: do you fall in love with your patients, or fall in love with your product or processes?

If you fall in love with your patients, instead of falling in love with your products or services, you give patients what they need, not what they want. This is the difference between a handyman and an architect. For example, when a part of a kitchen has broken down, people will go to a handyman to get it fixed. The handyman will give what the client wants. On the other hand, if the client goes to an architect, the architect may propose a completely new floor plan for the house. This may be exactly what the client needs.

The value distance between what a client wants and what a client needs is huge. In pharmaceutical care, examples of the difference between somebody who gives people what they want versus what they need are providing extended services to help clients beyond mere treatment support, understanding expertise outside the pharmacy field, and the willingness to give clients access to this expertise.

How to use power laws

The difference in performance between number one and number two in sports is often very small. However, the difference in prize money between number one and number two is huge. This is called a power law: Small differences in achievement may translate into huge differences in rewards.

The good news for pharmaceutical care providers who want to drive cultural transformation is that power laws often provide the easiest pathway to success. You do not need to become twice as good to double your results. You only need to become slightly better to create a vast difference. The three most promising areas for applying power laws are time, place, and knowledge.

- **Time** is your most important resource. You cannot save, stop, or get more of it; when it's gone, it's simply gone forever. Building a new future starts with the highest and best use of your time. These activities lie at the intersection between your skills, your passion, and the value you create for others. Which part of the pharmaceutical care provider blueprint allows you to expand your existing skills, ties into your deep passion, and creates the most value for your future clients?
- **Place** is the second area where power laws can be applied. For example, you can apply AI in the most brilliant way possible, but if your environment simply does not trust an algorithm's judgment, you will get nowhere. It's as futile as opening a

McDonald's franchise next to an all-you-can-eat restaurant. What would be the place where you are surrounded by clients who actually love what you do?

- **Knowledge** is the third area susceptible to power laws. For example, you command respect and a top salary if you are the only expert who knows how to shave off 10% of a pit stop time in a Formula One race. Ask yourself as a pharmaceutical care provider: Which piece of knowledge, if I decide to get it in the next few months, will really make a difference and set me apart from everyone else?

The value of strategic quitting

QR Code 21.2
Strategic quitting.

When designing a new future, the biggest pitfall is to simply add new goals on top of existing goals and activities. Typically, this excessive loading leads to overwork and stress, resulting in frustration and a deep failure to execute (as explained in Chapter 2); we call this an Expensive Old Organization. Instead, if you want to lead in digital transformation, one of the most important leadership behaviors is *strategic quitting*: You have to let go to reach out. Before starting a new project, ask yourself which activities you must quit first (see QR Code 21.2 for a verbal explanation).

If you want to apply strategic quitting, you must first understand your current highest and best use of your time. These are all activities that you're skilled at, passionate about, and create value for others. Then, everything else should be strategically quit. This approach will optimize your organization and release valuable resources to innovate.

The second step is to apply *strategic sacrifice*: Define which part of your work, which is currently your highest and best use of time, will no longer have a place in your future business. Then design a process to eliminate this part of your work as well, even if it is still valuable and important.

The area for pharmaceutical care providers where applying strategic quitting may be most effective is *irrelevant excellence*. Nothing is sadder than professionals becoming excellent at something that is rapidly becoming irrelevant.

How to take the first step and maintain momentum

After setting a goal to become a successful digital pharmaceutical care provider, the first step is to define exactly which behaviors will support you most to get there in the easiest way possible. Then role model these behaviors to transform your organizational culture. In summary, the six areas where new, consistent behaviors can make a huge impact are.

- Creating clarity around your medium- and long-term goals.
- Continuing efforts to measure progress on these goals.
- Playing to win: If the goals don't make you slightly uncomfortable, you're probably not thinking big enough.
- Falling in love with your patients: Ask yourself regularly how your goals will help improve the client's condition.
- Using the power laws of time, place, and knowledge.
- Letting go in order to reach out. A constant focus on strategically quitting irrelevant activities and strategically sacrificing actual valuable activities that are no longer future-proof will help you free up time, money, and energy.

How you spend your day defines how you will spend your life. Suppose after reading this book, you will execute three (small) actions every day to build the necessary high-performance culture to become a successful digital pharmaceutical care provider. In that case, you will have performed more than 1000 small actions after 1 year. This will dramatically impact your organization's culture and will most certainly set you apart from most of your peers. Information is overrated and is useless without action. Motion beats meditation every time. So what are you waiting for?

A number of reflections in this Chapter are taken from the books of the author [1,2].

 This means blended pharmaceutical care

- Suppose this book has inspired you to chase a future of blended pharmaceutical care by implementing digital health technology. In that case, you need to be aware of which behaviors will enable you to succeed in that ambition.
- A six-item blueprint of goal clarity, progress measurement, playing-mindset, customer orientation, power laws, and letting go may help to create a culture to increase the likelihood of success.
- By executing three (small) actions every day to build the necessary high-performance culture to become a successful digital pharmaceutical care provider, you will have performed more than 1000 small actions after 1 year.

References

[1] Rulkens PWP. The Power of preeminence: high performance principles to accelerate your business and career. 2nd ed. Vakmedianet Management; 2017.
[2] Rulkens PWP. How successful engineers become great business leaders. 1st ed. Business Expert Press; 2018.

CHAPTER 22

Final discussion: blending pharmaceutical care

Claudia Rijcken[1], Ardalan Mirzaei[2]
[1]Pharmi, Maastricht, The Netherlands; [2]School of Pharmacy, Faculty of Medicine and Health, The University of Sydney, Australia

The future belongs to those who believe in the beauty of their dreams.

Eleanor Roosevelt

Now that you have read the preceding chapters in this book, we assume you will be as inspired as the authors about how a health-tech convergence will create opportunities to improve our apothecary intelligence in years to come.

To a certain extent, this evolution resembles the future of cooking, where many examples show the growing effective integration of technology in kitchen and service models. For example, smart ovens, refrigerators, and dishwashers will offer new ways to monitor, control, and automate cooking tasks. In addition, online-ordered meal delivery services will become more common, making it easier for people to enjoy home-cooked meals without shopping for ingredients or planning menus. And artificial intelligence (AI)-powered food recognition and recommendation systems will become more prevalent, offering personalized suggestions for meals based on individual tastes and dietary needs. These technological advancements will continue to change how people cook, eat, and think about food, offering new opportunities for convenience, customization, and healthier eating habits.

As Massimo Bottura, Italian chef and restaurateur of a three-star Michelin restaurant, said it nicely: "I believe the future of cooking will be about creating healthy, delicious food in a sustainable, eco-friendly way. It's about using technology to reduce waste and make the most of every ingredient, while also celebrating the pleasures of the table."

This may be similar to how pharmacists make and provide pharmaceutical care in days to come: assuring sustainability, improving return of investment of medicine use, and optimizing the experience for both healthcare provider and patient.

Pharmaceutical Care in Digital Revolution. https://doi.org/10.1016/B978-0-443-13360-2.00039-3

In this chapter, some final reflections will be given to you on the general progress in blending digital health integration into pharmaceutical care.

Progress in digital health between the first edition (2019) and this second edition

Over the past 4 years, digital health has undergone tremendous growth and evolution. For example, the widespread adoption of telemedicine has provided patients with the convenience and accessibility of receiving medical consultations from their homes. This accessibility has been particularly important during the COVID-19 pandemic, where the need for remote consultations has increased dramatically.

Another major acceleration in digital health has been the broader use of electronic health records (EHRs). EHRs have improved the accuracy, efficiency, and accessibility of patient data, enabling healthcare providers to make informed decisions and provide better care. In many countries, focusing on interoperability improvement has augmented the value of the EHR.

The acceleration of interoperability in healthcare (as reflected in Chapter 8) has been seen in the last few years. It refers to the ability of different systems, devices, and software to work together and exchange information seamlessly. Interoperability supports care providers in eliminating errors and duplications in patient data and reduces the need for manual data entry.

Interoperability in healthcare is considered crucial for improving patient care, increasing efficiency, reducing errors, and promoting patient-centered care. In the next years, implementing interoperability solutions will be essential for advancing the quality and effectiveness of healthcare delivery in general and supporting apothecary intelligence specifically.

Also, in the last 4 years, AI and machine learning (see Chapter 11) have been increasingly used in healthcare. These technologies have improved the accuracy of diagnoses and predictions, leading to better patient outcomes. Radiology, oncology, and drug discovery are some examples of domains in healthcare that have been significantly disrupted by AI and will continue to be in days to come. Also, conversational AI support for both healthcare provider and patient has made a major development step in recent years, as could be seen in Chapter 12.

Moreover, wearable technology has become far more prevalent in the last years, empowering individuals to take control of their health and wellness by monitoring their biometric data. The recent evolution of wearable health technology has significantly impacted both the individual and the healthcare industry. It has empowered individuals to take control of their health and wellness and has provided healthcare providers with valuable data to inform better decision-making. Adequate home monitoring kept patients out of the hospital, which in COVID-times was crucial to warrant convenience, sustainability, and affordability. The future of wearable health technology is bright, and we can expect to see continued innovation and growth in this area.

Last but not least, genomics and precision medicine have been major focus areas in recent years. Improved personalized medicine has been and will be a game-changer in healthcare, providing patients with a tailored approach to their health and well-being. Rather than taking a one-size-fits-all approach, the approach considers an individual's unique genetic, environmental, and lifestyle factors to deliver the most effective and efficient care.

Personalized medicine, including the concepts of pharmacogenetics, eliminates the guesswork and trial-and-error approach of traditional medicine, providing patients with the peace of mind that they are receiving the most effective care for their specific needs. It also has the potential to reduce the risk of ineffective treatments and side effects, as well as improve patient compliance and satisfaction with their treatment. As our genome is increasingly better mapped and genetic tests are more affordable and accessible, pharmaceutical care is expected to adopt more individualized approaches in the upcoming years quickly.

The overpromised health technologies between the first edition (2019) and this second edition

In the previous edition of this book, there was a lot of excitement and hype surrounding certain health technologies that promised to revolutionize how we approach healthcare. However, as with any new and rapidly evolving field, there have been instances where certain technologies have been overpromised and have not lived up to their initial expectations.

While technology has the potential to bring about great change and improvements in healthcare, the conditions for success, as described in this book, are a complex and multifaceted field that often takes longer to develop and implement than initially anticipated. There are obstacles and challenges that arise during the development and implementation of these new technologies, such as regulatory hurdles, cost constraints, and technical limitations.

One technology that we expected 4 years ago to develop faster, given its potential, has been blockchain. The implementation of blockchain technology in healthcare has been a challenging process, with several obstacles standing in the way of widespread adoption.

One of the biggest reasons for the delay is the technical complexity of the technology itself. Blockchain is a rapidly evolving field, and developing and implementing blockchain-based solutions in healthcare requires a deep understanding of the technology and its potential applications.

Another factor contributing to the delay is the lack of standardization and interoperability across different blockchain platforms. This has made it difficult for healthcare organizations to adopt blockchain cohesively and consistently, leading to fragmentation and inefficiency in the healthcare system.

Privacy and security concerns have also been major roadblocks to implementing blockchain in healthcare. A patient's health information is secure and confidential by nature and thus requires a high level of trust in the technology and the systems that use it. As a result, ensuring blockchain-based solutions meet strict privacy and security standards has been a major challenge for healthcare organizations and developers. Furthermore, the turbulent times of the COVID-19 pandemic have seen rapid rises and decline in cryptocurrency, which uses blockchain technology. The deregulated nature of cryptocurrency has seen the collapse of some financial institutions leading to hefty losses for businesses and regular investors. These news-worthy events shine a negative light on the potential for blockchain technology, causing erosion in people's trust in the technology.

Despite these challenges, the potential benefits of blockchain in healthcare are significant, and many organizations are actively working to overcome these obstacles. With the right approach, blockchain has the potential to transform healthcare and improve patient outcomes, and it is exciting to see the progress that has been made in this field in recent years.

The very promises of the digital boom are also, paradoxically, undermining its future. Examples like the cases of IBM Watson [1] and Theranos [2] warrant sensitivity. Publicly traded companies recently valued in the billions are now trading for cents on the dollar. Some companies are overpromising and underdelivering, wasting billions that were earmarked to improve patient care and jeopardizing the already fragile trust of regulators and investors. Media hype compounded the problem as journalists trumpeted the fairy tale of health-tech unicorns and private companies with "game-changing" products to transform the healthcare system as we know it.

Nevertheless, the field of health technology is constantly evolving and changing, and what may have been seen as a disappointment in the past, with sensitivity and intelligent development, may still have the potential to develop and improve in the future.

The four questions in the foreword

We started this book off with some questions to a natural language program, asking it to provide a vision of future developments.

- What will the world look like in 10 years?
- Will the future of digital pharmaceutical care be impacted by the changes that happen in the next 10 years?
- As a pharmacist, should I be worried about the changes that are coming?
- As part of the foreword to the book pharmaceutical care in the digital revolution, do you have final words you would like to share with the readers?

Let's now finally reflect as professionals on these four questions, keeping the content of this book in mind.

What will the world look like in 10 years?

Without a doubt—as described in the first edition—we are in a transformation phase, and the future of blending our world with technology has not yet crystallized. As Lucien Engelen wrote in his book Augmented Health(Care), "We are just at the end of the beginning." Engelen addresses the fact that there are still many unanswered questions, for example, in the regulatory, legal, educational, and ethical domains.

Apart from these elements that need regulation and conceptual development (and will get a stronger foundation by experience), several risks need our priority focus in the next years. Topics like climate change-induced extreme weather events, widespread illness and death caused by pandemics, cyberattack-related damage to privacy and critical infrastructure, and political and economic instability are just a few examples of the many risks facing our future. However, our future sustainable world depends on our collective actions and decisions, openness to change, and flexibility in response to these trends.

If we act appropriately, our globe in 2033 may be drastically different from what it is today, with the effects of technological, social, and political developments shaping the global landscape.

In terms of technology, advancements such as AI, robotics, and biotechnology may have revolutionized how people live and work 10 years from now. Automation may have further transformed many global industries, increasing efficiency and productivity. Additionally, new roles for humans may have developed in 2033 to keep the blended society moving, as humans remain in the lead for keeping the system working. Finally, in 2033, the widespread use of renewable energy sources, such as wind and solar power, may have reduced greenhouse gas emissions and slowed the pace of climate change, thus, providing humankind with a safer outlook for living on the globe.

In terms of society, the world in 2033 may be more connected and diverse, with globalization and migration continuing to shape the cultural makeup of communities. In addition, advances in health care and medicine may have led to longer life expectancies and improved health outcomes. Furthermore, increased access to education and technology may have lifted many more people out of poverty.

Politically, the authors of this book would wish the world in 2033 to be more peaceful and cooperative, with increased efforts to resolve conflict through diplomacy and negotiations. However, new challenges may have arisen, such as the previously mentioned risk of cyberattacks and the proliferation of weapons of mass destruction. In addition, the rise of nonstate actors, such as transnational corporations and terrorist organizations, may have also complicated the global political landscape.

In summary, our world in 2033 will likely be shaped by a complex interplay of technological, social, and political developments (basically as it is now as well). Our pharmaceutical profession plays a crucial role in maintaining a sustainable future by taking several important steps to reduce its environmental impact. These steps include developing and producing medicines in an environmentally sustainable way, promoting the rational use of medicines to conserve resources, advocating for public policies that support sustainability in the healthcare sector, ensuring the responsible disposal of hazardous pharmaceutical waste, and researching and developing new drugs and technologies that are environmentally friendly. By taking these actions, the pharmaceutical profession helps to create a more sustainable future for both the planet and future generations.

Will the future of digital pharmaceutical care be impacted by the changes that happen in the next 10 years?

In the foreword, the future of digital pharmaceutical care was said to be heavily impacted by increased data collection methods, new chronic management tools, pattern and data analysis, and increased adoption rates of digital systems. Apparently, ChatGPT was right. These elements have all been discussed in the preceding chapters to enable pharmacists to glimpse the future wherever they are globally.

When observing the impressive content of this book, it is obvious that the technological advancements that impact our globe will inevitably and significantly impact our pharmacy profession. In addition, the combination of the increased number of patients with complex chronic conditions, and the reduced pharmaceutical care workforce, is fueling a transformation process toward new pharmaceutical care models, in which these technological advancements are crucial for building sustainability.

As much as the concepts of blending technology with human pharmaceutical care are extensively described in this book, effectively implementing these concepts requires a massive transformation process.

Creating such a transformation requires healthcare systems to analyze and plan in different steps globally. The first step is to define the desired blended pharmaceutical care model, which provides the direction and focus for the local, national, and even regional transformation process. Once that desired outcome is clear (this book may guide the framework), the next step is to understand the current state of pharmaceutical care, including any challenges and limitations that may need to be overcome. This, again, is a local, national, or international responsibility, where the analysis leads to an understanding and identification of the gap between the current state and the desired future outcome of how blended care is perceived.

The next step in the transformation process is developing a plan or strategy to close the current gap. The knowledge of the risks and opportunities of the current technologies available, the creation of the optimal environment for change as described in the conditional chapters in this book, and the mindset open for new system development are essential to driving this step into a plan that makes sense to build a sustainable future for our profession.

Once local, national, or international plans are drafted, the next years will be characterized by implementation, measuring, and in a data-driven way, ensuring that the transformation model is improved along the way. Finally, sustaining the changes is crucial to ensuring long-term success, as this helps to embed the new ways of working into our healthcare and educational systems' culture and practices.

How successful we will be, is highly dependent on the effective interplay of technological, social, and political developments. Of course, the priorities that regionally, nationally, and internationally are made determine whether healthcare funding can be guaranteed, whether transformation budgets are freed up, and whether education systems are adapted.

As a pharmacist, should I be worried about the changes that are coming?

It's understandable for any industry to feel uncertain about the future, especially with the rapid pace of change in technology and healthcare. However, the authors of this book trust that we have proven that change can also bring opportunities.

Pharmacy is an essential component of the healthcare system, and there will likely always be a need for trained professionals to dispense and manage medications. However, the pharmacist's role may evolve to include more patient-facing responsibilities, such as providing medication therapy and disease state management services.

Additionally, technological advancements, such as telepharmacy and automation, may change the way pharmacy services are delivered, as reflected in this book's chapters. Nevertheless, this could also lead to increased efficiency, higher work productivity, and satisfaction, more time for more focused professional care, and better patient outcomes.

It can be overwhelming to navigate the constant changes and advancements in the pharmaceutical care ecosystem. This emotion is a generally known phenomenon in the era that we live in, and the panacea is to take the time to process and adjust to the changing environment. The globe was not built as it is currently from day one, so evidence-based and gradually growing into new ways of working is the way to avoid worrying.

Pharmacists globally have a wealth of knowledge and experience, and together with their continuous dedication to providing the best care for patients, the profession is an inspiration to many within our population. Not in the least because citizens see the pharmacist as a profession with high ethical and moral standards.

The ethical role of a pharmacist remains unchanged in the technological era (see Chapter 19). As healthcare professionals, pharmacists are responsible for prioritizing patient safety and well-being, maintaining confidentiality, and promoting the appropriate use of medications.

In the technological era, pharmacists have access to more information and tools that can aid in their decision-making and improve patient care. However, with this increased access to information, pharmacists must also be mindful of privacy concerns and ensure that patient data is kept secure (see Chapter 17).

Pharmacists should also ensure that they are using technology ethically and responsibly. For example, pharmacists can judge any biases or limitations of the algorithms and decision-support tools they use and thus help patients make informed decisions.

Finally, as a professional, pharmacists will have to continue to educate themselves on emerging technologies and how they may impact their practice. As technology evolves, pharmacists as professionals have the moral obligation to be proactive in adapting their practice to ensure that they are providing the highest standard of care for their patients.

Doing so means there is no need to be scared of the future. On the opposite, there is a wealth of opportunities in front of us. Abraham Lincoln once said: "the best way to predict the future is to create it." And that is what it is. As long as we adjust, adapt, learn and move into new models like blended care, we will stay ahead and improve the lives of so many more patients.

As part of the final discussion of the book pharmaceutical care in digital revolution, do we have final words we would like to share with the readers?

Here, we would like to blend our author's human professional reflection with the answer that our large language model ChatGPT version 3.5 would envision.

So we asked an adjusted version of our fourth question in the foreword:

> *"ChatGPT, as part of the* **final discussion** *of the book pharmaceutical care in digital revolution, do you have any final words you would like to share with the readers?"*

As an AI language model, I do not have personal opinions or personal experiences, but here are some potential final words for the readers of "Pharmaceutical Care in the Digital Revolution."

- Technology is playing a significant role in the evolution of healthcare and pharmacy practice, and the use of digital tools has the potential to greatly improve patient outcomes and the efficiency of care delivery.
- However, it is crucial to carefully consider the ethical and privacy implications of utilizing personal health information and to ensure that appropriate measures are in place to protect patient confidentiality and data security.
- Additionally, it's essential to ensure that the implementation of technology in pharmacy practice is evidence-based and supported by robust research to ensure its effectiveness and safety.
- The integration of technology into pharmacy practice should also be done in a way that complements, rather than replaces, the human element of care, as the pharmacist—patient relationship remains a critical component of effective care delivery.
- Finally, it is important for pharmacists to stay up to date with the latest developments in technology and digital tools and to continuously educate themselves on their use and implementation in practice.

Well, even the yet sort of "toddler" version of ChatGPT (January 2023) seems to be rather knowledgeable in summarizing the content of this book.

Continuing to learn, adjust and improve in working with the blended care model will position the pharmacist as one of the key care providers of the future.

Investing by changing to innovative blended disease prevention programs by pharmacists is expected to reduce healthcare costs in the long term. By providing medication therapy management, health screenings, and education on healthy lifestyle choices, pharmacists can help prevent chronic diseases before they develop, leading to fewer hospitalizations and surgeries and lower healthcare costs. It will improve health outcomes as pharmacists can help prevent chronic diseases, leading to longer, healthier lives and avoiding complications associated with chronic conditions. And it can also positively impact society as a whole, as pharmacists can help prevent chronic diseases, which can reduce the burden on the healthcare system and improve the overall health of the population.

Final note

Integrating technology in pharmaceutical care can improve patient outcomes and make a real difference in people's lives. In the words of Steve Jobs: "Innovation distinguishes between a leader and a follower." By embracing technology, pharmacists can lead the way in providing the highest standard of care.

However, with great power comes great responsibility. Albert Einstein wisely noted: "Technology is a useful servant but a dangerous master." Pharmacists must use technology to respect patient privacy and ensure the secure handling of sensitive information. Pharmacists will have to remain focused on putting their patients first and using technology to enhance, not replace, the human element of care.

> *By blending patient-centered care with judicious use of technology, pharmacy practice becomes more valuable and sustainable.*

As Confucius once said: "Choose a job you love, and you will never have to work a day in your life." By using technology in a meaningful way, pharmacists can find fulfillment in their work and positively impact the lives of those they serve.

We wish you lots of luck and inspiration during your personal implementation of all the concepts that you've been able to absorb in this second edition of the book Pharmaceutical Care in Digital Revolution.

References

[1] Gagnon J. IBM Watson health's challenges tell us more about healthcare data than it does about AI. 2022 [cited 2023 17/02/2023]; Available from, https://www.forbes.com/sites/forbestechcouncil/2022/05/03/ibm-watson-healths-challenges-tell-us-more-about-healthcare-data-than-it-does-about-ai/?sh=4a75bf55b486.

[2] Laker B. Theranos founder Elizabeth Holmes jailed for 11 Years: four lessons for leaders. 2022. cited 2023 17/02/2023]; Available from, https://www.forbes.com/sites/benjaminlaker/2022/11/19/theranos-founder-elizabeth-holmes-jailed-for-11-years-four-lessons-for-leaders/?sh=477a573d6515.

Abbreviations

ACS	Acute Coronary Syndrome
ADHD	Attention-Deficit/Hyperactivity Disorder
AI	Artificial Intelligence
ANSI	American National Standards Institute
API	Application Programming Interface
AR	Augmented Reality
ASCO	American Society for Clinical Oncology
ATC Code	The Anatomical Therapeutic Chemical code
BCE	Beliefs, Concerns, and Expectations
BCIs	Behavior Change Interventions
BIDMC	Beth Israel Deaconess Medical Center
BMI	Body mass index
BPR	Business process reengineering
BYOhD	Bring Your Own health Device
CAGR	Compound Annual Growth Rate
CAR-T	Chimeric Antigen Receptor T-Cell
CBT	Cognitive Behavioral Therapy
CDA	Clinical Document Architecture
CDC	Centers for Disease Control and Prevention
CDISC	Clinical Data Interchange Standards Consortium
CDM	Chronic Disease Management
CDRH	Center for Devices and Radiological Health
CDSS	Clinical decision support systems
CE	Continuing Education
CEO	Chief Executive Office
CFR	Code of Federal Regulations
CGM	Continuous Glucose Monitor
CIA	Confidentiality, Integrity, and Availability
CMA	Continuous Medication Availability
COPD	Chronic Obstructive Pulmonary Disease
CPD	Continuing Professional Development
CPOE	Computerized Provider Order Entry
CRISPRs	Clustered Regularly Interspaced Short Palindromic Repeats
CRM	Customer Relationship Management
CTR	Clinical Trials Regulation
DbD	Digital by Design
DIKW	Data-Information-Knowledge-Wisdom
DNA	Deoxyribonucleic Acid
DPC	Digital Pharmaceutical Care
DSS	Decision Support Systems
DTx	Digital Therapeutics
ECG	Electrocardiogram

EEG	Electroencephalogram
EHD	Electronic Healthcare Data
EHDS	European Health Data Space
EHR	Electronic Health Record
EI	Emotional intelligence
EMA	European Medicines Agency
EMRs	Electronic Medical Records
EPRs	Electronic Pharmacy Records
ER	Emergency Room
ESS	Executive Support Systems
EU	European Union
FACT	Fairness, Accuracy, Confidentiality, and Transparency
FAIR	Findability, Accessibility, Interoperability, and Reuse
FAQs	Frequently Asked Questions
FDA	Food and Drug Administration
FHIRs	Fast Healthcare Interoperability Resources
GAS	Goal Attainment Scaling
GDP	Gross domestic product
GDPR	General Data Protection Regulation
GHTF	Global Harmonization Task Force
GP	general practitioners
GPAI	Global Partnership on AI
GPS	Global Positioning System
HIMSS	Healthcare Information and Management Systems Society
HIPAA	Health Insurance Portability and Accountability Act
HIT	Health Information Technology
HIV	Human Immunodeficiency Virus
HMRs	Home Medical Reviews
HTA	Health Technology Assessment
HUD	Heads-Up Display
IAPP	International Association of Privacy Professionals
ICD	International Statistical Classification of Diseases and Related Health Problems
ICER	Institute for Clinical and Economic Review
ICHOM	International Consortium for Health Outcomes Measurement
ID	Identification
IDC	International Data Corporation
IHI	Institute for Healthcare Improvement
IMDRF	International Medical Device Regulators Forum
IP	Internet Protocol
IPH	Institute of Positive Health
ISMS	Information Security Management System
ISO	International Organization for Standardization
IT	Information Technology
IV	Intravenous
KNMP	Royal Dutch Pharmacists Association
KP	Kaiser Permanente

KPIs	Key Performance Indicators
KWS	Knowledge Work Systems
LED	Light-Emitting Diode
LIDAR	Light Detection and Ranging
LMICs	Low- and Middle-Income Countries
MCO	Managed Care Organization
MDSAP	Medical Device Single Audit Program
MEMS	Micro-Electromechanical Systems
MIS	Management Information Systems
ML	Machine Learning
MPR	Medication Possession Ratio
MR	Mixed Reality
MRI	Magnetic Resonance Imaging
MTM	Medication Therapy Management
NCPDP	National Council for Prescription Drug Programs
NHS	National Health Service
NIST	National Institute of Standards and Technology
NLG	Natural Language Generation
NLP	Natural Language Processing
NSW	New South Wales
OBF	Outcome-Based Financing
OECD	The Organisation for Economic Co-operation and Development
OUD	Opioid Use Disorder
OWASP	The Open Worldwide Application Security Project
PASI	Psoriasis Area and Severity Index
PBM	Pharmacy Benefit Manager
PBRSAs	Performance-Based Risk-Sharing Arrangements
PC	Pharmaceutical Care
PCPs	Pharmaceutical Care Providers
PDC	Proportion of Days Covered
PDMPs	Prescription Drug Monitoring Programs
PDT	Prescribed DTx
PGx	Pharmacogenetics
PHA	Personal Health Application
PHC	Personalized Healthcare
PILs	Patient Information Leaflets
PIS	Pharmacy Information Systems
PREMs	Patient-Reported Experience Measures
PROMs	Patient-Reported Outcome Measures
PTSD	Posttraumatic stress disorder
QoL	Quality of Life
RAD	Reimaging Ambulatory Design
RCT	Randomized Clinical Trial
RFID	Radio Frequency Identification
RNA	Ribonucleic Acid
ROI	Return on Investment

RPM	Remote patient monitoring
RTPM	Real-Time Prescription Monitoring
RWE	Real-World Evidence
SBE	Simulation-based education
SMIs	Serious Mental Illnesses
SMS	Short Messaging System
SOCs	Service Organization Controls
SPCs	Summary of Product Characteristics
STEM	Science Technology Engineering Mathematics
SUD	Substance Use Disorder
TDF	Theoretical Domains Framework
TIA	Transfer Impact Assessment
TPS	Transaction Processing Systems
UCLA	The University of California, Los Angeles
UIs	User interfaces
UK	United Kingdom
UN	The United Nations
US	United States
USB	Universal Serial Bus
USD	United States Dollar
VAS	Visual Analogue Scale
VPAs	Virtual Personal Assistants
VR	Virtual Reality
VUIs	Voice-User-Interfaces
WEF	The World Economic Forum
WHO	World Health Organization

Appendix: Overview of laws, legislation, and standards referred to in Chapter 17

Rob Peters and Barry Meesters—updated by Anne Sophie Dil and Amy Eikelenboom

This appendix is an addendum to Chapter 17. In that chapter, we present the elements required to create a compliance blueprint (see Fig. A.1) and the related laws, legislation, and standards. In this appendix, we provide a more detailed view of the legislative landscape.

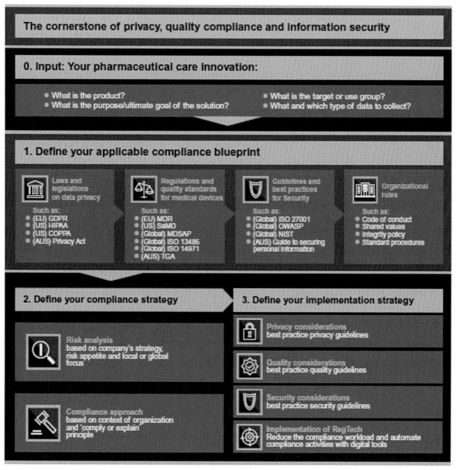

Figure A.1
The steps in a compliance blueprint.

The information in this appendix focuses only on the most common regulations related to privacy, quality, and security. More information on the organizational rules is included in Chapter 17.

General comments on the compliance blueprint

Variations in legislation among countries

Laws and regulations are changing rapidly as a response to technological advancement. A complete overview of all applicable requirements in all countries can, therefore, not be provided. The reader is advised to consult the website of local authorities to find out the current requirements applicable to their specific solution or situation.

Completeness of references

Please note that the legislation and guidelines listed in the chapter are nonexhaustive. We only described general requirements applicable in the United States, the EU, and Australia in 2022.

We recommend that one will always check on the most recent regulations.

More details on laws and legislation on data privacy

Chapter 17 refers to the following privacy laws and regulations:

- **EU privacy regulation:** General Data Protection Regulation (GDPR)
- **US privacy regulation:** Health Insurance Portability and Accountability Act (HIPAA)
- **US privacy regulation:** Children's Online Privacy Protection Act (COPPA)
- **Australian privacy regulation:** Privacy Act: Australian Privacy Principles

In the overview below, we deep-dive further in granular details of each individual regulation to data privacy.

EU privacy regulation: General data protection regulation

The European Union's General Data Protection Regulation 2016/679 aims to strengthen and unify data protection throughout the EU. Given it is a regulation, the GDPR applies to all member states directly and does not need to be transposed into national legislation. The GDPR, which entered into force in 2016, became applicable in May of 2018.

 Since the GDPR is a regulation, no local interpretations are necessary. Member state law can, however, build on the GDPR with specific requirements, such as for medical data.

The GDPR covers all personal data, defined "as any data from which a living individual is identified or identifiable, whether directly or indirectly." GDPR applies to all organizations established within or outside the EU that process EU residents' personal data.

A number of individual categories of personal data specifically related to health information and thus relevant for pharmaceutical care interactions are shown in Fig. A.2.

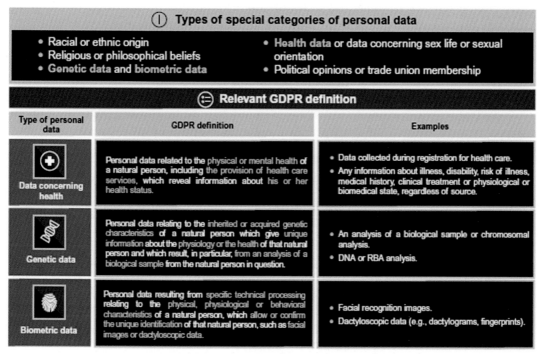

Figure A.2
Special categories of personal data.

US privacy regulation: Health insurance portability and accountability act

In the absence of single principal data protection legislation, the United States has a wide variety of sector-specific laws enacted. For healthcare, the Health Insurance Portability and Accountability Act applies. HIPAA Privacy rules ensure the confidentiality and security of protected health information (PHI) when that information is transferred, received, handled, or shared. The rules apply to healthcare providers and organizations and all their business associates and should help these parties develop and follow procedures related to the appropriate handling of PHI data, which includes, for example, paper, electronic, and *verbal* versions [1].

Under HIPAA, patient data are referred "protected health information (PHI)."This applies to all healthcare data. HIPAA defines PHI as any individually identifiable "past, present, and future information about mental and physical health and the condition of an individual, the provision of healthcare to an individual, and information related payments for healthcare."

Under HIPAA, the act is applicable to predefined (called covered) entities (such as a healthcare provider, physician, insurance company, and healthcare clearing house) and business associates. GDPR, however, applies to *all* organizations established within or *outside* the EU that process EU residents' personal data.

US privacy regulation: Children's online privacy protection act

The moment a digital solution is developed for or can be used by children under the age of 13 and is developed for use in US jurisdictions it falls under COPPA requirements.

The US Federal Trade Commission issued this act specifically to regulate and enforce the online collection of personal information about children under the age of 13 years.

The primary goal of COPPA is to give parents control over what information is collected online about their children. The act specifies what a healthcare provider (e.g., a pharmacist) must include in the mandatory privacy policy and how to seek verifiable consent from a parent or guardian before collecting personal information about children under the age of 13 years.

Furthermore, it is clearly defined which additional security measures must be taken and what the guidelines are for online marketing toward children's indications.

Under GDPR, the specific obligations related to processing data of children are included in the regulation. Similar to COPPA, the GDPR also defines children as a separate category of people who deserve specific protection from the unlawful processing of data.

Australian privacy regulation: Privacy act: Australian privacy principles

The original Privacy Act was passed in 1988 and went into effect in 1989. This Privacy Act has been amended several times. In 2019, the Australian Government announced a review of the Privacy Act 1988. The Privacy Legislation Amendment (Enhancing Online Privacy and Other Measures) Bill 2021 (the Online Privacy Bill) will give effect to the Australian Government's commitment to strengthen the Privacy Act 1988 [2].

Australia instituted the Health Records (Privacy and Access) Act in 1997, and the latest version became effective in August 2022 [3]. The main purposes of this dedicated act are to

- provide privacy rights in relation to personal health information;
- maintain integrity of records containing personal health information; and
- provide access to personal health information contained in health records.

Under the Privacy Act 1988, the Australian Information Commissioner issued several guidelines and documents to promote the understanding and awareness of the Australian Privacy Principles (APPs). Australian authorities have defined a total of 13 separate APPs starting from the principle of open and transparent management of personal information (APP 1) to the principal of correction of personal information (APP 13). The content and mandatory requirements of these APP guidelines can be found at www.oaic.gov.au/ agencies-and-organisations/app-guidelines [4].

More details on regulations and quality standards for medical devices

Chapter 17 noted the following relevant regulations and quality standards for medical devices as being relevant when working with digital pharmaceutical care solutions:

- **US Medical Devices Regulation:** Title 21 Code of Federal Regulations (CFR) Parts 800-1299 **Global Medical Device Single Audit Program** (MDSAP)
- **Global ISO 13485, medical devices**—Quality Management System—Requirements for regulatory purposes
- **Global ISO 14971, medical devices**—Application of risk management to medical devices
- **EU Medical Device Regulation (MDR)**

US medical devices regulation: Title 21 code of federal regulations (CFR) Parts 800-1299

The FDA makes a distinction between devices intended for wellness and devices intended for healthcare. The FDA does not regulate general wellness products, as strict as healthcare devices the moment they are intended for general use only and present a very low risk to users' safety. However, due to the increasing gray area between the wellness and healthcare applications entering the pharmaceutical care sector, we will focus first briefly on the criteria for wellness devices.

Wellness devices

In the Cures Act, the FDA describes a general wellness product as a device that helps maintain or encourage a general state of health and healthy lifestyle or that associates the role healthy lifestyle choices play in reducing the risk or impact of certain chronic diseases or conditions. To help clarify whether a pharmaceutical care innovation can be classified as a wellness product (and thus will not have to follow the regulations applied to medical devices), the FDA has provided a framework for such products, as shown in QR Code A.1 [5].

QR Code A.1

FDA wellness device regulation

However, as in many guidelines, there is room for interpretation, and the FDA strives to continuously improve those that it provides. The most recent version was issued in September 2019 [6]. This update specified and categorized activities that fall under the definition of wellness device:

Devices that do the following are classified as wellness devices:

- Provide administrative support for a healthcare facility;
- Maintain or encourage a healthy lifestyle;
- Serve as an electronic patient record; and
- Transfer and store data, convert formats, and display data and results.

Software as a medical Device

Since 2017, the US definition of Software as a Medical Device has been, "software intended to be used for one or more medical purposes that perform these procedures without being part of a hardware medical device" [7].

The guidelines set under the authority of the FDA define Software as a Medical Device [8] as:

- software used as a component, part, or accessory of a medical device;
- software that is itself a medical device;
- software used in the production of a device; and
- software used in implementing the device manufacturer's quality system.

Global medical device single audit program

The International Medical Device Regulators Forum (IMDRF) states that a global approach in auditing and monitoring of the manufacturing of medical devices (which could affect digital health software as well) could improve patient safety and optimize international scale up. The MDSAP program allows a single regulatory audit of a manufacturer's quality management system, which should satisfy the requirements of multiple regulatory jurisdictions.

These audits are conducted by auditing organizations authorized by the participating regulatory authorities to audit under MDSAP requirements.

The program became operational as of January 1, 2017. Currently, regulatory agencies from Canada, Brazil, Japan, Australia and the United States participate in MDSAP.

Global ISO 13485, Medical Devices—Quality Management Systems

The International Organization for Standardization (ISO) comprises well-known and globally recognized specifications, guidelines, and frameworks.

In 2017, the organization recognized 163 countries. The ISO is the world's largest developer of voluntary international standards and facilitates world trade by providing common standards among nations. Over 20,000 standards have been set, covering everything from manufactured products and technology to food safety, agriculture, and healthcare.

ISO 13485 is the global standard for medical device quality management systems. Regardless of their size and type, the moment organizations are involved with medical devices, the ISO 13485 standard provides valuable guidance. ISO 13485 is designed to be used by organizations involved in the design, production, installation, and delivery of medical devices and related services.

ISO 13485 is related to the MDSAP described earlier in this appendix. One aspect of MDSAP follows the standard of ISO 13485 which specifies requirements for a quality management system for medical devices. That is, ISO 13485 requires the pharmaceutical care stakeholder to demonstrate whether the quality system of the company or institute is effectively implemented and continuously maintained and improved.

ISO 13485 facilitates an effective quality management system, including the following key aspects:

- **Management responsibility:** Focuses on promotion and creating awareness of management's responsibility to comply with regulatory requirements and to have an effective and continuously maintained and improved quality management system.
- **Product safety:** Provides guidance for controls to ensure product safety in the quality management system and working environment.
- **Risk management:** Focuses on risk management activities during product development.
- **Requirements:** Provides guidance for requirements related to inspection, traceability, documentation, validation, and verification of effectiveness of corrective and preventive actions within the quality management system related to medical devices.

Compliance with ISO 13485 under the Medical Device Regulation is generally used to give substance to medical device requirements stemming from various regulations.

Global ISO 14971, medical devices: Application of risk management to medical devices

This standard (ISO 14971) specifies a process to identify the hazards associated with medical devices (including digital health software) in all stages of their lifecycle.

When developing a digital health innovation, the main items relevant to ISO 14971 for pharmaceutical care stakeholders are as follows:

- **Process:** Establish a process to manage and control the risks associated with your organization's medical devices.
- **Management:** Make sure that top management demonstrates a commitment to medical device risk management.
- **Qualifications:** Make sure that the people who perform risk management tasks have the knowledge and experience that are required to carry out the tasks that have been assigned to them.
- **Risk management plan:** Establish a risk management plan for each particular medical device under consideration, in use, or in development.

It is important that this plan is documented and includes (1) the risk analyses as performed, (2) the risk evaluations, (3) the mitigating risk controls implemented, (4) the evaluation of residual risks, and (5) the monitoring activities performed to make sure your risk management of the particular device is up to date.

EU medical software regulation: Medical device regulation

After being postponed by a year, the European Medical Devices Regulation became applicable in May, 2021.

The definition of a medical device in the MDR is any instrument, apparatus, appliance, software, implant, reagent, material, or other article to be used, stand-alone or in combination, for human beings for one or more of the following medical purposes:

- diagnosis, prevention, monitoring, prediction, prognosis, treatment of alleviation of disease
- diagnosis, monitoring, treatment, alleviation of, or compensation for, an injury or disability,
- investigation, replacement or modification of the anatomy or of a physiological or pathological process or state,
- providing information by means of *in vitro* examination of specimens derived from the human body, including organ, blood, and tissue donations.

Classification of medical devices under the EU MDR ranges from class I (low risk) up to class III (high risk).

⚠ Annex VIII to the EU MDR lists classification rules. These rules determine the classification a medical device will be assigned to. Rule 11 specifically relates to medical device software. When medical device software is intended to provide information used to make decisions for diagnostic or therapeutic purposes, it is minimally classified as class IIa.

Pharmaceutical care solutions with software implications are recommended to take into account new MDR classification and requirements immediately from the development phase on.

More details on guidelines and best practices for security

In Chapter 17, we wrote about how to support organizations in defining and implementing security measures and the general, globally accepted standards, guidelines, and best practices relevant for digital health compliance, such as

- ISO/IEC 27001 Information Security Management System (ISMS);
- Open Web Application Security Project (OWASP); and
- National Institute of Standards and Technology (NIST).

Let us deep-dive somewhat further into each of these individual standards and guidelines.

ISO/IEC 27001 information security management

This standard is the one best known in terms of providing requirements for an accurate and effective information security management system (ISMS). An ISMS is a systematic approach to managing sensitive company information in the most secure way. This risk-based system covers different topics and areas, such as people, processes, and IT systems. The standard is part of the ISO/IEC 27000 group, which focuses entirely on keeping information assets secure. To strengthen information security for personal health information specifically, ISO 27799 can be used to do so.

Open web application security project

The Open Web Application Security Project (OWASP) is a worldwide nonprofit organization focused on improving the security of software (in general) [9]. The organization provides practical information about application security to individuals, corporations, universities, government agencies, and many other organizations. OWASP is issuing software tools and knowledge-based documentation on how to improve security on a daily basis. The information is open-sourced and available, and all materials can be downloaded.

All software developers are supposed to know the best practices under OWASP. The organization published the "*Top 10 Most Mobile Risks*" and "*Top 10 Most critical Web Application Risks*," including the procedures to follow to mitigate those risks [9].

National institute of standards and technology

NIST [10] is a nonregulatory government agency that develops standards and guidelines for technology companies and also for federal agencies, to comply with several security legislation and requirements. Furthermore, NIST standards and guidelines assist in protecting information systems through cost-effective security measures and programs (see QR Code A.2).

Several national governments require that companies must comply with the NIST standards, although they are not actually legislation (but are accepted as guidelines in information security) [11].

QR Code A.2
Information about NIST standards.

In many cases, complying with NIST guidelines and recommendations will support being compliant with other regulations such as HIPAA. Also, complying with NIST standards means that the focus is not only on the security of a product but also on the security level of an entire organization.

References

[1] CDHCS. Health Insurance Portability and Accountability Act. 2023. https://www.dhcs.ca.gov/formsandpubs/laws/hipaa/Pages/1.00WhatisHIPAA.aspx.

[2] Australian Government Attorney-General's Department. Privacy. 2023. https://www.ag.gov.au/rights-and-protections/privacy.

[3] ACT Government. Health Records (Privacy and Access) Act 1997. 2022. https://www.legislation.act.gov.au/a/1997-125/.

[4] Commissioner, O.O.T.A.I. Australian Privacy Principles 2023.

[5] FDA. General Wellness: Policy for Low Risk Devices Draft Guidance for Industry and Food and Drug Administration Staff. 2019. https://www.fda.gov/downloads/Training/CDRHLearn/UCM569275.pdf.

[6] FDA. Changes to Existing Medical Software Policies Resulting from Section 3060 of the 21st Century Cures Act. 2019. https://www.fda.gov/media/106563/download.

[7] FDA. Digital Health Software Precertification Pilot Program. 2017. https://www.fda.gov/media/106563/download.

[8] FDA. General principles of software validation. 2002. https://www.fda.gov/regulatory-information/search-fda-guidance-documents/general-principles-software-validation.

[9] OWASP. OWASP foundation. 2020. https://wiki.owasp.org/index.php/Main_Page.

[10] NIST. NIST. 2018. https://www.nist.gov/.

[11] Lord N. What is NIST compliance?. In: Digital guardian; 2020. https://digitalguardian.com/blog/what-nist-compliance.

List of QR codes

In this digital age, where innovation and connectivity thrive, we have included a unique addition to the second edition—a collection of QR codes that serve as gateways to a world of supplemental content and immersive experiences. These QR codes, strategically placed throughout the pages of the book, aim to enhance your reading journey by seamlessly integrating the power of technology with the written word.

The inclusion of QR codes in this book represents a leap forward in bridging the gap between the physical and digital realms. Each code acts as a portal, unlocking a wealth of additional resources, multimedia content, and interactive features that enrich your understanding and provide a deeper level of engagement with the text.

To assist you in navigating this digital landscape, we have provided below a list of the specific content linked to each QR code found in the book. This will help you locate and access the desired content more efficiently, enhancing your reading experience and allowing you to fully immerse yourself in the digital extensions of our storytelling.

Chapter	QR Code name	Title	URL
Foreword	QR Code 1	ChatGPT | Open AI	https://pcindr.com/qrcode/p0c00qr01
1	QR Code 1.1	OECD health statistics	https://pcindr.com/qrcode/p1c01qr01
1	QR Code 1.2	EFPIA data center	https://pcindr.com/qrcode/p1c01qr02
2	QR Code 2.1	Example of combinatoric innovation in healthcare	https://pcindr.com/qrcode/p1c02qr01
2	QR Code 2.2	Institute of brilliant failures	https://pcindr.com/qrcode/p1c02qr02
3	QR Code 3.1	WEF global coalition for value in healthcare	https://pcindr.com/qrcode/p1c03qr01
3	QR Code 3.2	The value of medicines	https://pcindr.com/qrcode/p1c03qr02
4	QR Code 4.1	HIB: A form of social impact bond	https://pcindr.com/qrcode/p1c04qr01
5	QR Code 5.1	Askapatient	https://pcindr.com/qrcode/p1c05qr01
5	QR Code 5.2	DigitalMe	https://pcindr.com/qrcode/p1c05qr02
5	QR Code 5.3	MyHealthAppsblog	https://pcindr.com/qrcode/p1c05qr03

Chapter	QR Code name	Title	URL
6	QR Code 6.1	An explanation of adherence	https://pcindr.com/qrcode/p1c06qr01
7	QR Code 7.1	Consolidated telemedicine implementation guide	https://pcindr.com/qrcode/p2c07qr01
7	QR Code 7.2	Digital health intervention classification	https://pcindr.com/qrcode/p2c07qr02
7	QR Code 7.3	What is gamification?	https://pcindr.com/qrcode/p2c07qr03
8	QR Code 8.1	Internet of things explained	https://pcindr.com/qrcode/p2c08qr01
8	QR Code 8.2	Example of a personal health application	https://pcindr.com/qrcode/p2c08qr02
9	QR Code 9.1	Example of medication adherence innovation	https://pcindr.com/qrcode/p2c09qr01
9	QR Code 9.2	Example of an app library that provides resources for patients and clinician	https://pcindr.com/qrcode/p2c09qr02
10	QR Code 10.1	Applications of digital twin	https://pcindr.com/qrcode/p2c10qr01
11	QR Code 11.1	Can a computer pass for a human?	https://pcindr.com/qrcode/p2c11qr01
11	QR Code 11.2	Latest deep learning	https://pcindr.com/qrcode/p2c11qr02
11	QR Code 11.3	The hungry baby alarm	https://pcindr.com/qrcode/p2c11qr03
11	QR Code 11.4	The advent of AI in healthcare	https://pcindr.com/qrcode/p2c11qr04
11	QR Code 11.5	What's Kaggle	Kaggle	https://pcindr.com/qrcode/p2c11qr05
11	QR Code 11.6	Ethics in AI	https://pcindr.com/qrcode/p2c11qr06
12	QR Code 12.1	Demo movie digital pharmacist pharmi	https://pcindr.com/qrcode/p2c12qr01
12	QR Code 12.2	How real and virtual people connect in the metaverse	https://pcindr.com/qrcode/p2c12qr02
12	QR Code 12.3	Explanation of metaverse in healthcare by Bertalan Mesko	https://pcindr.com/qrcode/p2c12qr03
13	QR Code 13.1	VR to educate on the human body	https://pcindr.com/qrcode/p2c13qr01
13	QR Code 13.2	What is augmented reality?	https://pcindr.com/qrcode/p2c13qr02
13	QR Code 13.3	Difference between AR and VR	https://pcindr.com/qrcode/p2c13qr03
13	QR Code 13.4	Virtual reality to treat anxiety	https://pcindr.com/qrcode/p2c13qr04
13	QR Code 13.5	Example of AR smart packaging	https://pcindr.com/qrcode/p2c13qr05
13	QR Code 13.6	Example of VR/AR in healthcare education	https://pcindr.com/qrcode/p2c13qr06

Chapter	QR Code name	Title	URL
14	QR Code 14.1	History of pharmacy	https://pcindr.com/qrcode/p2c14qr01
14	QR Code 14.2	HIMSS international—interoperability in healthcare	https://pcindr.com/qrcode/p2c14qr02
14	QR Code 14.3	Spencer health	https://pcindr.com/qrcode/p2c14qr03
14	QR Code 14.4	Electronic health record data governance and data quality in the real world	https://pcindr.com/qrcode/p2c14qr04
14	QR Code 14.5	Health information privacy	https://pcindr.com/qrcode/p2c14qr05
14	QR Code 14.6	General data protection regulation GDPR	https://pcindr.com/qrcode/p2c14qr06
14	QR Code 14.7	Code grey: Lessons from a malware attack	https://pcindr.com/qrcode/p2c14qr07
15	QR Code 15.1	What are digital therapeutics?	https://pcindr.com/qrcode/p2c15qr01
16	QR Code 16.1	What is precision medicine	https://pcindr.com/qrcode/p2c16qr01
16	QR Code 16.2	Example of 3D printing	https://pcindr.com/qrcode/p2c16qr02
16	QR Code 16.3	Example of a social robot	https://pcindr.com/qrcode/p2c16qr03
16	QR Code 16.4	Example of a humanoid robot	https://pcindr.com/qrcode/p2c16qr04
16	QR Code 16.5	Mabu	https://pcindr.com/qrcode/p2c16qr05
16	QR Code 16.6	Blockchain explained	https://pcindr.com/qrcode/p2c16qr06
17	QR Code 17.1	Data protection	https://pcindr.com/qrcode/p3c17qr01
17	QR Code 17.2	Cybersecurity	https://pcindr.com/qrcode/p3c17qr02
18	QR Code 18.1	The human game	https://pcindr.com/qrcode/p3c18qr01
18	QR Code 18.2	Moral choices of driverless cars	https://pcindr.com/qrcode/p3c18qr02
19	QR Code 19.1	The future of jobs	https://pcindr.com/qrcode/p3c19qr01
19	QR Code 19.2	Overview of pharmacy informatics	https://pcindr.com/qrcode/p3c19qr02
19	QR Code 19.3	Gaming to train communication skills	https://pcindr.com/qrcode/p3c19qr03
20	QR Code 20.1	Power of why	https://pcindr.com/qrcode/p4c20qr01
21	QR Code 21.1	Why the majority is always wrong	https://pcindr.com/qrcode/p4c21qr01

Chapter	QR Code name	Title	URL
21	QR Code 21.2	Strategic quitting	https://pcindr.com/qrcode/p4c21qr02
Appendix	QR Code A1.1	FDA wellness device regulation	https://pcindr.com/qrcode/p0cA1qr01
Appendix	QR Code A1.2	Information about NIST standards	https://pcindr.com/qrcode/p0cA1qr02

Index

'*Note:* Page numbers followed by "f" indicate figures and "t" indicate tables.'

Printed in the United States
by Baker & Taylor Publisher Services